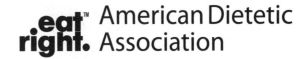

American Dietetic
Association

Managing Obesity

A Clinical Guide

Second Edition

Cathy A. Nonas, MS, RD, CDE, and
Gary D. Foster, PhD
Editors

Diana Faulhaber, Publisher
Elizabeth Nishiura, Production Manager

The views expressed in this publication are those of the authors and do not necessarily reflect policies and/or official positions of the American Dietetic Association. Mention of product names in this publication does not constitute endorsement by the authors or the American Dietetic Association. The American Dietetic Association disclaims responsibility for the application of the information contained herein.

10 9 8 7 6 5 4 3 2

Library of Congress Cataloging-in-Publication Data

Managing obesity: a clinical guide / Cathy A. Nonas and Gary D. Foster, editors. — 2nd ed.
    p. ; cm.
Includes bibliographical references and index.
ISBN 978-0-88091-425-3
1. Obesity—Treatment. I. Nonas, Cathy. II. Foster, Gary D., 1959– III. American Dietetic Association.
[DNLM: 1. Obesity--therapy. 2. Diet Therapy--methods. 3. Health Behavior. 4. Patient Education as Topic. WD 210 M2673 2009]
RC628.M348 2009
616.3'9806—dc22

                                      2009016971

To Mark

 —Cathy A. Nonas

To my wife, Kathleen, and our children, Katie, Ryan, and Kevin

 —Gary D. Foster

CONTENTS

Section 1: Assessment and Treatment

Section 2: Special Issues

Lawrence J. Appel, MD, MPH
Professor of Medicine, Epidemiology and
    International Health (Human Nutrition)
Johns Hopkins Medical Institutions

Jeannette M. Beasley, PhD, MPH, RD
Postdoctoral Fellow
Group Health Center for Health Studies
Fred Hutchinson Cancer Research Center

Christina K. Biesemeier, MS, RD, FADA
Director, Clinical Nutrition
Vanderbilt University Medical Center

Susan Bowerman, MS, RD, CSSD
Lecturer, Department of Food Science and
    Nutrition
California Polytechnic State University,
    San Luis Obispo

Jennie Brand-Miller, PhD, FAIFST
Professor of Human Nutrition
Institute of Obesity, Nutrition and Exercise
The University of Sydney

George A. Bray, MD
Boyd Professor and Chief, Division of Clinical
    Obesity and Metabolism
Pennington Biomedical Research Center

Stacy A. Brethauer, MD
Staff Surgeon
Bariatric and Metabolic Institute
Cleveland Clinic

Ruth Ann Carpenter, MS, RD
Lead Integrator
Health Integration, LLC

Sue Cummings, MS, RD
Clinical Programs Coordinator
MGH Weight Center
Massachusetts General Hospital

Nichola J. Davis, MD, MS
Assistant Professor of Medicine
North Bronx Healthcare Network
Albert Einstein College of Medicine

Thomas A. Farley, MD, MPH
Director, Prevention Research Center
Tulane University School of Public Health &
    Tropical Medicine

Eileen G. Ford, MS, RD
Program Director
Center for Obesity Research & Education
Temple University

John P. Foreyt, PhD
Professor of Medicine
Director, Behavioral Medicine Research Center
Baylor College of Medicine

Gary D. Foster, PhD
Professor of Medicine and Public Health
Director, Center for Obesity Research &
    Education
Temple University School of Medicine

Molly Gee, MEd, RD
Project Leader
Behavioral Medicine Research Center
Baylor College of Medicine

David Heber, MD, PhD, FACP, FACN
Professor of Medicine and Public Health and
    Director, UCLA Center for Human Nutrition
David Geffen School of Medicine at UCLA

Frank B. Hu, MD, PhD
Associate Professor of Nutrition and
    Epidemiology
Harvard School of Public Health
Associate Professor of Medicine
Harvard Medical School

Carmen R. Isasi, MD, PhD
Assistant Professor, Department of
    Epidemiology & Population Health
Albert Einstein College of Medicine

John M. Jakicic, PhD
Professor and Chair, Department of Health and
    Physical Activity
University of Pittsburgh School of Education

Shiriki K. Kumanyika, PhD, MPH, RD
Professor of Epidemiology in Biostatistics and
    Epidemiology
Professor of Epidemiology in Pediatrics
    (Nutrition Section)
University of Pennsylvania School of Medicine

Robert F. Kushner, MD
Professor, Department of Medicine
Northwestern University Feinberg School of
    Medicine

Jennifer C. Lovejoy, PhD
Vice President, Clinical Development and
    Support
Free and Clear, Inc, Seattle

David S. Ludwig, MD, PhD
Associate Professor of Pediatrics, Harvard
    Medical School
Director, Optimal Weight for Life (OWL)
    Program
Children's Hospital Boston

Angela Makris, PhD, RD
Independent Weight Management Consultant

Kate Marsh, MNutrDiet, AdvAPD, CDE
Director, Northside Nutrition and Dietetics

Pam Michael, MBA, RD
Director, Nutrition Services Coverage
American Dietetic Association

Cathy A. Nonas, MS, RD, CDE
Assistant Clinical Professor
Mt. Sinai School of Medicine, NYC

Suzanne Phelan, PhD
Assistant Professor of Kinesiology
California Polytechnic State University

Rebecca M. Puhl, PhD
Research Scientist
Director of Research
Rudd Center for Food Policy & Obesity at
    Yale University

Rebecca Reeves, DrPH, RD
Assistant Professor of Medicine
Managing Director, Behavioral Medicine
    Research Center
Baylor College of Medicine

Leigh Rosen, MUEP
Project Manager
Center for Clinical Epidemiology and
    Biostatistics
University of Pennsylvania

Donna H. Ryan, MD
Professor
Associate Executive Director for Clinical
    Research
Pennington Biomedical Research Center

Philip R. Schauer, MD
Professor of Surgery
Lerner College of Medicine
Director, Advanced Laparoscopic &
    Bariatric Surgery
Cleveland Clinic

CONTRIBUTORS

Sara Solomon, MPH, RD
Health Promotion Coordinator
Center for Obesity Research & Education
Temple University

Amy Virus, RD
Sr. Health Services Coordinator
Center for Obesity Research & Education
Temple University

Rena R. Wing, PhD
Professor of Psychiatry and Human Behavior
Brown Medical School
Director, Weight Control and Diabetes
    Research Center

Anne Wolf, MS, RD
Instructor of Research
Department of Public Health Sciences
University of Virginia School of Medicine

Judith Wylie-Rosett, EdD, RD
Professor and Division Head for Behavioral &
    Nutritional Research
Department of Epidemiology & Population
    Health
Professor, Department of Medicine
Albert Einstein College of Medicine

REVIEWERS

Abbe Breiter, MS, RD
Consultant
Coral Springs, FL

Patti Landers, PhD, RD
Department of Nutritional Sciences
University of Oklahoma Health Sciences Center
Normal, OK

Louise Peck, PhD, RD, CD
University of Washington
Seattle, WA

Helen M. Seagle, MS, RD
Kaiser Permanente
Denver, CO

Laurie Tansman, MS, RD, CDN
The Mount Sinai Hospital
New York, NY

ACKNOWLEDGMENTS

We would like to thank each of the contributors for crafting state-of-the-art accounts about the research and treatment of obesity. Their enthusiasm and willingness to help write a clinically based book on obesity were central to this undertaking.

From the American Dietetic Association, we would like to thank Elizabeth Nishiura for shepherding this book in a superb manner. Thanks also go to Aurora Nonas-Barnes for helping so diligently with the permissions and Toni Darden-Brown for editorial assistance. We are also very grateful to Christine Reidy, executive director, Commission on Dietetic Registration, for having the vision to start a Weight Management Certificate Course. It was that course and its faculty that gave us the idea for this book.

We would like to acknowledge all of our patients who have shared their struggles about weight management, and taught us so much over the years. They are the reason for this book. Likewise, we thank each of our colleagues who continue in the battle to treat overweight and obesity more effectively. This book incorporates many of their teachings.

Cathy A. Nonas and Gary D. Foster, editors

INTRODUCTION

We are pleased to be editing a second edition of *Managing Obesity: A Clinical Guide*. The first edition, published in 2004, seemed to meet the need for a resource that combined authoritative research briefings with practical advice about bringing empirically supported treatments to life. In this edition, we have more than updated this important information; we have also added new chapters on issues such as pregnancy and menopause, weight bias, and reimbursement.

In the first edition, we included a number of sections that discussed the clinical care of the obese individual in both outpatient and inpatient settings. This information remains important, but not much has changed. We have added some important new information about the Nutrition Care Process, but we have not repeated sections that we thought could be read in the original edition and remain current today.

On the other hand, in the last edition, we devoted only one chapter to dietary approaches for obesity management. Over the years, it has become clear that all diets that create an energy deficit result in weight loss, and most approaches are associated with improvements in health. The Achilles' heel of any dietary approach is adherence, which remains less than optimal for most hypocaloric regimens. Therefore, in this second edition of the book, different dietary approaches are explored in greater detail. To that end, we asked experts who have been instrumental in the development and/or evaluation of various dietary approaches to write separate sections about each one: meal replacements (Chapter 2), low-glycemic index/load diets (Chapter 3), Mediterranean/DASH diets (Chapter 4), and low-carbohydrate diets (Chapter 5). In addition, each of the diet-focused chapters includes a section written by a clinical expert on implementing these approaches in the real world. As reviewed in the first edition, no matter which approach is used, it is important to keep in mind several principles: (*a*) flexibility; (*b*) nutritional status; (*c*) health outcomes; (*d*) weight-loss outcomes; and (*e*) the client's perspective.

In Section 1 of this edition, we have once again structured chapters to present a brief, authoritative research overview followed by a discussion of practical applications that translates science into real-life scenarios. In this section, we have updated the assessment, physical activity, behavior therapy, and weight maintenance chapters (Chapters 1, 6, 7, and 10, respectively) because these topics remain vital to any successful weight-management strategy. The medication chapter (Chapter 8) has been rewritten to include the most up-to-date information about Food and Drug Administration approvals and nonapprovals as well as what may be in store in the future. The surgery chapter (Chapter 9) has been expanded to include more information on the different kinds of surgery, the recommendations for weight loss before surgery, and postoperative micro- and macro-nutrient needs.

Finally, we have added an entirely new section on special issues. Chapters 11 through 16 address six topics not explicitly covered in the first edition that we believe are critical to better understanding and treating those who suffer from obesity.

It would be remiss not to bring public health issues to the forefront. The chapter on obesity and public health (Chapter 11) highlights that the individual is not the only focal point. Public health efforts help change the environment, making the difficult work of eating better and moving more a bit easier.

As efforts to secure insurance coverage for the treatment of obesity continue, the chapter on economics of obesity (Chapter 12) underscores both the significant costs of obesity and its associated diseases and the issues of billing for a nonreimbursable disease. This up-to-date information is vital to any clinician who treats obesity.

As Chapter 13 explains, cultural mores—such as beliefs about body size, dietary preferences, and physical activity—are critical to consider in the clinical arena. Discrimination and prejudice related to obesity (Chapter 14) is another topic to which our field has not paid enough attention. Greater focus on these issues will result in increased sensitivity among clinicians and more compassionate care for those we treat.

We have also included a chapter on prevention of obesity in school settings (Chapter 15). Given the serious and refractory nature of obesity and the limited reach of any clinic-based treatment, prevention is a key to reducing overall obesity prevalence. In schools, we have an opportunity to change an environment in which children spend a great percentage of their time, potentially reducing the risk of obesity and promoting a lifetime of healthy behaviors.

Finally, Chapter 16 discusses the distinct weight-management challenges that face women from puberty to menopause. Helping to prevent weight gain during these particular life stages, and helping women to understand they are not alone, is vital to the long-term health of women as they age.

It takes tremendous effort to defend against an environment that promotes individuals to eat more and move less. This biological and behavioral battle must be approached from both an individual and a public health perspective. It is heartening to see progress. Obesity prevalence remains high, but recent reports show a flattening in prevalence for both adults and children (1). There is a growing national movement to increase physical activity in schools and to promote more community gardens and bring farm food back to the neighborhood. At least six cities/counties—New York City, Kings County (WA), Multnomah County (OR), San Francisco, Santa Clara county (CA), and Philadelphia—and one state (California) have mandated that calorie information be easily available in chain restaurants. On the individual side, there are encouraging signs that the toolbox for treating obesity, from diet to surgery, is getting larger and making long-term intervention possible. Recent research by Wing and her colleagues in the *New England Journal of Medicine* has shown remarkable rates of weight maintenance after weight loss (2). Finally, it is important to remind ourselves and our clients that small weight losses bring large improvements in health and quality of life.

We hope that this second edition of *Managing Obesity: A Clinical Guide* offers a more holistic view of obesity with a clear focus on how to best treat this serious, prevalent, and refractory disease. Most importantly, we hope this book offers encouragement to all of you working on the frontlines of the obesity pandemic. Although we have much more to do, we are moving on the right track.

Cathy A. Nonas and Gary D. Foster

CHAPTER 1

ASSESSMENT OF THE OBESE INDIVIDUAL

PART A: OVERVIEW

ROBERT F. KUSHNER, MD

INTRODUCTION

When we think of assessment of the overweight and obese individual, it is typically defined as recording anthropometric measurements, such as calculating body mass index (BMI) from height and weight data, measuring waist circumference or waist-to-hip ratio, taking a diet and weight history, noting obesity-related comorbid conditions, and summing up the problem. That is all true. However, a skilled and experienced clinician knows that these necessary components of the assessment are only part of the evaluation process. Listening to the client to ascertain her perceptions and world view and characterizing her personality are equally important. For example, whether the client answers questions methodically and analytically or through a stream of tears provides valuable insight. Whether the client comes to the first visit prepared with any pre-visit questionnaires and forms completed or arrives unprepared with no forms completed is also a useful diagnostic observation. Furthermore, it is important to set the stage by establishing the right tone, style, and empathy during the first encounter with the client. Developing a concerned and trusting therapeutic relationship is essential to the treatment that will follow. In other words, a skillful assessment is characterized not only by what the clinician *does*, but also *how* the clinician acts and interprets information. It is this "relationship-centered" encounter that will, in part, determine treatment outcomes. This is the art of an effective and informative obesity assessment. This chapter will highlight key aspects of the obesity assessment as an introduction to the next chapter on practical applications.

REFLECTIONS FROM THE MEDICAL PROFESSION

Why is obesity assessment given so much attention in this book? The answer is simple—it is infrequently done in medical practice. Therefore, whether the registered dietitian

(RD) is seeing a client primarily for overweight, obesity, weight gain, or an obesity-related comorbid condition, it is highly likely that the client has not had a thorough obesity-focused assessment by their health care practitioner. Furthermore, be prepared for your client to harbor a wide range of attitudes and biases about the medical profession when it comes to addressing obesity. Although overweight or obesity represents one of the most common chronic medical problems seen by the primary care physician and is associated with an increased risk of multiple health problems, obesity is underrecognized and undertreated in the primary care setting. Survey studies conducted among patients and physicians uniformly demonstrate that physicians are failing to adequately identify overweight and mildly obese individuals, although there is greater recognition for moderate to severe obesity in patients, particularly when accompanied by comorbid conditions. In general, fewer than half of obese adults are being advised to lose weight by health care professionals. In a survey study by Potter et al (1) of more than 400 adult patients attending two primary care practices, the most common weight-loss approach physicians used for overweight patients was not bringing up the subject at all—a "don't ask, don't tell" strategy was noted by 61% of the patients.

The low rates of identification and treatment of obesity are thought to be due to multiple factors, including lack of reimbursement, limited time during office visits, lack of training in counseling, competing demands, or low confidence in ability to treat and change patient behaviors. And when obesity is addressed, many patients feel demeaned by their physician for having no willpower or just not trying hard enough.

Despite the low rates of evaluation, physicians are being encouraged to identify, assess, and treat obesity. The US Preventive Services Task Force (2,3) and other societies and organizations (4–10) have endorsed periodic measurement of height and weight for all patients as a useful screening tool. Additionally, the US Department of Health Services Agency for Healthcare Research and Quality (AHRQ) checklist for health recommends that all men and women have their BMI calculated to screen for obesity (11). Thus, clients coming to the RD for obesity counseling may or may not have been adequately screened and counseled by their physicians. As part of the dietary assessment process, it is therefore helpful to determine what the client has been told and whether any recommendations were made by the health care provider.

KEY COMPONENTS OF THE OBESITY-FOCUSED HISTORY

Information from the history should address the following questions:

- What factors contribute to the client's obesity?
- How is the obesity affecting the client's health?
- What is the client's level of risk regarding obesity?
- What are the client's goals and expectations?
- Is the client motivated to enter a weight management program?
- What level of support does the client have at home to make changes?
- What kind of help does the client need?

Specific information pertinent to an obesity-focused history includes the following:

- The chronological history of weight gain (age at onset, description of weight gain [and loss] and inciting events, weight pattern [progressive weight gain, weight cycling])
- Family history of obesity
- Endocrine disorders causing obesity (polycystic ovarian syndrome [PCOS], hypothyroidism, hypothalamic tumors, genetic syndromes)
- Response to previous weight loss attempts
- Lifestyle history (client's current diet and physical activity patterns along with existing or potential barriers to change)
- Social history (issues that are supportive of or interfere with a weight loss plan)
- Psychiatric/psychological history (emotional triggers to eating, such as loneliness, boredom, stress, low self-esteem, social isolation, depression, binge eating disorder [BED])
- Medication history (to uncover possible drug-induced weight gain as well as medications interfering with weight loss)

Table 1.1 provides a list of medications that are associated with weight gain due to increased body fat. Drug-induced weight gain is an extremely important consideration. Often, the physician can either reduce the medication or prescribe a substitute medication that is weight-neutral or even promotes weight loss. If the client is taking one of those medications, and the initial history reveals weight gain secondary to taking the prescribed drug, then suggest that the client return to the prescribing physician for reassessment.

In the end, the purpose of gathering this information is to form an impression of the client, to identify the factors that have led to and are sustaining his or her body weight. Determination of these factors is vital because it will lead to targeted and individualized treatment. Quite simply, every person has his or her own story to tell, usually a mix of

TABLE 1.1
Drugs That May Induce Weight Gain

Drug Category	Examples
Antidepressants	• Tricyclic antidepressants (TCAs): amitriptyline, imipramine, nortriptyline • Selective serotonin reuptake inhibitors (SSRIs): paroxetine • Monoamine oxidase inhibitors (MAOIs): phenelzine, tranylcypromine • Miscellaneous: mirtazepine
Mood stabilizers	• Lithium
Typical antipsychotics	• Chlorpromazine, haloperidol
Atypical antipsychotics	• Clozapine, olanzapine, risperidone
Anti-epileptics	• Valproate, gabapentin, carbamazepine
Diabetes medication	• Insulin • Sulfonylureas: glyburide, glipizide • Thiazolidinediones: pioglitazone, rosiglitizone
Steroid hormones	• Prednisone, medroxyprogesterone

social, behavioral, cultural, psychological, and medical factors. This author has used a lifestyle patterns approach as a means of synthesizing information from the history and developing a personalized treatment plan (12,13). Based on empirical observations, these patterns or habits have been categorized into distinct eating, exercise, and coping lifestyle patterns. By listening for and identifying patterns during the assessment, the clinician is able to validate the client's habits, beliefs, and attitudes and begin planning for treatment.

To expedite the historical portion of the assessment, many clinicians use a self-administered history questionnaire that can be either mailed to the client before the initial visit or completed in the waiting room. An example of a patient history questionnaire can be obtained from the American Medical Association's Assessment and Management of Adult Obesity: A Primer for Physicians (14).

ASSESSING MEDICAL CONDITIONS

It is essential to know the client's conditions and diseases that are directly or indirectly related to obesity. Box 1.1 (15) lists the nine organ systems and more than 40 medical conditions associated with obesity. It can be conveniently used as a checklist during the review of systems section of the medical history and when developing an obesity-related medical problem list.

Although individuals vary, the number and severity of organ-specific comorbid conditions usually rises with increasing levels of obesity (15). Often clients with obesity will be referred for counseling for a comorbid condition, such as type 2 diabetes mellitus, coronary heart disease, hypertension, or hyperlipidemia, as the chief disorder. During the assessment, the clinician should evaluate the duration, severity, and control of the comorbid condition(s). In addition, questions about the client's perception of the condition and self-care behaviors are informative in planning obesity treatment. Examples of useful questions include the following:

- "Do you think that your weight affects your health or medical condition? If so, how?"
- "What have you done to control the medical condition?"
- "Do you monitor your medical condition and take medication as prescribed?"

Poor self-care behaviors or low confidence in one's ability to manage the condition need to be explored further because they may translate into difficulties in obesity care. When possible, pertinent laboratory and diagnostic tests should be requested from the client's health care provider on a periodic basis because these will be used to guide treatment.

EXAMINATION OF THE OBESE CLIENT

According to the National Heart Lung and Blood Institute guidelines, assessment of risk status due to overweight or obesity is based on the client's BMI, waist circumference, and comorbid conditions (4). As previously discussed, a list of medical problems can be

Box 1.1
Obesity-Related Organ Systems Review

Cardiovascular
- Hypertension
- Congestive heart failure
- Cor pulmonale
- Varicose veins
- Pulmonary embolism
- Coronary artery disease

Respiratory
- Dyspnea
- Obstructive sleep apnea
- Hypoventilation syndrome
- Pickwickian syndrome
- Asthma

Endocrine
- Metabolic syndrome
- Type 2 diabetes
- Dyslipidemia
- Polycystic ovarian syndrome (PCOS)/androgenicity
- Amenorrhea/infertility/menstrual disorders

Gastrointestinal
- Gastroesophageal reflux disease (GERD)
- Non-alcoholic fatty liver disease (NAFLD)
- Cholelithiasis
- Hernias
- Colon cancer

Musculoskeletal
- Hyperuricemia and gout
- Immobility
- Osteoarthritis (knees and hips)
- Low back pain

Genitourinary
- Urinary stress incontinence
- Obesity-related glomerulopathy
- renal disease (ESRD)
- Hypogonadism (male)
- Breast and uterine cancer
- Pregnancy complications

Psychological
- Depression/low self-esteem
- Body image disturbance
- Social stigmatization

Integument
- Striae distensae (stretch marks)
- Stasis pigmentation of legs
- Lymphedema
- Cellulitis
- Intertrigo, carbuncles
- Acanthosis nigricans
- Acrochordon (skin tags)
- Hidradenitis suppurativa

Neurologic
- Stroke
- Idiopathic intracranial hypertension
- Meralgia paresthetica
- Dementia

Source: Data are from reference 15.

obtained by taking a thorough history or having the client use the items in Box 1.1 as a checklist. In contrast, height, weight, and waist circumference will need to be measured by the clinician.

Body Mass Index

The classification of obesity by BMI replaces previous weight-height terminology such as percent ideal or desirable body weight. BMI is recommended because it provides an estimate of body fat and is related to risk of disease. A desirable or healthful BMI is 18.5

to 24.9, overweight is a BMI of 25 to 29.9, and obesity is BMI of 30 or more. Obesity is further subdefined into class I (30.0–34.9), class II (35.0–39.9), and class III (≥40). Although "morbid obesity" is still listed in the ICD-9-CM for coding purposes, it is currently being replaced by other descriptive terms, including class III obesity, extreme obesity, or clinically severe obesity.

Waist Circumference

Abdominal fat is clinically defined as a waist circumference of 102 cm or more (≥40 inches) in men and 88 cm or more (≥35 inches) in women. According to the *Practical Guide to the Identification, Evaluation, and Treatment of Overweight and Obesity in Adults* (16):

> To measure waist circumference, locate the upper hip bone and the top of the right iliac crest. Place a measuring tape in a horizontal plane around the abdomen at the level of the iliac crest. Before reading the tape measure, ensure that the tape is snug, but does not compress the skin, and is parallel to the floor. The measurement is made at the end of a normal expiration.

Overweight individuals with waist circumferences exceeding these limits should be urged more strongly to pursue weight reduction because an enlarged waist categorically increases disease risk for each BMI class. Measuring and documenting waist circumference in clients with a BMI less than 35 is important because abdominal fat independently contributes to the development of comorbid diseases, particularly metabolic syndrome.

WORKING WITH THE CLIENT'S HEALTH CARE PROVIDER

Whether the clinician works in a health care provider's office, in a hospital outpatient setting, or has her own practice, it is important that the RD functions as part of an integrative team. Interdisciplinary teams are an important component of the chronic care model (17,18). In this model, team members come from different professions and each member contributes his or her expertise to the care of the client. In a delegative model, one team member (usually the primary care physician) leads the team and retains overall responsibility for patient care. For this cooperation to exist, communication channels need to be established and sustained. This can be accomplished by developing assessment and treatment forms that are sent by mail, fax, or e-mail along with periodic informal telephone calls.

The most important aspect of an integrated team is to share a common philosophy of care. Be sure to document when attempts to reach the physician were made and whether you discussed with the client the need for a follow-up visit to monitor potential changes in the risk profile.

SUMMARY

Assessment of the overweight and obese individual is the first and indispensable component of the obesity care process. According to the chronic care model, good outcomes are the result of productive interactions between an informed, engaged client (and their family or caregivers) and a prepared, proactive practice team. This communication leads to a continuous healing relationship. By establishing a trustworthy and caring rapport on the first assessment visit, the clinician will be able to obtain the necessary information to guide the client's treatment course.

References

1. Potter MB, Vu JD, Groughan-Minhane M. Weight management: what patients want from their primary care physicians. *J Fam Pract*. 2001;50:513.

2. US Preventive Services Task Force. Screening for obesity in adults: recommendations and rationale. *Ann Intern Med*. 2003;139:930–932.

3. McTigue KM, Harris R, Hemphil B, Lux L, Sutton S, Bunton AJ, Lohr KN. Screening and interventions for obesity in adults: summary of the evidence for the U.S. Preventive Services Task Force. *Ann Intern Med*. 2003;139:933–949. (Appendix tables are available at: http://www.annals.org.)

4. National Heart, Lung, and Blood Institute. Clinical guidelines on the identification, evaluation, and treatment of overweight and obesity in adults. The evidence report. *Obes Res*. 1998;6(suppl):51S–209S.

5. Guzman SE, American Academy of Family Physicians Panel on Obesity. Practical advice for family physicians to help overweight patients. Leawood, KS: AAFP; 2003. https://secure.aafp.org/catalog/viewProduct.do?productId=709&categoryId =2. Accessed February 2, 2009

6. Nawaz H, Katz DL. American College of Preventive Medicine practice policy statement. Weight management counseling of overweight adults. *Am J Prev Med*. 2001;21:73–78.

7. Lyznicki JM, Young DC, Riggs JA, Davis RM; Council on Scientific Affairs, American Medical Association. Obesity: assessment and management in primary care. *Am Fam Physician*. 2001;63:2185–2196.

8. Cummings S, Parham ES, Strain GW. Position of the American Dietetic Association: weight management. *J Am Diet Assoc*. 2002;102:1145–1155.

9. National Task Force on the Prevention and Treatment of Obesity. Medical care for obese patients: advice for health professionals. *Am Fam Physician*. 2002;65: 81–88.

10. Eyre H, Kahn R, Robertson RM. Preventing cancer, cardiovascular disease, and diabetes. A common agenda for the American Cancer Society, the American Diabetes Association, and the American Heart Association. *Circulation*. 2004;109:3244–3255.

11. US Department of Health Services Agency for Healthcare Research and Quality (AHRQ). Screening for obesity in adults. http://www.ahrq.gov/clinic/3rduspstf/obesity/obeswh.htm. Accessed February 2, 2009.

12. Kushner RF, Kushner N. *Dr. Kushner's Personality Type Diet*. New York, NY: St. Martin's Griffin Press; 2004.

13. Kushner RF, Kushner N, Jackson Blatner D. *Counseling Overweight Adults: The Lifestyle Patterns Approach and Toolkit*. Chicago, IL: American Dietetic Association; 2009.

14. Kushner RF. Roadmaps for Clinical Practice: Case Studies in Disease Prevention and Health Promotion—Assessment and Management of Adult Obesity: A Primer for Physicians. Chicago, IL: American Medical Association; 2003. http://www.ama-assn.org/ama/pub/category/10931.html. Accessed November 10, 2008.

15. Kushner RF, Roth JL. Assessment of the obese patient. *Endocrinol Metab Clin N Am*. 2003;32:915–934.

16. National Heart, Lung, and Blood Institute (NHLBI) and North American Association for the Study of Obesity (NAASO). *Practical Guide to the Identification, Evaluation, and Treatment of Overweight and Obesity in Adults*. Bethesda, MD: National Institutes of Health; 2000. NIH pub 00-4084.

17. Bodenheimer T, Wagner EH, Grumbach K. Improving primary care for patients with chronic illness. *JAMA*. 2002;288:1775–1779.

18. Wagner E. The role of patient care teams in chronic disease management. *BMJ*. 2000;320:569–672.

PART B: PRACTICAL APPLICATIONS

CHRISTINA K. BIESEMEIER, MS, RD, FADA

INTRODUCTION

No one would dispute that a paramount skill in patient/client relations is the ability of the clinician to meet the client where the client is and to move toward client-centered goals at the speed the client is willing to go. That said, these individualized goals need to be couched within a set of standard, evidence-based guidelines that are integral to appropriate nutrition care. The American Dietetic Association's four-step cycle of care, the Nutrition Care Process (NCP), in combination with the Adult Weight Management Evidence Based Practice Guideline (AWM), provides that necessary guidance for managing overweight and obese clients (1,2). The NCP offers a standardized framework in which to provide patient care; it does not suggest that all clients receive the same care. The NCP incorporates medical nutrition therapy, but it also can be used to guide nutrition education and other preventive care. The NCP relies on evidence-based practice—that is, the integration of the best available evidence with professional expertise and client values to improve outcomes (3). The AWM summarizes evidence-based care for ambulatory adults with overweight and obesity.

NCP STEP 1: NUTRITION ASSESSMENT

2. nutrition diagnosis
3. nutrition intervent
4. monitoring 1 evalion

Critical thinking skills are imperative throughout the four steps of the NCP. In the first step of the NCP, nutrition assessment, the registered dietitian (RD) completes two activities: (*a*) collects timely and appropriate data and (*b*) analyzes and interprets the collected data, using relevant norms and evidence-based standards (1). The clinician identifies discrepancies between the client's data and the norms and standards—ie, situations when the client's data are either above or below the norms and standards.

Data are collected from the referral form, the medical record, and the client and/or caregivers. Measurements are obtained by other providers or by the RD at the time of the initial appointment. Ideally, the client completes history forms and keeps a record of food intake before the initial appointment, to make maximum use of face-to-face time during the appointment to fill in any gaps in data, collect measurements, and discuss priorities and goals for intervention.

Data are organized into five broad categories (see Table 1.2). Categories of data are discussed in more detail in the following sections.

Client History

The RD evaluates the client's medical history from a nutrition perspective and identifies obesity-related conditions and medical risk factors that indicate a need for more in-depth nutrition therapy. Refer to Box 1.1 in Part A of this chapter or the *Clinical Guidelines on the Identification, Evaluation, and Treatment of Overweight and Obesity in Adults* (4) for medical conditions associated with obesity.

TABLE 1.2
Nutrition Assessment Data

Category	Examples
Client history	• Personal history • Client and family medical histories • Social history
Food/nutrition-related history	• Food and nutrient intake • Medications and dietary supplements • Physical activity and function • Client perceptions and beliefs—goals and stage of readiness to make changes; self-efficacy; HRQoL and NQoL
Biochemical data, medical tests, and procedures	• Laboratory test results • Measured resting metabolic rate • Metabolic profile
Nutrition-focused physical findings	• Blood pressure • Heart rate
Anthropometric measurements	• Physical measurements • Body mass index • Waist circumference

Abbreviations: HRQoL, Health-related Quality of Life; NQoL, Nutrition Quality of Life.

During the review of the medical history, the RD identifies possible medical causes for overweight or obesity and rules out contraindications for weight reduction. Contraindications to weight loss intervention include pregnancy and lactation; medical conditions that might be negatively affected by energy restriction (eg, cancer during active treatment with surgery, chemotherapy, or radiation therapy); and uncontrolled psychiatric conditions (eg, clinical depression, anorexia nervosa, bulimia nervosa, anxiety disorder, or binge eating disorder), especially when clients are not in active treatment (2). Box 1.2 lists selected tools that the RD can use to screen for possible psychiatric conditions and to identify clients who might benefit from referral to other providers for psychological intervention. (For more information on these types of tools, refer to reference 5.) The RD should remain within his/her scope of practice, based on education, experience, competency, state licensure, and institutional policies.

The RD also collects and evaluates the client's family and social history, including family health history; family history of overweight, obesity, and/or eating disorders; personal events and stressors; and support systems.

Food/Nutrition-related History

The RD collects several types of data in this section of the nutrition assessment, including:

- Food intake
- Weight history
- Diet experience
- Exercise/physical activity history
- Medication and herbal supplement intake
- Client knowledge, beliefs, and attitudes

The RD can use a variety of tools and resources to collect food and nutrition history data, based in part on the practice setting, educational level of the client, the client's ability to use computer technology, and available time. Evaluation of food intake can range from simple (eg, number of servings from each food group) to complex (eg, computer analysis of macronutrients and micronutrients). A weight history provides data on usual

---

Box 1.2
Screening Tools for Psychological/Psychiatric Conditions

Beck Depression Inventory-II: Self-administered, 21 items; measures characteristics of depression.
Questionnaire on Eating and Weight Pattern—Revised: Measures characteristics of overeating and loss of control.
On-Line Tool: LEARN Program (http://www.TheLifestyleCompany.com): Includes depression and binge-eating questionnaires, stress management assessment, and readiness test.

weight, patterns of gain and loss, situations associated with weight change, preferred weight, and reason(s) for this preference. A dieting history provides data on the number and types of diets followed in the past, as well as information on success, perceptions of what worked and did not work, and reasons why or why not.

In the physical activity history, the RD determines the frequency, duration, and intensity of current activity; the amounts of lifestyle activity, sedentary time, and screen time; the role that activity has played in previous weight-loss attempts; and whether the client is doing self-monitoring of activity. When clients are not physically active, the RD assesses attitudes about activity and uses the Physical Activity Readiness Questionnaire (PAR-Q) to determine need for a medical clearance to participate in physical activity (6). Because physical activity is an essential component of any comprehensive weight-management program the RD may prefer to obtain a medical clearance for physical activity for all clients referred for weight-management treatment, rather than adding a second step in the referral process. (See Chapter 6 for more information on PAR-Q and physical activity.)

The food/nutrition-related history includes a review of prescription and nonprescription medications, including those used for the treatment of overweight and obesity, and dietary supplements. It can be helpful to ask the client to bring all medications and supplements to the first appointment so that a complete list of medications can be made. The RD evaluates reasons for medication and supplement use (eg, weight loss, improved performance, or correction of nutrient deficits and deficiencies) and evaluates the impact of medications on weight status.

The food/nutrition-related history also includes collecting and evaluating data related to the client's perceptions and beliefs about weight and weight management, readiness to make changes in individual health and eating behaviors, and ability to cope with stress and maintain changes in behaviors over time. Box 1.3 lists questions the RD might ask during this component of the assessment.

The RD also assesses the client's baseline quality of life. A valuable tool to use in this section of the assessment is the Nutrition Quality of Life (NQoL), a tool that measures the impact of medical nutrition therapy (MNT) on a client's quality of life in six areas: food impact, self image, psychological factors, social/interpersonal, physical, and self-efficacy (7). The NQoL was developed using focus group research with clients and the RDs who provided MNT to these clients. It has content validation, reliability testing,

---

Box 1.3

Questions on Readiness to Change and Self-Efficacy

- Why is the client seeking treatment now?
- What are the client's goals for treatment?
- What does the client think weight management will achieve?
- How motivated or interested is the client in making changes? How ready is the client to commit time, energy, and resources to weight loss?
- How confident is the client in his/her ability to make desired changes?
- What barriers does the client foresee to weight loss?

and an analysis of sensitivity to change over time. Until full validation is complete, the NQoL developers suggest using the tool in a yes/no format, an example of which is available in the Web Learning Resource Center at the AWM Certificate Course link on the Weight Management Dietetic Practice Group Web site (http://www.wmdpg. org) (8).

Biochemical Data, Medical Tests, and Procedures

The types of laboratory data and results from medical tests required for nutrition assessment depend on the client's degree of overweight/obesity, risk factor profile, and the type and intensity of medical or surgical treatment planned for the client. At a minimum, the RD needs a baseline lipid profile and fasting blood glucose for each client. Box 1.4 lists other laboratory and medical tests that may be useful, depending on the client's condition.

Nutrition-focused Physical Findings

Baseline blood pressure and heart rate are needed. Serial blood pressure measurements should be monitored for clients on weight-loss or antihypertensive medications. Serial heart rate monitoring is important for clients on low- and very-low-calorie diets because the rate of weight loss increases the risk of cardiac abnormalities.

Anthropometric Measurements

According to the AWM Practice Guideline and the National Heart, Lung, and Blood Institute (NHLBI) Guidelines, BMI, and waist circumference should be used to classify overweight and obesity, estimate risk for disease, and identify treatment options (2,4). This recommendation was made because BMI and waist circumference are highly corre-

---

Box 1.4
Additional Laboratory Tests and Procedures

Laboratory values
- Insulin
- Thyroid stimulating hormone
- Electrolytes
- Uric acid
- Liver function tests
- Hemoglobin A1C
- Urinalysis (ketones)

Medical tests
- Electrocardiogram (EKG) (to evaluate arrhythmias, obtain exercise clearance, evaluate cardiovascular disease status/risk)
- Tests to evaluate sleep apnea and dyspnea

TABLE 1.3

Classification of Overweight and Obesity by BMI, Waist Circumference, and Associated Disease Risk

Classification	BMI	Health Risk Relative to BMI and WC	
		Men: WC ≤ 40 in Women: WC ≤ 35 in	Men: WC > 40 in Women: WC > 35 in
Underweight	< 18.5	—	—
Normal	18.5–24.9	—	Increased
Overweight	25.0–29.9	Increased	High
Obesity class I	30.0–34.9	High	Very high
Obesity class II	35.0–39.9	Very high	Very high
Extreme obesity (obesity class III)	≥ 40	Extremely high	Extremely high

Abbreviations: BMI, body mass index; WC, waist circumference.
Source: Adapted from reference 4.

lated with obesity or fat mass and the risk of other diseases. In addition, both measurements are simple to obtain, inexpensive, and noninvasive. Table 1.3 (4) shows classifications of weight based on BMI and disease risk based on BMI and waist circumference.

BMI presumes an accurate measurement of weight and height, using scales with adequate weight capacity and a wall-mounted stadiometer to measure height. BMI has limitations, including an insensitivity to small changes in weight; possible overestimation of body fat in athletes, individuals with a muscular build, and those with edema; and possible underestimation of body fat in older individuals and clients who have lost muscle mass (4).

The NHLBI recommends measurement of waist circumference at the ileac crest, although there is no universally accepted site for this measurement (9). In addition, although waist circumference can be used to identify cardiometabolic risk beyond BMI alone, a waist circumference measurement is not likely to affect the clinical management of clients if BMI and other risk factors have already been determined (9). For this reason, a 2007 consensus statement recommended the following use of waist circumference (9):

• To determine need for risk-factor evaluation in individuals with normal BMI
• To determine disease risk in individuals with BMI < 35, because disease risk is very high or extremely high for BMI ≥ 35 regardless of waist circumference
• To monitor response to diet and physical activity because regular aerobic exercise can cause a reduction in both waist circumference and cardiometabolic risk without a change in BMI

Body fat composition can be determined. However, the National Institutes of Health and the World Health Organization have not established guidelines for assessment of body fat composition due to the lack of consistency and reliability in measurement techniques (4,10). In addition, measurement equipment is costly and not readily available in most practice settings, making this parameter an impractical one for most RDs.

Cardiometabolic Risk

It is important for the RD to evaluate the client's risk factors to determine his/her cardiometabolic risk profile—ie, the risk of disease and the likelihood of complications and death from these diseases. The RD can assess disease risk either by performing a Disease Risk Assessment (risk for diabetes mellitus, cardiovascular disease, and/or hypertension) or by determining whether the client meets the criteria for metabolic syndrome (risk for diabetes mellitus and cardiovascular disease) (10). Box 1.5 (11) lists the criteria for metabolic syndrome.

The RD can assess the likelihood of disease complications and mortality risk by determining either the client's Obesity Health Risk or his/her "hard coronary heart disease" (hard CHD) risk (ie, risk for a myocardial infarction and death from CHD within the next 10 years) (4,11). According to the Obesity Health Risk, clients who are obese with coronary heart disease, atherosclerotic disease, type 2 diabetes mellitus, and/or sleep apnea are at very high risk for complications and mortality. Those who are obese with three or more specified risk factors are at high risk of disease complications (4).

Hard CHD risk is based on Framingham data and establishes three levels of risk. Individuals with existing CHD, other clinical forms of atherosclerotic disease, and diabetes are at the highest risk level, more than 20% hard CHD risk. Individuals with zero or one specified risk factor are likely to be at low CHD risk, less than 10% risk in the next 10 years. A risk assessment is needed to determine risk for individuals with two or more risk factors (11).

Information about cardiometabolic risk is not intended to frighten clients. However, this information puts the data in perspective for both the RD and the client, clarifies health status and priorities, and provides a basis for building motivation to change behaviors.

Comparative Standards: Energy Requirements

Total energy expenditure (TEE) is composed of resting metabolic rate (RMR; 65%–70% of TEE), physical activity level (20%–30% of TEE), and the thermic effect of food

---

Box 1.5
Criteria for Metabolic Syndrome

Any three of the following risk factors:

- Abdominal obesity defined by waist circumference: men > 40 in (102 cm); women > 35 in (88 cm)
- Triglycerides ≥ 150 mg/dL
- High-density lipoprotein: men < 40 mg/dL; women < 50 mg/dL
- Blood pressure ≥ 130 mmHg systolic, ≥ 85 mmHg diastolic
- Fasting glucose ≥ 100 mg/dL

Source: Adapted from reference 11.

Box 1.6
Mifflin-St. Jeor Equations for Estimating Resting Metabolic Rate (RMR)

Men: RMR (kcal/d) = 10 × Wt (kg) + 6.25 × Ht (cm) − 5 × Age (y) + 5

Women: RMR (kcal/d) = 10 × Wt (kg) + 6.25 × Ht (cm) − 5 × Age (y) − 161

Source: Data are from reference 12.

(approximately 10% of TEE) (12). According to the AWM Practice Guideline, when possible, estimated energy needs should be based on a measured RMR obtained by either direct or indirect calorimetry (2).

When RMR cannot be measured, the AWM Practice Guideline (2) recommends use of the Mifflin-St. Jeor equation (13) for estimating RMR in overweight and obese ambulatory clients, using actual body weight in calculations (see Box 1.6) (2). A systematic review of the literature determined that in ambulatory patients the Mifflin-St. Jeor equation (using actual weight) estimated RMR closest to the measured RMR. In 70% of patients, this equation came within ±10% of measured RMR. For the remaining 30%, there was a 21% underestimation and a 9% overestimation (2).

RMR, whether measured or estimated, is used to determine the energy requirement. For example:

Energy Expenditure = RMR × Physical Activity Factor (PAF)

This equation incorporates an activity factor. One set of activity factors that can be used as a reference is published in the Dietary Reference Intakes for energy expenditure (12):

- ≥ 1.0 < 1.4 (sedentary)
- ≥ 1.4 < 1.6 (low active)
- ≥ 1.6 < 1.9 (active)
- ≥ 1.9 < 2.5 (very active)

The RD uses the client's energy requirement to evaluate overall energy intake in the context of recent weight changes, make nutrition diagnoses, and determine the client's nutrition prescription. Nine of 10 individuals do not know the correct number of calories they should eat each day. Therefore, it is helpful to share this information with the client (14).

NCP STEP 2: NUTRITION DIAGNOSIS

In the second step of the NCP, nutrition diagnosis, the RD identifies the client's nutrition problems based on discrepancies between his/her actual data or measurements, collected during the nutrition assessment, and relevant norms and evidence-based standards. A nutrition diagnosis is a specific nutrition problem that can be resolved or improved through nutrition intervention by the RD (1). Signs and symptoms are clustered together; and a problem is identified and given a label from the ADA's International Dietetics and Nutrition Terminology (IDNT) (15). The RD determines the root cause or etiology of the nutrition problem, which becomes the focus of nutrition interventions that are carried out in the next step of the NCP.

PES Statements

The RD's critical thinking often follows a flow from signs and symptoms to problem to etiology; however, the nutrition diagnosis is written in a problem, etiology, signs and symptoms format known as a PES statement, with connecting phrases between the three components of the statement. Box 1.7 provides a template of this format. Box 1.8 provides a sample process and two PES statements.

Types of Nutrition Diagnoses

Nutrition diagnoses are organized into three domains: intake, clinical, and behavioral-environmental. Box 1.9 provides a list of common nutrition diagnoses for clients with overweight and obesity (15).

The *International Dietetics & Nutrition Terminology (IDNT) Reference Manual* has a reference sheet for each nutrition diagnosis that includes a definition of the problem, a

---

Box 1.7
PES Format

Nutrition diagnostic (*problem*) label: _____

Related to (*etiology*): _____

As evidenced by (*signs and symptoms*): _____

Box 1.8
Examples of PES Statements

- Excessive energy intake related to reduction in physical activity after injury to right foot and increased consumption of evening snacks while watching TV as evidenced by self-report of change in activity and intake patterns and weight gain of 20 pounds over past 4 months.
- Involuntary weight gain related to reduction in physical activity after injury to right foot and increased consumption of evening snacks while watching TV as evidenced by self-report of change in activity and intake patterns and weight gain of 20 pounds over past 4 months.

Box 1.9

Common Nutrition Diagnoses in Overweight and Obesity

IDNT

- NI-1.5: Excessive energy intake
- NI-2.2: Excessive oral food/beverage intake
- NC-3.3: Overweight/obesity
- NC-3.4: Involuntary weight gain
- NI-4.3: Excessive alcohol intake
- NI-51.2: Excessive fat intake
- NI-53.2: Excessive intake of carbohydrate
- NC-2.2: Altered nutrition-related lab values
- NB-1.1: Food, nutrition, and nutrition-related knowledge deficit
- NB-1.3: Not ready for diet/lifestyle change
- NB-1.4: Self-monitoring deficit
- NB-1.5: Disordered eating pattern
- NB-1.6: Limited adherence to nutrition-related recommendations
- NB-2.1: Physical inactivity

---

list of possible etiologies, and the signs and symptoms of the problem, outlined in the five data categories described previously in this chapter. In selecting a specific diagnosis, at least one sign or symptom listed on the problem's reference sheet must be present, although preferably a cluster of signs and symptoms from the reference sheet can be identified. The RD may make one nutrition diagnosis or several, depending on the complexity of the client's clinical situation. Each nutrition diagnosis is written in a PES statement, although nutrition diagnoses with the same etiology may be written in a single PES (15).

Strategies for Success

RDs may find it helpful to study the IDNT reference sheets for common nutrition diagnoses to become familiar with their signs and symptoms (15). Some RDs have made personal reference sheets for the diagnoses they commonly use for quick review during office visits, to ensure accuracy of their diagnoses. RDs can use the Nutrition Assessment Matrix in the Nutrition Care Process section of the ADA Web site (http://www.eatright.org) to determine possible diagnoses for the signs and symptoms they have identified (16).

In terms of how to use the NCP while providing seamless client care, it can be helpful to complete the nutrition assessment step in an initial "intake" appointment, which allows the RD time to review the data and make nutrition diagnoses before beginning work with the client on interventions. When time is limited, collecting as much data as possible prior to the appointment allows the RD some critical thinking time in advance of meeting with the client. Another option is to complete the nutrition assessment in the first segment of the appointment and then have the client read informational materials or watch a video for a few minutes while the RD reviews the data, makes nutrition diagnoses, and prepares a "results report" that summarizes the client's results and normative data and standards.

NCP STEP 3: NUTRITION INTERVENTION

In step 3 of the NCP, nutrition intervention, the RD and the client plan the nutrition intervention and the plan is implemented. In planning the nutrition intervention, the RD works with the client to prioritize the identified nutrition diagnoses. Once priority nutrition problems are determined, the RD and client work together to formulate goals and expected outcomes; select nutrition interventions directed at reducing or eliminating the etiologies of the identified nutrition diagnoses; and define a process for monitoring and evaluation. The RD develops the client's nutrition prescription and shifts the emphasis from data collection and analysis to focus on the client's priorities, preferences, and readiness to change.

To assist in prioritizing the client's nutrition diagnoses, the RD summarizes the identified nutrition problems, shares evidence-based treatment priorities, and determines where the client wants to start. To identify evidence-based treatment priorities, the RD considers the client's comorbidities and risk factors. For example, for a client with an elevated low-density lipoprotein (LDL) cholesterol level, the Adult Treatment Panel (ATP) III Guidelines recommend starting nutrition therapy by reducing saturated fat, *trans* fat, and cholesterol intake and increasing physical activity, followed by increasing intake of soluble fiber and plant sterols and stanols at the second appointment. Weight management is a component of recommended treatment, but according to these guidelines this should be deferred until the third appointment (11). In contrast, for clients with metabolic syndrome, weight reduction and increased physical activity are first-line treatments, followed by treatment of associated lipid and non-lipid risk factors (11).

The client's BMI also provides direction about treatment options. Table 1.4 (4) illustrates how BMI can be used to determine the appropriateness of weight loss vs weight-loss maintenance, and whether the weight-loss medications and weight-loss surgery are considerations. Using a "results report" is an effective way of presenting information to the client in an objective manner, allowing the RD to facilitate the client's sharing of priorities and goals related to the results presented.

Goals are set to reduce or improve the signs and symptoms of identified nutrition diagnoses. Goals should be specific, measurable, action-oriented, realistic, and timed ("SMART"). According to the AWM Practice Guideline, when the client desires weight loss, individualized weight-loss goals are set to reduce body weight at an optimal rate of 1 to 2 pounds per week for the first 6 months to achieve an initial weight loss of up to 10% of baseline weight (2). Depending on the client's preferences and health priorities, weight maintenance and weight-loss maintenance may also be appropriate goals.

In determining goals for treatment, the RD should consider level of disease risk and comorbidities. For example, a client's LDL cholesterol goal depends on his/her hard-CHD risk category, and blood pressure targets for hypertension are lower when the client has diabetes mellitus and/or chronic kidney disease. In addition, smaller step-goals that lead to larger overall goals may be more realistic and less daunting for clients.

The RD develops a nutrition prescription that states the energy, nutrient, and food group recommendations that will support achievement of the stated goals. An individualized diet that is 500 to 1,000 kcal less than estimated energy needs, as determined in the nutrition assessment, is the basis of the dietary component of a comprehensive weight-management program and should result in the desired 1 to 2 pounds of weight loss per week (2).

TABLE 1.4

Use of BMI to Select Weight Management Intervention Strategies[a]

| | BMI | | | | |
Treatment	25–26.9	27–29.9	30–34.9	35–39.9	> 40
Diet, physical activity, and behavior therapy[b]	Yes with comorbidities	Yes with comorbidities	Yes[c]	Yes[c]	Yes[c]
Pharmacotherapy[d]		Yes with comorbidities	Yes[c]	Yes[c]	Yes[c]
Weight-loss surgery				Yes with comorbidities	Yes[c]

Abbreviation: BMI, body mass index.

[a]Prevention of weight gain with lifestyle therapy is indicated in any individuals with a BMI ≥ 25, even without comorbidities; weight loss is not necessarily recommended for those with a BMI of 25 to 29.9 or a high waist circumference, unless they have two or more comorbidities.

[b]Combined therapy with a low-calorie diet, increased physical activity, and behavior therapy provides the most successful intervention for weight loss and weight maintenance.

[c]"Yes" represents the use of indicated treatment regardless of comorbidities.

[d]Consider pharmacotherapy only if a patient has not lost 1 pound per week after 6 months of combined lifestyle therapy.

Source: Adapted from reference 4.

The RD presents nutrition interventions that target the cause or etiology of the priority nutrition problems for consideration. The RD and the client discuss the pros and cons of these interventions, and decide which interventions to include in the action plan. The action plan details the small steps the client will take during the interval before the next appointment to meet the agreed-upon goals. The program for weight loss and weight maintenance should be comprehensive, including diet and nutrition interventions, physical activity, and behavior therapy. Comprehensive programs are more successful than programs that focus on a single mode of treatment (2).

According to the IDNT, interventions are organized into four categories: food and/or nutrient delivery, nutrition education, nutrition counseling, and coordination of nutrition care (15). A comprehensive weight-management program often includes interventions from each category, sometimes at each appointment and sometimes distributed over several appointments.

Nutrition diagnoses from the intake or clinical domains lend themselves to treatment by interventions from the food and/or nutrient delivery category. Examples of this type of intervention, supported by recommendations from the AWM Practice Guideline (2), are meal distribution of four to five meals/snacks throughout the day; portion control; incorporation of one to two meal replacements into the meal plan; changes in the macronutrient content of meal plans (eg, using low-fat or low-carbohydrate meal plans); and, under specific circumstances, use of a very–low-calorie diet. Much of this book (Chapters 2–5) is devoted to describing food and/or nutrient delivery interventions.

Nutrition diagnoses and etiologies related to knowledge deficit are treated by nutrition education interventions, either brief or comprehensive. Nutrition education is distinguished from nutrition counseling. Nutrition education emphasizes instruction or training of the client in a skill or sharing knowledge that can be used to manage or

---

Box 1.10
Nutrition Education Standardized Language

Definition of nutrition education: Formal process to instruct or train a patient in a skill or to impart knowledge to help patient voluntarily manage or modify food choices and eating behavior to maintain or improve health. Nutrition education may be initial/brief or comprehensive.
    International Dietetics and Nutrition Terminology (IDNT) nutrition education terms include the following:

- Purpose of nutrition education
- Priority modifications
- Recommended modifications
- Survival information

- Advanced or related topics
- Results interpretations
- Skill development

Source: Data are from reference 15.

modify food choices and eating behaviors (15). Box 1.10 (15) lists examples of nutrition education interventions.

Nutrition diagnoses and etiologies related to lifestyle and habits, such as ability to cope, solve problems, maintain positive self-talk, accept feelings, and set and work toward priorities, are treated by nutrition counseling interventions. Nutrition counseling is a supportive process, characterized by a collaborative counselor-client relationship that involves setting priorities, establishing goals, and creating an individualized action plan. It acknowledges and fosters the client's responsibility for self-care. Nutrition counseling is based on one or more theoretical approaches and incorporates strategies to promote behavior change (15). Box 1.11 (15) lists nutrition counseling theoretical approaches and strategies.

During nutrition counseling, the RD's role is to be a care manager and reflective listener. As a care manager, the RD defines options, facilitates the client's access to information, promotes skill-building, and assists the client in evaluating the benefits and costs of options. The RD is not a "fixer," problem-solver, advice-giver, or persuader. The client is responsible for making decisions.

The RD uses coordination of nutrition care interventions when he/she participates in team meetings or rounds (for example, case rounds to discuss selection of clients for bariatric surgery); collaborates with the client's providers; and refers the client to other providers, another RD with a different expertise, and/or community agencies and programs.

NCP STEP 4: MONITORING AND EVALUATION

In step 4 of the NCP, monitoring and evaluation, the RD monitors plan implementation and progress made by the client. Some monitoring and evaluation may take place during nutrition education and counseling, such as evaluating improvement in type and amount of knowledge to correct a knowledge deficit, while much of it may occur in follow-up

Box 1.11
Nutrition Counseling Standardized Language

Definition of nutrition counseling: Supportive process, characterized by a collaborative counselor-patient relationship to set priorities, establish goals, and create an individualized action plan that acknowledges and fosters responsibility for self-care to treat an existing condition and promote health.

International Dietetics and Nutrition Terminology (IDNT) nutrition counseling terms include the following:

- Theoretical basis or approach:
  - Cognitive-behavioral theory
  - Health belief model
  - Social learning theory
  - Transtheoretical model/stages of change

- Strategies:
  - Motivational interviewing
  - Goal-setting
  - Self-monitoring
  - Social support
  - Stress management
  - Stimulus control
  - Cognitive restructuring
  - Relapse prevention
  - Rewards/contingency management

Source: Data are from reference 15.

appointments. At follow-up appointments, the RD gathers new data related to the signs and symptoms of the original nutrition diagnoses, including weight, waist circumference, lipid and blood glucose results, blood pressure, intake, and quality of life. The RD also determines if the client has implemented the agreed-upon action plan and evaluates the progress made toward goals.

When implementation of the intervention plan has not occurred, the RD works with the client to identify barriers to implementation and facilitates the client's problem-solving to overcome these barriers. As needed, the intervention plan is revised and new goals are set. Table 1.5 lists the four types of IDNT outcomes that the RD monitors and evaluates in this step of the NCP and provides examples. Each outcome is measured against criteria, such as the client's goal, his/her nutrition prescription, baseline status or status at the previous appointment, or a normative value or standard (15). The RD is also alert for changes in status that indicate the need to refer the client for care by another provider.

SUMMARY

The RD works with clients who are overweight and obese, using the ADA's Nutrition Care Process and the American Dietetic Association Evidence Based Adult Weight Man-

TABLE 1.5

Monitoring and Evaluation Standard Terminology

Categories	Examples of Indicators
Food/nutrition-related history outcomes:	
• Energy intake	• Total energy intake
• Food and beverage intake	• Amount of food
	• Types of food/meals
	• Meal/snack pattern
	• Diet Quality Index: Healthy Eating Index
	• Food variety
• Bioactive substance intake	• Alcohol intake: drink size/volume
	• Alcohol intake: Frequency
• Macronutrient intake	• Total fat
	• Total carbohydrate
	• Total protein
• Micronutrient intake	• Vitamin D
Beliefs and attitudes	• Self-efficacy
Food and nutrition knowledge	• Area of knowledge
	• Level of knowledge
Beliefs and attitudes	• Motivation
	• Readiness to change nutrition-related behaviors
Behavior	• Self-reported adherence score
	• Self-monitoring at agreed upon rate
	• Self-management as agreed upon
Nutrition-related client-centered measures	• NQoL responses
Physical activity and function	• Consistency
	• Frequency
	• Duration
	• Intensity
	• Strength
Anthropometric measurements	• Weight
	• Weight change
	• BMI
	• Body compartment estimate: waist circumference
Biochemical data, medical tests, and procedures	• Glucose, fasting
	• Cholesterol, serum
Nutrition-focused physical findings	• Blood pressure
	• Heart rate

Abbreviations: NQoL, Nutrition Quality of Life; BMI, body mass index.
Source: Data are from reference 15.

agement Nutrition Practice Guideline. The RD initiates the NCP with an individualized nutrition assessment to collect data and determine the client's energy and nutrient requirements. Collected data are compared with evidence-based norms and standards, and the RD identifies discrepancies in data. In the second step of the NCP, the RD makes nutrition diagnoses, written as PES statements, based on the discrepancies in data that have been identified. Step 3 of the NCP involves working with the client to prioritize nutrition diagnoses, set goals, develop a nutrition prescription, and plan interventions to reduce or resolve the client's nutrition diagnoses. In the last step of the NCP, monitoring and evaluation, the RD collects new data, confirms implementation of the intervention plan, and evaluates effectiveness of interventions in meeting goals and resolving nutrition diagnoses. Revisions in goals and the plan are made as needed. The RD provides client-centered nutrition care, keeping the client's values, goals, and priorities at the center of the Nutrition Care Process.

References

1. American Dietetic Association Nutrition Care Process and Model. http://www.eatright.org (members-only section). Accessed September 27, 2008.
2. American Dietetic Association Evidence Analysis Library: Adult Weight Management Evidence Based Practice Guideline. http://www.adaevidencelibrary.com. Accessed December 13, 2007.
3. American Dietetic Association Scope of Dietetic Practice Framework: Definition of Terms. Updated August 2007. http://www.eatright.org/cps/rde/xchg/ada/hs. xsl/home_13663_ENU_HTML.htm. Accessed December 13, 2007.
4. National Heart, Lung, and Blood Institute. *Clinical Guidelines on the Identification, Evaluation, and Treatment of Overweight and Obesity in Adults.* Bethesda, MD: National Institutes of Health; 1998. NIH publication 98-4083.
5. Allison DB. *Handbook of Assessment Methods for Eating Behaviors and Weight-Related Problems: Measures, Theory, and Research.* Thousand Oaks, CA: Sage Publications; 1995.
6. Canadian Society for Exercise Physiology. PAR-Q and You. http://www.csep.ca/ communities/c574/files/hidden/pdfs/par-q.pdf. Accessed December 13, 2007.
7. Barr J, Schumacher G. Using focus groups to determine what constitutes quality of life in clients receiving medical nutrition therapy: first steps in the development of a nutrition quality-of-life survey. *J Am Diet Assoc.* 2003;103:844–851.
8. Weight Management Dietetic Practice Group Web site. http://www.wmdpg.org. Accessed September 27, 2008.
9. Klein S, Allison DB, Heymsfield SB, Kelley DE, Leibel RL, Nonas C, Kahn R. Waist circumference and cardiometabolic risk: a consensus statement from Shaping America's Health. Association for Weight Management and Obesity Prevention, NAASO, the Obesity Society, American Society for Nutrition, American Diabetes Association. *Obesity.* 2007;15:1061–1067.
10. Loan V. The how and why of body composition assessment. In: Berdanier CD. *Handbook of Nutrition and Food.* Boca Raton, FL: CRC Press; 2002:637–656.
11. Executive summary of the Third Report of the National Cholesterol Education Program (NCEP) Expert Panel on Detection, Evaluation, and Treatment of High Blood Cholesterol in Adults (Adult Treatment Panel III). *JAMA.* 2001;285:2486–2497.
12. Institute of Medicine. *Dietary Reference Intakes for Energy, Carbohydrate, Fiber, Fat, Fatty Acids, Cholesterol, Protein, and Amino Acids.* Washington, DC: National Academy Press; 2002.
13. Mifflin MD, St. Jeor ST, Hill LA, Scott BJ, Daugherty SA, Koh YO. A new predictive equation for resting energy expenditure in healthy individuals. *Am J Clin Nutr.* 1990;51:241–247.
14. International Food Information Council (IFIC) Foundation. 2007 Food and Health Survey. http://ific.org/research/upload/2007Survey-FINAL.pdf. Accessed December 13, 2007.
15. *International Dietetics & Nutrition Terminology (IDNT) Reference Manual: Standardized Language for the Nutrition Care Process.* 2nd ed. Chicago, IL: American Dietetic Association; 2009.
16. Nutrition assessment matrix. http://www.eatright.org (members-only section). Accessed September 27, 2008.

CHAPTER 2

DIET—MEAL REPLACEMENTS

PART A: OVERVIEW

DAVID HEBER, MD, PHD, FACP, FACN

INTRODUCTION

The pandemic in obesity and type 2 diabetes is continuing to increase. Although vital environmental changes are needed, it is also true that this major global health problem requires new approaches to make diet and lifestyle change more effective. Research has shown repeatedly that meal replacements are a safe and effective weight-management strategy among subjects with obesity and/or type 2 diabetes because they increase compliance to dietary regimens (1–5). Meal replacements have also shown efficacy in weight maintenance. In a 4-year study, after an initial 3-month period of weight loss using two meal replacements per day, participants were able to maintain weight while consuming one meal replacement daily (2).

WEIGHT-LOSS TREATMENT AND DIABETES

The rationale for weight-loss treatment is that it improves the health profile. This improvement is particularly profound with diabetes. Although the long-term health benefits of weight loss in obese individuals with type 2 diabetes have not been clearly defined, several clinical trials have found short-term benefits of weight loss on glycemic control. Agurs-Collins (6) found that weight loss through diet and exercise was significantly greater at 6 months when compared with a control group who received standard diabetes care. The mean amount of weight loss (–2.4 kg) in the intervention group resulted in a significant decrease in hemoglobin A1C of 2.4%. Heller et al (7) reported similar results in a randomized study in which a weight loss of 5 kg was achieved through diet, resulting in a significant 2% reduction in A1C at 6 months.

USE OF MEAL REPLACEMENTS TO TREAT CLIENTS WITH OBESITY AND TYPE 2 DIABETES

Our own research has shown that use of meal replacements in obese clients with type 2 diabetes can improve dietary adherence and is a safe and viable strategy for weight reduction, resulting in beneficial changes in measures of glycemic control, inflammation, and a reduction in the need for diabetes medications (3). In one study, we compared the effects of a soy-based meal replacement (MR) plan vs an individualized diet plan (IDP), as recommended by the American Diabetes Association, on weight loss and metabolic profile (3). In this prospective study, 104 subjects were randomly assigned to the two treatments for a total of 12 months. In all, 77 of the 104 subjects completed the study. The weight loss observed in the group treated with meal replacements was 4.57% ± 0.81% and was significantly greater than the weight loss observed in the IDP group, which was 2.25% ± 0.72%. Because the two groups were prescribed the same number of calories, the difference was due to enhanced compliance in the MR group. Initial fasting plasma glucose levels were not different in the two groups. By 6 months, fasting plasma glucose levels were significantly reduced in MR group at 126.4 ± 4.9 mg/dL compared with the IDP group at 152.5 ± 6.6 mg/dL ($P < .0001$). Controlling for baseline levels, A1C level improved by 0.49 ± 0.22% for those in the MR group when compared with the IDP group ($P < .05$). A greater number of subjects in MR group had a significant reduction in their dosage of reduced sulfonylureas ($P < .0001$) and metformin ($P < .05$) as compared with the IDP group. High-sensitivity C-reactive protein (hs-CRP) decreased by 26.3% ($P = .019$) in the MR group vs 7.06% ($P = .338$; not significant) in the IDP group at 6 months. This study demonstrated that MR is a viable strategy for weight reduction in obese clients with type 2 diabetes, resulting in beneficial changes in measures of glycemic control and reduction of medications.

The dropout rate in this study was 26% over the study period, with most of the dropouts occurring at the screening and initial visits (3). Most of the subjects who dropped out did so because they were not randomly assigned to the MR group although they had hoped to be, or because they realized the time commitment of the study was not manageable with their work schedules. The dropout rate decreased to 6% after the initial dropout in the first month of the study. Overall, the meal replacements were very well tolerated.

Meal plans that use two portion-controlled meal replacement shakes and two snacks with only one conventional food meal over the course of the day may improve food-choice behavior. Further, the use of meal replacements may increase the accuracy of calorie-counting and estimation of portion size. In addition, meal replacements help provide structure to a meal plan and in the course of time may help form more healthful eating patterns (8,9).

A meta-analysis of studies using meal replacements indicated that weight-loss plans that include meal replacements are more effective than conventional diets (10), or at least as effective as a conventional low-fat strategy. The use of meal replacements for weight loss is a popular strategy because shakes and nutrition bars can be incorporated easily into the lifestyles of those attempting weight loss (11). Individuals who include meal replacements into their dietary regimen are able to include self-help strategies for treatment and prevention of obesity in addition to using meal replacements (12).

The National Institutes of Health multicenter trial Look AHEAD examining outcomes of weight management in type 2 diabetes has included the use of meal replacements as a prominent strategy. The primary objective of the Look AHEAD clinical trial (13) is to assess the long-term effects (up to 11.5 years) of an intensive weight-loss program delivered over 4 years in approximately 5,000 overweight and obese individuals with type 2 diabetes. The Look AHEAD lifestyle intervention of diet modification and increased physical activity is designed to induce a minimum weight loss of 7% of initial body weight during the first year. Individual participants are encouraged to lose 10% (or more) of their initial body weight. The intervention uses a portion-controlled diet during the initial phase of weight loss, consisting of two meal replacement products, one portion-controlled snack, and a self-selected meal each day. At week 20, participants are prescribed one meal replacement per day and two meals of self-selected foods are allowed. The maintenance dietary protocol for years 2 through 4 allows for continued use of one meal replacement per day.

Based on the these research efforts, it is now clear that the use of meal replacement shakes has attained greater recognition as an alternative strategy for managing weight in clients with type 2 diabetes.

References

1. Heber D, Ashley JM, Wang HJ, Elashoff RM. Clinical evaluation of a minimal intervention meal replacement regimen for weight reduction. *J Am Coll Nutr.* 1994;13:608–614.
2. Flechtner-Mors M, Ditschuneit-HH, Johnson TD, Suchard MA, Adler G. Metabolic and weight loss effects of long-term dietary intervention in obese subjects. Four year results. *Obes Res.* 2000;8:399–402.
3. Li Z, Hong K, Saltsman P, DeShields S, Bellman M, Thames G, Liu Y, Wang HJ, Elashoff R, Heber D. Long-term efficacy of soy-based meal replacements vs an individualized diet plan in obese type II DM patients: relative effects on weight loss, metabolic parameters, and C-reactive protein. *Eur J Clin Nutr.* 2005;53:411–418.
4. Allison DB, Gadbury G, Schwartz LG, Murugesan R, Kraker JL, Heshka S, Fontaine KR, Heymsfield SB. A novel soy-based meal replacement formula for weight loss among obese individuals: a randomized controlled clinical trial. *Eur J Clin Nutr.* 2003;57:514–522.
5. Noakes M, Foster PR, Keogh JB, Clifton PM. Meal replacements are as effective as structured weight-loss diets for treating obesity in adults with features of metabolic syndrome. *J Nutr.* 2004;134:1894–1899.
6. Agurs-Collins TD, Kumanyika SK, Ten Have TR, Adams-Campbell LL. A randomized controlled trial of weight reduction and exercise for diabetes management in older African-American subjects. *Diabetes Care.* 1997;20:1503–1511.
7. Heller SR, Clarke P, Daly H, Davis I, McCulloch DK, Allison SP, Tattersall RB. Group education for obese patients with type 2 diabetes: greater success at less cost. *Diabet Med.* 1988;5:552–556.
8. Ashley JM, St. Jeor ST, Perumean-Chaney S, Schrage J, Bovee V. Meal replacements in weight intervention. *Obes Res.* 2001;9(suppl 4):312S–320S.
9. Wing RR, Jeffry RW, Burton LR, Thorson C, Nissinoff KS, Baxter JE. Food provision vs structured meal plans in the behavioral treatment of obesity. *Int J Obes Relat Metab Disord.* 1996;20:56–62.
10. Heymsfield SB, van Mierlo C, van der Knaap HCM, Heo M, Frier HI. Weight management using a meal replacement strategy: meta and pooling analysis from 6 studies. *Int J Obes.* 2003;27:537–549.
11. Levy AS, Heaton AW. Weight control practices of U.S. adults trying to lose weight. *Ann Intern Med.* 1993;119:661–666.

12. Rothacker DQ, Blackburn GL. Obesity prevalence by age group and 5-year changes in adults in rural Wisconsin. *J Am Diet Assoc.* 2000;100:784–790.

13. Ryan DH, Espeland MA, Foster GD, Haffner SM, Hubbard VS, Johnson KC, Kahn SE, Knowlder WC, Yanovsky SZ, Look AHEAD Research Group. Look AHEAD (Action for Health in Diabetes): design and methods for a clinical trial of weight loss for the prevention of cardiovascular disease in type 2 diabetes. *Control Clin Trials.* 2003;24:610–628.

PART B: PRACTICAL APPLICATIONS

SUSAN BOWERMAN, MS, RD, CSSD

INTRODUCTION

Health care providers often find themselves frustrated when their overweight and obese clients claim to be adhering to diet plans, yet they are not losing weight. Clients also become frustrated when the scale refuses to budge, particularly when they believe they are putting forth their best efforts. Inaccurate calorie-counting and underestimation of portion sizes are two common problems that can impede weight loss. The use of meal replacements, which are structured to provide a percentage of macro- and micronutrients within a defined calorie limit, has a proven track record as a valuable tool for treatment of overweight and obesity.

PROBLEMS WITH PORTION CONTROL AND HIDDEN CALORIES

Although portion control is one of the primary strategies in calorie control, many dieters lack the time or the inclination to weigh and measure foods. Others may weigh and measure foods for a time but then stop, believing they are able to estimate portions and calories fairly well. Dieters are often unaware of how large their portions are, and they may not understand that even "low-calorie" foods add to the day's intake. Finally, food records can be inaccurate because dieters may neglect to record some items, believing their calorie value is too small to matter or forgetting that the food was eaten. Even the most avid record keepers may forget to account for cream in coffee, spreads on breads or vegetables, mayonnaise or cheese on sandwiches, and dressings on salads.

There is much evidence that food consumed away from home poses more problems for dieters. Studies have shown that eating food away from home increases calorie consumption and that calorie-counting is virtually impossible for most consumers, including registered dietitians (1–5). In one study by Burton et al (5), participants underestimated calorie levels by more than 600 kcal. Wansink et al (6) found that foods with a

TABLE 2.1

Small Changes in the Meal Plan Can Add Significant Calories

Meal Plan (Calories)	Actual Food Choice (Calories)	Difference in Energy Intake
Salad greens with 3 oz grilled chicken and nonfat dressing **(350 kcal)**	Restaurant Chinese chicken salad **(1,000 kcal)**	650 kcal
3 oz cooked top sirloin steak, 1 cup green beans, ½ cup brown rice **(325 kcal)**	5 oz cooked t-bone steak, 1 cup green beans with a pat of butter, ¾ cup white rice **(665 kcal)**	340 kcal
1 cup flaked cereal, 1 cup nonfat milk **(170 kcal)**	1 cup granola, 1 cup 2% milk **(570 kcal)**	400 kcal
Sandwich with two slices whole-grain bread, 3 oz turkey, mustard, lettuce, and tomato **(300 kcal)**	Sandwich with two slices white bread, 5 oz roast beef, mayonnaise, lettuce, and tomato **(520 kcal)**	220 kcal
One slice of cheese and vegetable pizza; tossed salad with light dressing; unsweetened iced tea **(450 kcal)**	One slice of pepperoni pizza; tossed salad with regular dressing; lemonade **(850 kcal)**	400 kcal
1 cup nonfat cottage cheese, 1 cup sliced strawberries, 1 slice whole-grain toast **(275 kcal)**	1 cup regular cottage cheese, 8 oz orange juice, one slice toast with 1 Tbsp strawberry jam **(475 kcal)**	200 kcal

connotation of being healthy caused consumers to significantly underestimate calories, naming this effect the "halo" effect. It is therefore not hard to imagine that a few minor mistakes by a patient/client who tries to follow a 1,200-kcal diet may make the difference between losing and maintaining weight. Table 2.1 illustrates how easily calories can add up when unintentional changes are made to the food plan and why meal replacements create an opportunity for a dieter to adhere to prescribed guidelines.

PARTIAL VS TOTAL MEAL REPLACEMENT PLANS

Presently, there are no standard definitions of meal replacement or partial meal replacement plans; however, there are some differences. Partial meal replacements tend to be sold over-the-counter (OTC) whereas total meal replacements are usually medically supervised. Partial meal replacements are part of a low-calorie diet (LCD) that supplies at least 1,200 kcal/d and consists of a combination of meal replacements and regular food, whereas total meal replacements tend to used in very-low-calorie diets (VLCDs) that supply no more than 800 kcal/d.

LOW-CALORIE DIETS USING PARTIAL MEAL REPLACEMENTS

Partial meal replacement plans typically replace two meals per day with guidelines for one sensible, healthful meal, usually lunch or dinner. These OTC meal replacements are not intended as total diet replacements because their single meal nutrition relies on the premise that much of the protein and other nutrients will be included in the regular food meal—thus, the rationale for selling them as replacements for only one or two daily meals. All LCD meal replacement regimens should incorporate whole fresh fruits and vegetables and whole grains among regular food choices to provide additional phytonutrients, vitamins, minerals and fiber. As with all diets, a daily, multiple vitamin/mineral supplement is also appropriate.

Although most of the research has been done using liquid meal replacements, these OTC meal replacements can conceivably encompass a wide range of food products, including beverages, prepackaged shelf-stable and frozen entrees, soups, hot cereals, and meal or snack bars. OTC meal replacements are generally reasonably priced and therefore can be prescribed to a lower-income population. In a study by Huerta et al (7), meal replacements were a successful tool for weight loss in comparison to usual care in an indigent population in a Los Angeles free clinic setting.

OTC meal replacements can be used as the sole energy source for a meal or in combination with other foods that are specifically prescribed to go along with the meal (eg, a frozen meal plus a salad). OTC meal replacements are often prescribed with snacks that consist of measurable foods such as fruits, vegetables, or snack bars. OTC meal replacements have been studied for three decades with significant weight-loss success. In 1993, Jeffery and associates (8) compared the use at a weight-loss center of prepackaged meals vs financial incentives for weight loss and found that the prepackaged meals were associated with greater weight loss. In this study, 202 obese men and women were randomly assigned to receive either standard behavioral treatment (SBT), SBT with the provision of prepackaged meals, SBT with financial incentive, or SBT with both provision of meals and financial incentives. After 18 months, weight loss with the provision of food was more successful than either SBT or financial incentives. Food provision also enhanced attendance, completion of food records, quality of the diet, and nutrition knowledge. Furthermore, subjects who received the prepackaged meals were more apt to record food intake and were more apt to record food intake accurately.

Although most studies of meal replacements used liquid meals, studies using foods have similar findings. In a study of Special K brands (Kellogg's, Battle Creek, MI) by Van der Wal et al (9), using different cereal products twice each day as meal replacements, subjects lost more than 3 kg over 4 weeks. Hannum et al (10) compared 60 healthy women (BMI 26 to 40) randomly assigned to either a 1,365-kcal regular-food diet or a 1,365-kcal diet using frozen Uncle Ben's Rice Bowls (Mars NA, Inc, Mt Olive, NJ) for two meals per day. In 8 weeks, participants in the meal replacement group lost more weight and had more significant improvements in glucose and insulin than the conventional-diet group (10).

Some clients may not perceive meal replacements as "real" food. In fact, meal replacements are often higher in healthful nutrients than the "real" foods that people may choose on their own (eg, fast-food hamburgers and french fries, which are high in saturated fat). There are a variety of meal replacement products available, as well as recipes for preparing homemade meal replacement protein shakes. Therefore, health care providers can stress that meal replacements provide nutrition, and their convenience and availability may make them an appropriate choice for people with busy lifestyles.

What are the Benefits to the Client?

Several studies have shown that metabolic risk factors improve through the use of meal-replacement products, exceeding the changes achieved by dietary change alone (even structured low-energy diets) (11,12). Partial meal replacements also have particular benefits for clients with diabetes (13,14). Soon after the diet is initiated, glucose control improves due to energy restriction. In recent randomized controlled trials conducted in individuals with hypertension, dyslipidemia, or type 2 diabetes, those who received meal replacements lost more weight at the end of 1 year and had improved lipid profiles and hs-CRP than those randomly assigned to a standard exchange-system diet (13,15).

As noted previously, meal replacements are available over-the-counter, and they can be used with minimal supervision (16). However, they are more effective when used as part of a more comprehensive program in which clients have regular follow-up (17).

Most studies show greater client satisfaction and lower dropout rates with partial meal replacements than with other diets, possibly because the use of meal replacements results in less hunger (18). Meal replacements have also been shown to be effective in people from low socioeconomic backgrounds (7), who are more likely to be overweight and hence in greater need of weight-loss treatments (19).

Although the sugar content of many commercial meal-replacement products has fostered concern about their use in management regimens for obese clients with type 2 diabetes, data suggest that these concerns may be unfounded (20,21). As with any diet designed for the person with type 2 diabetes, the meal plan must be tailored to the needs and requirements of the individual, and clients should be monitored by their health care provider in conjunction with the registered dietitian (RD).

What to Look for in a Meal Replacement

When counseling clients, advise them to select a meal replacement shake, bar, soup, or frozen meal that does not exceed approximately 300 kcal. That way, fruits and vegetables can be added to the meal and the calories will still be within reason.

The percentage of calories from fat should be no more than 30% of total calories. Most shakes, bars, and soups will be much lower than this, but advise clients to read labels carefully on frozen meals.

Some clients may need to restrict sodium in the diet, and should be advised to read labels for sodium content, particularly in frozen meals and soups. Shakes, bars, and soups that are designed to be full meal replacements should be vitamin- and mineral-fortified, and it is helpful if they provide at least 5 g fiber.

Frozen entrées as meal replacements will not be vitamin- and mineral-fortified, but they will generally match calorie and fat recommendations. Additional vegetables and salad can be added to the entrée, shake, bar, or soup to complete the meal.

Because clients will most likely purchase the meal replacement at a neighborhood store, it is helpful to suggest that they try several meal-replacement products until they find those that appeal to them. Some clients will have to match appeal with affordability, and meal replacements offer a variety of choices. Finally, you may wish to provide clients with recipes to create their own meal replacements using nonfat milk or soy milk, protein powder, and fruit (22).

Meal replacements are not contraindicated for those with common comorbidities of obesity, such as diabetes or heart disease. However, food sensitivities such as lactose intolerance and food allergies need to be considered when choosing specific products.

Box 2.1
1,200-Calorie Meal Plan

Breakfast: Meal replacement + a piece of fruit
Lunch: Meal replacement + large mixed green and vegetable salad with light dressing
Afternoon snack: Choose one small protein snack such as a protein snack bar, 1/2 cup cottage cheese, string
   cheese with a few whole-grain crackers, and a small piece of fruit
Dinner: 4 oz baked or broiled chicken or fish; large green salad with light dressing; 1 cup steamed vegetables;
   1/2 cup brown rice or whole-grain pasta, *or* 1 small baked potato with skin

---

Meal Plans Using Meal Replacements

Most meal replacements and frozen portion-controlled meals contain 300 kcal or fewer. Rounding out the meal with vegetables and salads, and fruit for dessert, creates a nutritious and satisfying meal for approximately 450 kcal. See Box 2.1 for a sample 1,200-calorie menu using meal replacements twice per day. The meals are supplemented with fruit at breakfast and with vegetables and salad at lunch and dinner, with fruit for dessert.

People who complain that preparing the proper foods for a weight-loss diet is too time consuming may find the simplicity of this plan appealing because the meal replacement takes care of the entrée. Adding the vegetables and fruits can also be simplified. Whole pieces of fruit, precut melons, prewashed salad greens and carrots, and washed and cut vegetables ready for steaming are all widely available in most supermarkets. A variety of fat-free salad dressings and seasoned vinegars complete the shopping list. If the average person eats 21 meals and 14 snacks per week, replacing 10 meals per week with a structured meal replacement can result in substantial calorie control.

In summary, for many clients, OTC meal replacements provide a simple, nutritious, and inexpensive way for patients/clients to follow a lower-calorie diet successfully. In a meta-analysis of weight-loss studies 1 year or longer (23), meal replacements were associated with an average weight loss of more than 6 kg. Meal replacements can provide good nutrition, can serve as a healthful alternative when only unhealthful items are available, and are an appropriate alternative to skipping meals.

VERY-LOW-CALORIE DIETS

As noted earlier in this chapter, VLCDs provide 800 or fewer kcal per day. Therefore, clients on a VLCD are medically monitored and usually participate in comprehensive multidisciplinary programs in which care is provided by a physician, often in conjunction with an RD, psychologist, and/or exercise physiologist (24–26).

VLCD programs are appropriate for clients with a BMI of 30 or more and with obesity-related comorbidities. Close medical monitoring is important for all clients, but clients with diabetes are a special population because significant decreases in blood glucose can occur in a very short time, within 4 to 10 days after initiation of a VLCD, often before significant weight loss has occurred (27–29).

VLCDs are designed to produce rapid weight loss while preserving lean body mass. This is accomplished by providing dietary protein typically in the range of 70 to 100 g per day, or 0.8 to 1.5 g per kilogram of ideal body weight (19,24). Protein is generally obtained from a whey, soy, and/or egg white protein powder, which is mixed with water and consumed as a liquid diet. Clients typically consume a minimum of five packets per day, and many programs also offer a range of products for use on a VLCD plan, such as shakes, soups, hot cereals, and bars.

Most of the available VLCD meal-replacement products supply approximately 100 kcal and 15 g protein per serving, up to 80 g carbohydrate per day, and 15 g fat per day. Clients also take a daily multiple vitamin-mineral supplement, an additional 2 to 3 g potassium, and are encouraged to consume 2 liters of noncaloric fluids daily (24).

Recently, more attention has been given to the fiber content of VLCDs. Because of the absence of nonenergy bulking agents in the products used in VLCDs, constipation is one of the most common adverse effects. In the past, addition of fiber was limited because of technological problems involved in producing a palatable drink. Currently, several soluble and insoluble fibers that do not adversely affect taste are available.

Clients must drink at least 2 liters of noncaloric liquid per day to compensate for decreased food intake and to avoid dehydration. Water is the preferred choice. Caffeinated drinks should be limited or avoided. They may increase dehydration and clients may be more sensitive to the effects of caffeine.

VLCDs are usually prescribed for 12 to 16 weeks, at which point a re-entry diet of part formula and part food is prescribed until the client is weaned off all formula (30). The goal is to slowly reintroduce enough healthful calories to equal 1,200 to 1,500 kcal/d. Refeeding generally takes 4 to 6 weeks but varies among clients. Energy intake is increased by 100 to 150 kcal/d. For example, in the first week, the client might reduce one packet of formula per day, replacing it with 3 ounces of white meat chicken and 1/2 cup of steamed vegetables. Alternatively, the number of packets of formula might remain the same, but the formula could be blended with a banana, or a small meal of protein and vegetables could be prescribed in addition to the formula to increase calorie intake. Eventually, as the stomach gets used to regular food, salads and other raw vegetables as well as seasonings are reintroduced.

Weight gain is common after VLCDs are stopped, and some researchers therefore consider VLCDs to be too expensive for the relatively modest long-term outcomes (31,32), particularly when compared with the success of more easily used OTC meal replacements. However, the jury is still out. VLCDs have a very rapid effect on health profiles, and the individual clinician may decide that the expense and the greater initial weight loss are beneficial for a patient.

SUMMARY

Contemporary lifestyles may affect compliance with a traditional calorie-counting approach. Convenience foods often lack a nutrient balance, and clients may have increased difficulty maintaining a diet while away from home. Additionally, complex diet plans may be time-consuming or difficult to follow on a daily basis.

People who use insulin or other hypoglycemic medications face additional challenges to dietary management because a quick meal or snack is often necessary to prevent nocturnal or daytime hypoglycemia, to spread the nutritional load, or to match the energy demand of exercise.

The use of meal replacements is one method that can enhance dietary adherence to result in successful weight loss. OTC meal replacements can provide practical convenience to clients, and the use of such therapy to promote weight loss on a daily basis is endorsed by professional societies, including the American Diabetes Association (33) and the Canadian Diabetes Association (34).

References

1. Binkley JK, Eales J, Jekanowski M. The relation between dietary change and rising US obesity. *Int J Obesity*. 2000;24:1032–1039.
2. Young L, Nestle M. Portion sizes and obesity: responses of fast-food companies. *J Public Health Policy*. 2007;28:238–248.
3. Niemeier HM, Raynor HA, Lloyd-Richardson EE, Rogers ML, Wing RR. Fast food consumption and breakfast skipping: predictors of weight gain from adolescence to adulthood in a nationally representative sample. *J Adolesc Health*. 2006;39:842–849.
4. Carels RA, Konrad K, Harper J. Individual differences in food perceptions and calorie estimation: an examination of dieting status, weight and gender. *Appetite*. 2007;49:450–458.
5. Burton S, Creyer EH, Kees J, Huggins K. Attacking the obesity epidemic: the potential health benefits of providing nutrition information in restaurants. *Am J Public Health*. 2006;96:1669–1675.
6. Wansink B. *Mindless Eating*. New York, NY: Bantam Books; 2006:187.
7. Huerta S, Li Z, Li HC, Hu MS, Heber D. Feasibility of a partial meal replacement plan for weight loss in low-income patients. *Int J Obes Relat Metab Disord*. 2004;12:1575–1579.
8. Jeffery RW, Wing RR, Thornson C, Burton LR, Raether C, Harvey J, Mullen M. Strengthening behavioral interventions for weight loss: a randomized trial of food provision and monetary incentives. *J Consult Clin Psychol*. 1993;61:1038–1045.
9. Vander Wal JS, McBurney MI, Cho S, Dhurandhar N. Ready-to-eat cereal products as meal replacements for weight loss. *Int J Food Sci Nutr*. 2007;58:331–340.
10. Hannum SM, Carson L, Evans EM, Canene KA, Petr EL, Bui L, Erdman JW Jr. Use of portion-controlled entrees enhances weight loss in women. *Obes Res*. 2004;12:538–546.
11. Ditschuneit HH, Flechtner-Mors M. Value of structured meals for weight management: risk factors and long-term weight maintenance. *Obes Res*. 2001;9(suppl 4):S284–S289.
12. Quinn Rothacker D. Five-year self-management of weight using meal replacements: comparison with matched controls in rural Wisconsin. *Nutrition*. 2000;16:344–348.
13. Li Z, Hong K, Saltsman P, DeShields S, Bellman M, Thames G, Liu Y, Wang HJ, Elashoff R, Heber D. Long-term efficacy of soy-based meal replacements weight

loss, metabolic parameters, and C-reactive protein. *Eur J Clin Nutr*. 2005;59:411–418.

14. Hensrud DD. Dietary treatment and long-term weight loss and maintenance in type 2 diabetes. *Obes Res*. 2001;9(suppl 4):S348–S353.

15. Ditschuneit HH, Frier HI, Flechtner-Mors M. Lipoprotein responses to weight loss and weight maintenance in high-risk obese subjects. *Eur J Clin Nutr*. 2002;56:264–270.

16. Winick C, Rothacker DQ, Norman RL. Four worksite weight loss programs with high-stress occupations using a meal replacement product. *Occup Med (Lond)*. 2002;52:25–30.

17. Ashley JM, St Jeor ST, Perumean-Chaney S, Schrage J, Bovee V. Meal replacements in weight intervention. *Obes Res*. 2001;9(suppl 4):S312–S320.

18. Rothacker DQ, Watemberg S. Short-term hunger intensity changes following ingestion of a meal replacement bar for weight control. *Int J Food Sci Nutr*. 2004;55:223–226.

19. National Health and Medical Research Council. *National Clinical Guidelines for Weight Control and Obesity Management*. Canberra, Australia: Commonwealth Department of Health and Ageing; 2002.

20. Flechtner-Mors M, Ditschuneit HH, Johnson TD, Suchard MA, Adler G. Metabolic and weight-loss effects of long-term dietary intervention in obese patients: four-year results, *Obes Res*. 2000;8:399–402.

21. Yip I, Go VL, DeShields S, Saltsman P, Bellman M, Thames G, Murray S, Wang HJ, Elashoff R, Heber D. Liquid meal replacements and glycemic control in obese type 2 diabetes patients. *Obes Res*. 2001;9(suppl 4):S341–S347.

22. Heber D. *The L.A. Shape Diet*. New York, NY: Harper-Collins; 2004.

23. Franz MJ, VanWormer JJ, Crain AL, Boucher JL, Histon T, Caplan W, Bowman JD, Pronk NP. Weight-loss outcomes: a systematic review and meta-analysis of weight-loss clinical trials with a minimum of 1-year follow-up. *J Am Diet Assoc*. 2007;107:1755–1767.

24. National Task Force on the Prevention and Treatment of Obesity, National Institutes of Health. Very low-calorie diets. *JAMA*. 1993;270:967–974.

25. National Heart, Lung, and Blood Institute. Clinical guidelines on the identification, evaluation, and treatment of overweight and obesity in adults: the evidence report. *Obes Res*. 1998;6(suppl 2):51S–209S.

26. Wadden TA, Van Itallie TB, Blackburn GL. Responsible and irresponsible use of very-low-calorie diets in the treatment of obesity. *JAMA*. 1990;263:83–85.

27. Henry RR, Scheaffer L, Olefsky JM. Glycemic effects of intensive caloric restriction and isocaloric refeeding in noninsulin-dependent diabetes mellitus. *J Clin Endocrinol Metab*. 1985;61:917–925.

28. Kelley DE, Wing R, Buonocore C, Sturis J, Polonsky K, Fitzsimmons M. Relative effects of calorie restriction and weight loss in noninsulin-dependent diabetes mellitus. *J Clin Endocrinol Metab*. 1993;77:1287–1293.

29. Markovic TP, Jenkins AB, Campbell LV, Furler SM, Kraegen EW, Chisholm DJ. The determinants of glycemic responses to diet restriction and weight loss in obesity and NIDDM. *Diabetes Care*. 1998;21:687–694.

30. Wadden TA, Berkowitz RI. Very-low-calorie diets. In: Fairburn CG, Brownell KD, eds. *Eating Disorders and Obesity: A Comprehensive Handbook.* 2nd ed. New York, NY: Guilford Press; 2005:534–538.

31. Vogels N, Westerterp-Plantenga MS. Successful long-term weight maintenance: a 2-year follow-up. *Obesity.* 2007;15:1258–1266.

32. Tsai AG, Wadden TA. Systematic review: an evaluation of major commercial weight loss programs in the United States. *Ann Intern Med.* 2005;142:56–66.

33. American Diabetes Association. Evidence-based nutrition principles and recommendations for the treatment and prevention of diabetes and related complications. *Diabetes Care.* 2003;26(suppl 1):S51–S61.

34. Canadian Diabetes Association Clinical Practice Guidelines Expert Committee. Clinical practice guidelines for the prevention and management of diabetes in Canada. *Can J Diabetes.* 2003;27(suppl 2):S1–S140.

CHAPTER 3

DIET—GLYCEMIC INDEX AND GLYCEMIC LOAD

PART A: OVERVIEW

JENNIE BRAND-MILLER, PHD, FAIFST, AND DAVID S. LUDWIG, MD, PHD

INTRODUCTION

Weight loss can be achieved by any means of energy restriction, but the challenge is to achieve sustainable weight loss and prevent weight "creep" without increasing the risk of chronic disease. The modest success of low-fat diets has prompted research on alternative dietary strategies. Conventional high-carbohydrate diets, even when high in fiber, can increase postprandial glycemia and insulinemia and compromise weight control via mechanisms relating to appetite stimulation, fuel partitioning, and metabolic rate. Postprandial hyperglycemia is recognized as an important risk factor for type 2 diabetes and cardiovascular disease (1–3), and many diabetes associations now recommend the judicious use of low-glycemic index (GI) carbohydrate foods (4–10). There are no known adverse effects of low-GI diets, and their safety, palatability, and low cost give them advantages over low-fat and low-carbohydrate diets. For these reasons, low-GI diets can be considered for the management of obesity and prevention of obesity-related complications.

GLYCEMIC INDEX

The concept of GI was originally introduced as an alternative to the sugar/starch distinction for improving glycemic control in the management of diabetes. Carbohydrate content is the most important determinant of glycemia, but even in equal amounts, the carbohydrates in some foods have more glycemic potential than others. In essence, GI ranks the postprandial impact of different foods, gram for gram of available carbohydrate. The carbohydrates in most fruits, nonstarchy vegetables, pasta, legumes, nuts, and dairy products tend to have a low GI, whereas those in potatoes, breads, and breakfast cereals often have a high GI. Within most food groups, there are examples of both high- and low-GI products.

The GI of a food is influenced by many factors, including the type of monosaccharide (eg, fructose vs glucose), the type of starch (eg, amylose vs amylopectin), the degree of gelatinization of the starch, the type of fiber (eg, viscous or not), the method of processing (eg, high-pressure extrusion vs home cooking), and the presence of large amounts of fat or protein. Technological advances in food processing and increased dependence on convenient, instant, and precooked foods have together resulted in faster rates of carbohydrate digestion and absorption. A food's GI cannot be predicted from its composition or appearance, and many highly processed "whole grain" foods have a high GI. Modern diets dominated by high-GI foods have significant implications for the pathogenesis of diabetes and obesity.

GLYCEMIC LOAD

When foods contribute large amounts of carbohydrate to the diet, their GI is of greater consequence. *Glycemic load* (GL) is defined as the GI multiplied by the amount of available carbohydrate in grams, and this concept captures both the quantity and quality of the carbohydrate. In the context of mixed meals, knowledge of GL of the composite foods allows precise prediction of the magnitude of the glycemic and insulin response (11). High intake of saturated fat is known to increase low-density lipoprotein (LDL) cholesterol concentration in blood, but it is less well recognized that diets with a high GL (both high in carbohydrate and high in GI) can worsen many of the features of metabolic syndrome, including insulin resistance, postprandial hyperglycemia, dyslipidemia (hypertriglyceridemia, low high-density lipoprotein [HDL] cholesterol), and hypercoagulatory states (12–14).

Dietary GL can be reduced in various ways—by substituting low-GI carbohydrates for high-GI versions (without changing total carbohydrate), by reducing overall carbohydrate intake, or by a combination of both approaches. For many people, replacing high-GI carbohydrate sources with low-GI sources is relatively simple and has advantages over making major changes to macronutrient distribution. The traditional Mediterranean diet, vegetarian diets based on legumes, and the traditional diets of many indigenous people have a low GI and low GL.

THE RATIONALE FOR LOW-GI DIETS IN OBESITY

Reducing the magnitude of fluctuations in blood glucose can influence weight loss and weight control via several mechanisms, including effects on appetite, fat oxidation, and metabolic rate. Low-GI foods and meals have been associated with increased satiety, reduced hunger, or lower subsequent voluntary food intake (15–20), but not all studies have shown differences. Higher satiety may be related to a specific effect of slowly digested starch on gut-brain signaling (eg, higher cholecystokin levels), rather than the glycemic response per se. However, large spikes in blood glucose, followed by dynamic decreases of sufficient magnitude to elicit a counter-regulatory hormone response, may also stimulate appetite in the body's attempt to reestablish euglycemia. During both low- and high-intensity exercise, low-GI meals increase fat oxidation and encourage use of fat rather than carbohydrate as the source of fuel (21–24). Higher rates of fat oxidation and/or less dependence on carbohydrate would be expected to facilitate weight loss over the long-term. Carefully controlled trials indicate that the reduction in energy expenditure that normally occurs during active weight loss is of lesser magnitude in people following low-GI/GL diets (16,25). In animals predisposed to type 2 diabetes, long-term feeding of high-GI starches produced glucose intolerance and disrupted beta cell architecture (26). Even when matched for body weight, rats and mice fed high-GI diets have higher fat mass and less lean mass than macronutrient-matched low-GI diets. Studies in animals may not always be extrapolated to humans, but they suggest that the rate of carbohydrate digestion and absorption per se influences weight gain and body composition.

Observational studies in large cohorts provide evidence that the self-selected diets with a low GI minimize weight gain over the long-term (27–29). Ma et al (27) found higher body mass index (BMI) was independently associated with higher dietary GI but not with carbohydrate intake or GL. A Danish study (30) found that high-GI diets were associated with increases in fat mass and waist circumference in women, especially sedentary women, but no relationship was observed in men. Although some observational studies have found no associations, methodological issues, including misclassification and underreporting, would tend to bias to the null hypothesis (31).

RANDOMIZED CONTROLLED TRIAL EVIDENCE FOR GI IN THE MANAGEMENT OF OBESITY

Intervention studies that are adequately powered with careful attention to treatment fidelity provide the most convincing evidence that low-GI diets promote faster weight loss or greater body fat loss than conventional diets. Among 129 overweight young adults, an ad libitum low-GI diet was shown to be almost twice as effective as a conventional low-fat diet in achieving weight loss of 5% or more by 12 weeks (32). Women experienced more benefits than men, losing 80% more body fat compared with those on the conventional diet. In the same study, cardiovascular risk factors, particularly LDL cholesterol, were most improved on the high-carbohydrate, low-GI diet, an effect also noted by others even in the absence of differences in weight loss (33). Similarly, overweight and obese adults on a reduced-GL diet lost more weight over 12 weeks than those on an energy-restricted reduced-fat diet, and the participants on the reduced-GL diet showed a trend to better weight-loss maintenance and higher HDL cholesterol levels at 36 weeks (34).

In the longest randomized controlled trial to date, Ebbeling et al (35) found a strong diet-phenotype interaction for weight loss on low-GI/GL diets. Both weight loss (6 months) and weight maintenance (18 months) were greater on the low-GL diet in those individuals who showed a high 30-minute insulin response at the beginning of the diet. Others have made similar observations (36). Together, these findings suggest that individuals with either high insulin secretion or insulin resistance have the most to gain by adopting low-GI diets for weight loss.

Low-GI diets have also proven effective in children, vegetarians, and individuals with diabetes. A 12-month study (with 6 months of intense intervention) in 16 obese adolescents found a greater reduction in BMI and body fat on an ad libitum reduced-GL diet compared with a reduced-fat, energy-restricted diet (37). A study by Barnard and colleagues (38) showed greater weight loss and improved glycemic control among individuals with type 2 diabetes on low-GI vegan diets. In pregnancy, low-GI diets have been shown to reduce weight gain compared with high-GI diets with similar energy and macronutrient content (39). Finally, offspring of women who followed a low-GI diet during pregnancy had a lower ponderal index and were much less likely to be large-for-gestational age than babies born to women consuming a conventional healthful diet (40).

Not all studies have shown superior weight loss with a low-GI diet when compared with other dietary modifications (32,33,41). In hindsight, this inconsistency in findings might be traced to differences in phenotype and insulin sensitivity among subjects as demonstrated by Ebbeling et al (35) or lack of fidelity in intervention delivery. Although additional high-quality, long-term studies are needed, a Cochrane review and meta-analysis (42) concluded that body weight, total fat mass, BMI, total cholesterol, and LDL cholesterol all decreased significantly more on low-GI diets than on conventional diets.

References

1. Ludwig D. The glycemic index. Physiological mechanisms relating to obesity, diabetes and cardiovascular disease. *JAMA*. 2002;287:2414–2423.

2. Jenkins DJ, Kendall CW, Augustin LS, Franceschi S, Hamidi M, Marchie A, Jenkins AL, Axelsen M. Glycemic index: overview of implications in health and disease. *Am J Clin Nutr*. 2002;76(suppl):266S–273S.

3. Aston LM. Glycaemic index and metabolic disease risk. *Proc Nutr Soc*. 2006;65: 125–134.

4. FAO/WHO Joint Expert Consultation. *Carbohydrates in Human Nutrition*. Geneva, Switzerland: Food and Agriculture Organisation, Food and Nutrition; 1998. FAO Food and Nutrition paper 66.

5. Perlstein R WJ, Hines C, Milsavljevic M. Dietitians Association of Australia review paper: glycaemic index in diabetes management. *Aust J Nutr Diet*. 1997;54:57–63.

6. Canadian Diabetes Association. Guidelines for the nutritional management of diabetes mellitus in the new millennium. A position statement by the Canadian Diabetes Association. *Can J Diabetes Care*. 2000;23:56–69.

7. Recommendations for the nutritional management of patients with diabetes mellitus. *Eur J Clin Nutr*. 2000;54:353–355.

8. Diabetes Australia—NSW. GI Symbol Program. http://www.diabetesnsw.com.au/ diabetes_prevention/glycemicindex.asp. Accessed February 4, 2009.

9. Connor H, Annan F, Bunn E, Frost G, McGough N, Sarwar T, Thomas B; Nutrition Subcommittee of the Diabetes Care Advisory Committee of Diabetes UK. The implementation of nutritional advice for people with diabetes. *Diabet Med*. 2003;20:786–807.

10. Nutrition Subcommittee of the Diabetes Care Advisory Committee of Diabetes UK. The implementation of nutritional advice for people with diabetes. *Diabet Med*. 2003;20:786–807.

11. Wolever T, Yang M, Zeng X, Atkinson F, Brand-Miller J. Food glycemic index, as given in glycemic index tables, is a significant determinant of glycemic responses elicited by composite breakfast meals. *Am J Clin Nutr*. 2006;83:1306–1312.

12. Liu S. Lowering dietary glycemic load for weight control and cardiovascular health: a matter of quality. *Arch Intern Med*. 2006;166:1438–1439.

13. Halton TL, Willett WC, Liu S, Manson JE, Albert CM, Rexrode K, Hu FB. Low-carbohydrate-diet score and the risk of coronary heart disease in women. *N Engl J Med*. 2006;355:1991–2002.

14. Mozaffarian D, Rimm E, Herrington D. Dietary fats, carbohydrate, and progression of coronary atherosclerosis in postmenopausal women. *Am J Clin Nutr*. 2004;80:1175–1184.

15. Ludwig D, Majzoub J, Al-Zahrani A, Dallal G, Blanco I, Roberts S. High glycemic index foods, overeating, and obesity. *Pediatrics*. 1999;103:E26.

16. Agus M, Swain J, Larson C, Eckert E, Ludwig D. Dietary composition and physiologic adaptations to energy restriction. *Am J Clin Nutr*. 2000;71:901–907.

17. Warren J, Henry J, Simonite V. Low glycemic index breakfasts and reduced food intake in preadolescent children. *Pediatrics*. 2003;112:414–419.

18. Roberts S. High-glycemic index foods, hunger, and obesity: is there a connection? *Nutr Rev*. 2000;58:163–169.

19. Ludwig DS, Pereira MA, Kroenke CH, et al. Dietary fiber, weight gain, and cardiovascular disease risk factors in young adults. *JAMA*. 1999;282:1539–1546.

20. Jimenez-Cruz A, Gutierrez-Gonzalez AN, Bacardi-Gascon M. Low glycemic index lunch on satiety in overweight and obese people with type 2 diabetes. *Nutr Hosp*. 2005;20:348–350.

21. Febbraio M, Keenan J, Angus D, Campbell S, Garnham A. Preexercise carbohydrate ingestion, glucose kinetics, and muscle glycogen use: effect of the glycemic index. *J Appl Physiol*. 2000;89:1845–1851.

22. Stevenson E, Williams C, Nute M. The influence of the glycemic index of breakfast and lunch on substrate utilization during the postprandial periods and subsequent exercise. *Br J Nutr*. 2005;93:885–893.

23. Wu CL, Nicholas C, Williams C, Took A, Hardy L. The influence of high-carbohydrate meals with different glycemic indices on substrate utilisation during subsequent exercise. *Br J Nutr*. 2003;90:1049–1056.

24. Wee SL, Williams C, Tsintzas K, Boobis L. Ingestion of a high-glycemic index meal increases muscle glycogen storage at rest but augments its utilization during subsequent exercise. *J Appl Physiol*. 2005;99:707–714.

25. Pereira M, Swain J, Goldfine A, Rifai N, Ludwig D. Effects of a low-glycemic load diet on resting energy expenditure and heart disease risk factors during weight loss. *JAMA*. 2004;292:2482–2490.

26. Pawlak DB, Kushner J, Ludwig D. Effects of dietary glycaemic index on adiposity, glucose homoeostasis, and plasma lipids in animals. *Lancet*. 2004;364:778–785.

27. Ma Y, Olendzki B, Chiriboga D, Hebert JR, Li Y, Li W, Campbell M, Gendreau K, Ockene IS. Association between dietary carbohydrates and body weight. *Am J Epidemiol*. 2005;161:359–367.

28. Murakami K, Sasaki S, Okubo H, Takahashi Y, Hosoi Y, Itabashi M. Dietary fiber intake, dietary glycemic index and load, and body mass index: a cross-sectional study of 3931 Japanese women aged 18–20 years. *Eur J Clin Nutr*. 2007;61:986–995.

29. Hare-Bruun H, Flint A, Heitmann BL. Glycemic index and glycemic load in relation to changes in body weight, body fat distribution, and body composition in adult Danes. *Am J Clin Nutr*. 2006;84:871–879; quiz 952–953.

30. Hare-Bruun H, Flint A, Heitmann B. Glycemic index and glycemic load in relation to changes in body weight, body fat distribution, and body composition in adult Danes. *Am J Clin Nutr*. 2006;84:871–879.

31. Lau C, Toft U, Tetens I, Richelsen B, Jørgensen T, Borch-Johnsen K, Glümer C. Association between dietary glycemic index, glycemic load and body mass index: is underreporting a problem? *Am J Clin Nutr*. 2006;84:641–645.

32. McMillan-Price J, Petocz P, Atkinson F, O'Neill K, Samman S, Steinbeck K, Caterson I, Brand-Miller J. Comparison of 4 diets of varying glycemic load on weight loss and cardiovascular risk reduction in overweight and obese young adults: a randomised controlled trial. *Arch Intern Med*. 2006;166:1466–1475.

33. Sloth B, Krog-Mikkelsen I, Flint A, Tetens I, Björck I, Vinoy S, Elmståhl H, Astrup A, Lang V, Raben A. No difference in body weight decrease between a low-glycemic-index and a high-glycemic-index diet but reduced LDL cholesterol after 10-wk ad libitum intake of the low-glycemic-index diet. *Am J Clin Nutr*. 2004;80:337–347.

34. Maki KC, Rains TM, Kaden VN, Raneri KR, Davidson MH. Effects of a reduced-glycemic-load diet on body weight, body composition, and cardiovascular disease risk markers in overweight and obese adults. *Am J Clin Nutr*. 2007;85:724–734.

35. Ebbeling CB, Leidig MM, Feldman HA, Lovesky MM, Ludwig DS. Effects of a low-glycemic load vs low-fat diet in obese young adults: a randomized trial. *JAMA*. 2007;297:2092–2102.

36. Pittas A, Das S, Hajduk C, Golden J, Saltzman E, Stark PC, Greenberg AS, Roberts SB. A low-glycemic load diet facilitates greater weight loss in overweight adults with high insulin secretion but not in overweight adults with low insulin secretion in the CALERIE Trial. *Diabetes Care*. 2005;28:2939–2941.

37. Ebbeling C, Leidig M, Sinclair K, Hangen J, Ludwig D. A reduced-glycemic load diet in the treatment of adolescent obesity. *Arch Pediatr Adolesc Med*. 2003;157:773–779.

38. Barnard ND, Cohen J, Jenkins DJ, Turner-McGrievy G, Gloede L, Jaster B, Seidl K, Green AA, Talpers S. A low-fat vegan diet improves glycemic control and cardiovascular risk factors in a randomized clinical trial in individuals with type 2 diabetes. *Diabetes Care*. 2006;29:1777–1783.

39. Clapp J. Diet, exercise, and feto-placental growth. *Arch Gynecol Obstet*. 1997;261:101–107.

40. Moses RG, Luebcke M, Davis WS, Coleman KJ, Tapsell LC, Petocz P, Brand-Miller JC. Effect of a low-glycemic-index diet during pregnancy on obstetric outcomes. *Am J Clin Nutr*. 2006;84:807–812.

41. Ebbeling C, Leidig M, Sinclair K, Seger-Shippee L, Feldman H, Ludwig D. Effects of an ad libitum reduced glycemic load diet on cardiovascular disease risk factors in obese young adults. *Am J Clin Nutr*. 2005;81:976–982.

42. Thomas DE, Elliott EJ, Baur L. Low glycaemic index or low glycaemic load diets for overweight and obesity. *Cochrane Database Syst Rev*. 2007:CD005105.

PART B: PRACTICAL APPLICATIONS

KATE MARSH, M NUTR DIET, ADVAPD, CDE

Critics of the glycemic index claim that it is too hard to understand, but, in practice, changing to a low-GI diet is relatively easy for most people. There is no need to eliminate any foods or food groups; one just needs to make better choices within food groups. In many cases, it simply comes down to swapping one food for another (see Table 3.1).

To a large extent, following a low-GI diet means eating fewer processed foods, which is something that as practitioners we are likely to recommend to anyone who is trying to lose weight. Unlike some other popular diets, a low-GI eating plan has the advantage of many health benefits, including a reduced risk of type 2 diabetes, cardiovascular disease, and some types of cancer, and no known detrimental health effects.

In children with type 1 diabetes, a low-GI diet resulted in better blood glucose control without an increased risk of hypoglycemia or weight gain when compared with traditional carbohydrate counting. Furthermore, the children and their parents preferred the low-GI diet, finding it easier to follow (1). In a study to determine whether parents of overweight children age 5 to 12 years could reduce the GI of their child's diet after receiving brief instructions and a handout from their pediatrician, all of the parents in the study described the diet as easy to understand, and two-thirds of them reported that their child was generally able to follow the diet (2). Finally, a study of pregnant women found that those assigned to a low-GI diet reported that the diet was "easier" compared with those assigned to the conventional (low-sugar/high-fiber) diet (3).

When counseling clients to change to a low-GI diet, it is best to start by focusing on the carbohydrate foods that make up a regular part of their diet, and switching these to lower GI choices. One way to check for the GI in foods is the Glycemic Index and GI Database (http://www.glycemicindex.com). For example, if your clients eat white rice (GI 80–90 for most varieties) and processed breakfast cereals on most days, you could suggest they try serving more pasta (GI 45) prepared from dry noodles in place of rice and change their processed breakfast cereal to old-fashioned oatmeal. If clients eat large

TABLE 3.1

High– vs Low–Glycemic Index (GI) Carbohydrate Foods

High-GI Food	Low-GI Alternatives
Bread, white or whole meal	Bread high in whole grains; sourdough and pumpernickel breads
Processed breakfast cereals	Unrefined cereals, such as rolled oats or natural muesli, or a low-GI processed cereal, such as those containing psyllium husks
Plain cookies or crackers	Cookies made with dried fruit, oats, and whole grains
Cakes and muffins	Cakes and muffins made with fruit, oats, oat bran, rice bran, and psyllium husks
Potato	Baby new potatoes; sweet potatoes, taro , yam, and corn; mashed potatoes made with half cannellini beans
Rice	Longer grain varieties such as basmati; pearled barley, quinoa, pasta, or noodles

amounts of white bread and potatoes, you could suggest that they change to a stone-ground whole-grain bread and have more orange sweet potatoes, yams, or corn instead of potatoes. Not all food choices need to be low-GI—switching just half of the carbohydrate foods your client eats in a day from high- to low-GI choices or including one low-GI food at each meal is of benefit.

It is important to explain to clients that GI, like any single dietary factor, should not be used in isolation when making healthful food choices—this is a topic that confuses some people. Some low-GI foods are obviously not the most nutritious choices because of their high content of saturated fat (eg, ice cream, pizza, and potato chips), whereas some high-GI foods may still be acceptable because of their relatively high-nutrient and low-energy content (eg, watermelon). GI should be used to select foods within a healthful diet that is also low in saturated fat and high in dietary fiber. In this way, a low-GI diet fits closely with general healthful eating recommendations, including eating more fruits, vegetables, and whole-grain breads and cereals.

In GI testing, each food is assigned a number representing its effect on blood glucose relative to oral glucose. However, there is no need to counsel clients to learn these numbers, nor is counting or calculation required. For most people, the descriptions "low," "medium," and "high" (where low is a GI < 55; medium GI = 55–70; and high GI ≥ 70 on the glucose = 100 scale) are sufficient to guide the transition to a low-GI diet. For the person who is eating mostly high-GI foods, simply substituting low- or medium-GI alternatives can substantially reduce the overall GI of their diet, with resulting beneficial effects.

CASE STUDIES

To explore the practical application of GI in more detail, let us consider how nutrition counseling about a low-GI diet could be done with two illustrative clients, Robert and Karen. Some of this advice is generic; ideally, however, the name of branded products with proven low GI should be specified. RDs can play an important role in encouraging food manufacturers to provide GI values on food labels.

Case Study 1: Robert

Robert is a 45-year-old businessman who was referred by his doctor for weight loss. He has a BMI of 35; waist circumference of 43 inches; increased blood fats, blood pressure, and fasting blood glucose levels; and a strong family history of type 2 diabetes. He lives alone and works long hours in a stressful job. Robert does not enjoy cooking for himself and is usually too busy, relying heavily on convenience and take-out meals. Although he is motivated to make some changes because of his fear of developing diabetes, Robert is also concerned about feeling hungry (which has been his experience when trying to diet in the past) and about having to spend a lot of time cooking and shopping. See Box 3.1 for a typical 1-day food record and nutritional analysis.

You start by explaining to Robert the benefits of lifestyle changes for reducing diabetes risk, citing the results of the Diabetes Prevention Program (DPP) and the Finnish Diabetes Prevention Study (DPS) (4,5). This certainly gets his interest, and he is

Box 3.1
Typical 1-Day Food Record for Robert Before Nutrition Counseling

Breakfast: Coffee and bagel with cream cheese
Morning snack: Cappuccino and two store-bought cookies
Lunch: Ham and cheese on a white roll, sugar-sweetened soft drink
Afternoon snack: Potato chips
Dinner: Large steak, mashed potato, peas, and two slices of white bread with butter
Evening snack: Rice crackers

Nutritional analysis: 2450 kcal; 97 g fat (35% of kcal), 48 g saturated fat (18% of kcal); 134 g protein (22% of kcal); 254 g carbohydrate (42% of kcal); 22 g fiber.
Glycemic index = 69; glycemic load = 147.

keen to know exactly what sort of changes he needs to make to achieve this potential risk reduction.

Before you make any recommendations, you want to find out a few things from Robert:

- Is his intake of fruit and vegetables low because he does not like these foods or just because he does not shop for and prepare them?
- Are there many foods he does not like eating?
- Would he be willing to have breakfast at home and/or take lunch from home rather than relying on take-out?
- Are the cookies and chocolate he snacks on at work chosen mostly for convenience, and if so could he take some healthful snacks to work with him?

You find out that he likes most foods and reports being willing to make any necessary changes as long as it does not take too much time to prepare and he is not left hungry. He agrees he could manage to have breakfast at home before he leaves for work and also feels he could take in some healthful snacks to prevent him heading for the cookie jar. But he still wants to buy his lunch and does not want to do any "fancy" cooking at night. You help him establish a revised eating plan (Box 3.2).

Although these changes will substantially increase his intake of vegetables, fruits, and whole grains, Robert is encouraged that this new eating plan does not seem difficult or time-consuming. Also, in making these changes, the GI of Robert's diet has been substantially reduced, without even mentioning the term *glycemic index* to him. Glycemic index is something you can explain to him in more detail at a subsequent consultation, once he has made these initial changes.

As Robert's case highlights, even if the concept of GI seems too confusing for some clients, or is not their first priority, it is easy to focus on low-GI foods because they typically fit in with the other healthful eating recommendations. There is actually no need even to mention the term *glycemic index*—you could instead just talk about eating more unprocessed foods (eg, stone-ground, whole-kernel breads instead white bread, steel-cut or old-fashioned oatmeal in place of puffed and flake cereals, and fresh fruit in place of starchy snacks), which is a concept that is easy for most people to understand.

Box 3.2
Revised 1-Day Meal Plan for Robert

Breakfast: Two slices of stone-ground (low-GI) whole-grain bread with one poached egg and a grilled tomato, coffee with nonfat milk
Morning snack: Fruit and cappuccino with low-fat milk
Lunch: Low-GI whole grain roll with turkey, lettuce, and tomato; small fruit juice
Afternoon snack: Low-fat yogurt
Pre-dinner snack: Handful of dry-roasted nuts
Dinner: Small lean steak; corn on the cob, carrots, beans, and peas (frozen and cooked in the microwave); two slices of low-GI, whole grain bread with olive oil spread
Evening snack: Frozen berries with low-fat ice cream

Nutritional analysis: 1,830 kcal; 64 g fat (31% of kcal), 13 g saturated fat (6% of kcal); 95 g protein (22% of kcal); 204 g carbohydrate (47% of kcal); 33 g fiber.
Glycemic index = 46; glycemic load = 73.

Case Study 2: Karen

Karen is a 30-year-old woman with polycystic ovary syndrome (PCOS) and obesity (BMI = 31). She has struggled with her weight since puberty and has been dieting on-and-off for "most of her life" with little success. Her most recent laboratory report indicates dyslipidemia (high triglycerides and low HDL cholesterol levels), normal fasting blood glucose, and increased fasting insulin levels. She was prescribed metformin 3 months ago and since that time has been exercising regularly and following a low-fat diet. However, she has only lost 2 kg and is finding the diet hard to maintain because of constant hunger. Karen has also been experiencing symptoms of hypoglycemia and complains of feeling tired all the time. Her current diet and nutritional analysis are outlined in Box 3.3.

Box 3.3
Typical 1-Day Food Record for Case Study of Karen Before Nutrition Counseling

Breakfast: Bowl of bran flakes with low-fat milk
Morning snack: Apple
Lunch: Whole-grain roll with tuna, salad greens, and avocado
Afternoon snack: Rice cakes with low-fat cottage cheese and tomato
Dinner: Lean pork and vegetable stir-fry with brown rice
Evening snack: Cantaloupe and low-fat yogurt

Nutritional analysis: 1,550 kcal; 46 g fat (27% of kcal), 13 g saturated fat (7.5% of kcal); 88 g protein (24% of kcal); 186 g carbohydrate (50% of kcal); 24 g fiber.
Glycemic index = 63; glycemic load = 105.

Box 3.4
Revised 1-Day Meal Plan for Case Study of Karen

Breakfast: Steel-cut oatmeal (winter) or muesli (summer) with strawberries and low-fat milk
Morning snack: Apple
Lunch: Stone-ground (low-GI), whole grain bread with tuna, salad greens, and avocado
Afternoon snack: Low-GI whole grain crackers with cottage cheese and tomato
Dinner: Lean pork and vegetable stir-fry with pasta
Evening snack: Pear and low-fat yogurt

Nutritional analysis: 1,530 kcal; 45 g fat (28% of kcal), 12.5 g saturated fat (7.5% of kcal); 90 g protein (25%); 176 g carbohydrate (47%); 32 g fiber.
Glycemic index = 45; glycemic load = 70.

With her history of insulin resistance, difficulties losing weight with a traditional low-fat diet, and symptoms of hypoglycemia, Karen would be particularly suited to a low-GI eating plan. But before you begin educating her on such a diet, you will want to find out:

- Has she heard of GI and does she understand what it means?
- Has she ever tried a low-GI eating plan in the past?
- Does she understand the implications of insulin resistance and how dietary changes might help reduce her insulin levels and thereby improve her chances of weight loss?

After exploring these issues, you educate Karen about a low-GI diet, explaining the benefits it could provide to her and discussing the basics of the diet, focusing on the idea of substitution. You suggest some modifications to Karen's current diet that will help to reduce the GI (and the GL) of her meals and snacks without requiring any substantial increase in shopping or food-preparation time. See Box 3.4 for Karen's new meal plan.

As the nutritional analysis demonstrates, this new meal plan is similar in energy and macronutrient composition to Karen's original eating style. However, the GI and GL were substantially lowered by making a few small changes to Karen's diet.

SUMMARY

The role of the GI in weight control is still vigorously debated among scientists. Nonetheless, at the present time, the demonstrated advantages of low-GI/GL diets over low-fat and low-carbohydrate diets make them "best practice" in the management of obesity and its comorbidities. For successful weight loss, our goal as practitioners is to help people adhere to an eating plan that is healthful, satisfying, and sustainable in the long-term. A low-GI diet meets all of these criteria and has the advantage of having no detrimental effects while also fitting closely with general healthful eating recommendations. When explained in simple terms and used within the context of a healthful diet, GI is an easy concept for most people to understand.

References

1. Gilbertson H, Brand-Miller J, Thorburn A, Evans S, Chondros P, Werther G. The effect of flexible low glycemic index dietary advice versus measured carbohydrate exchange diets on glycemic control in children with type 1 diabetes. *Diabetes Care.* 2001;24:1137–1143.

2. Young PC, West SA, Ortiz K, Carlson J. A pilot study to determine the feasibility of the low glycemic index diet as a treatment for overweight children in primary care practice. *Ambul Pediatr.* 2004;4:28–33.

3. Moses RG, Luebcke M, Davis WS, Coleman KJ, Tapsell LC, Petocz P, Brand-Miller JC. Effect of a low-glycemic-index diet during pregnancy on obstetric outcomes. *Am J Clin Nutr.* 2006;84:807–812.

4. Diabetes Prevention Program Research Group. Reduction in the incidence of type 2 diabetes with lifestyle intervention or metformin. *N Engl J Med.* 2002;346:393–403.

5. Tuomilehto J, Lindstrom J, Eriksson JG, Valle TT, Hämäläinen H, Ilanne-Parikka P, Keinänen-Kiukaanniemi S, Laakso M, Louheranta A, Rastas M, Salminen V, Uusitupa M; Finnish Diabetes Prevention Study Group. Prevention of type 2 diabetes mellitus by changes in lifestyle among subjects with impaired glucose tolerance. *N Engl J Med.* 2001;344:1343–1350.

CHAPTER 4

DIET—DASH (DIETARY APPROACHES TO STOP HYPERTENSION) AND MEDITERRANEAN

PART A: OVERVIEW

JEANNETTE M. BEASLEY, PHD, MPH, RD, AND

LAWRENCE J. APPEL, MD, MPH

Clinically important outcomes associated with weight loss include reduced blood pressure, lower low-density lipoprotein (LDL) cholesterol, and improved insulin sensitivity. In clinical trials, the Dietary Approaches to Stop Hypertension (DASH) diet (1,2) and Mediterranean (3) diets improve cardiovascular risk factors independent of weight loss. Such diets might also be beneficial in controlling weight; however, evidence is limited. Both diets emphasize plant-based foods and are rich in nutrients associated with lower weight—ie, fiber and whole grains (4). Furthermore, neither diet is a particularly low fat—Mediterranean-style diets are often high in total fat (sometimes > 40% of energy), whereas the DASH diet is a moderate-fat diet (27% of energy). Some research suggests higher adherence with moderate-fat dietary patterns compared with low-fat diets, presumably because moderate-fat diets are more palatable and have fewer restrictions (5). The 2005 Dietary Guidelines for Americans advocate the DASH diet because it meets each of the major nutrient recommendations and has well-documented beneficial effects on blood pressure and LDL cholesterol (4). For these reasons, the DASH and Mediterranean diets are reasonable to prescribe for individuals who are attempting to control their weight.

THE DASH DIET

The DASH trial tested whether modification of whole dietary patterns would affect blood pressure (1). In contrast to most diet–blood pressure trials, the DASH trial was a feeding study. Participants (n = 459, 29% hypertensive, 60% African-American) were randomly assigned to one of the following diets: (*a*) the DASH diet, (*b*) a control diet, or (*c*) a diet rich in fruits and vegetables but otherwise similar to the control diet.

The DASH diet emphasized fruits, vegetables, and low-fat dairy products; included whole grains, poultry, fish and nuts; and was reduced in red meat, sweets, and sugar-containing beverages (6). This diet was rich in potassium, magnesium, calcium, and fiber; moderate in total fat (27% of energy); and reduced in saturated fat (6% of energy) and cholesterol (150 mg); it was also slightly increased in protein (18% of energy). The control diet had a nutrient composition typical of that consumed by many Americans; its potassium, magnesium, and calcium levels were comparatively low, and its macronutrient profile and fiber content corresponded to average US consumption. The third arm of the DASH trial, the fruits and vegetables diet, was rich in potassium, magnesium, and fiber but otherwise similar to the control diet. All three diets contained similar amounts of sodium (approximately 3,000 mg/d).

Among all participants, the DASH diet significantly reduced mean systolic blood pressure by 5.5 mmHg and mean diastolic blood pressure by 3.0 mmHg. The fruits and vegetables diet also significantly reduced blood pressure but to a lesser extent, approximately 50% of the effect of the DASH diet. The effects occurred rapidly and were apparent after 2 weeks (see Figure 4.1) (1). In subgroup analyses, the DASH diet significantly ($P < .05$) lowered blood pressure in all major subgroups (men, women, African-Americans, non-African-Americans, and subjects with and without hypertension) compared with the control diet (1). Compared with the control diet, the DASH diet also reduced LDL cholesterol and homocysteine.

Results from the DASH trial have important public health and clinical implications. It has been estimated that a population-wide reduction in blood pressure of the magnitude observed in DASH could reduce stroke incidence by 27% and incidence of coronary heart disease (CHD) by 15%. Further reduction in CHD risk might be anticipated from the net changes in lipids. Evidence from prospective observational studies corroborates this notion (7).

The Optimal Macronutrient Intake Trial to Prevent Heart Disease (OMNI-Heart) extended results from the DASH trial by investigating whether partial replacement of carbohydrate with protein (approximately half from plant sources) or unsaturated fat (predominantly monounsaturated fat) would further reduce blood pressure and improve blood lipids (8). In this randomized, three-period, crossover feeding trial, partial replacement of carbohydrate with either unsaturated fat or protein from mixed sources decreased systolic blood pressure by 1 mmHg in prehypertensive individuals and by 3 mmHg in those with hypertension, improved blood lipid profiles, and reduced estimated cardiovascular risk (9).

Findings from the OMNI-Heart trial support the notion individuals have considerable flexibility in selecting heart-healthy diets that also consider comorbidities and taste preferences. For example, the diet rich in unsaturated fat closely resembles a Mediterranean-style diet, which is characteristically higher in fat, especially monounsaturated fat, and rich in fruits and vegetables. This diet might also appeal to people with diabetes, who are commonly advised to reduce their intake of carbohydrate.

THE MEDITERRANEAN DIET

The Mediterranean "diet" is not a single plan. Rather, this term is a general descriptive term applied to diets consumed in several regions close to the Mediterranean Sea.

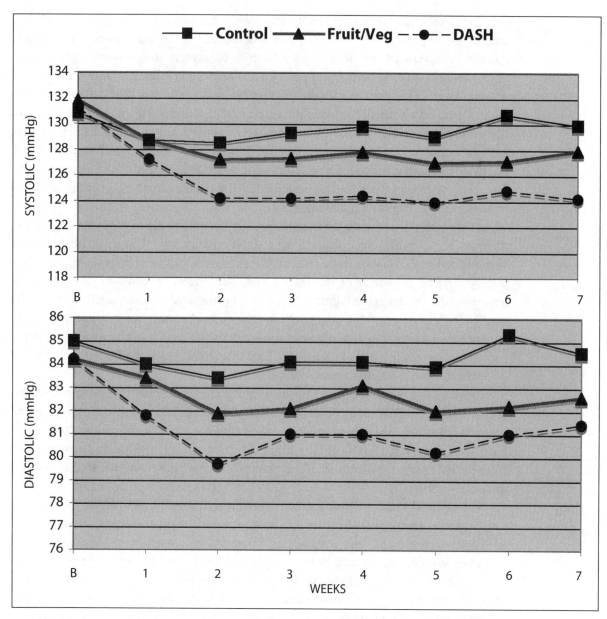

FIGURE 4.1 Effects of control, fruits and vegetables, and DASH diets on blood pressure: results from the DASH trial. Reprinted with permission from Appel LJ, Moore TJ, Obarzanek E, Vollmer WM, Svetkey LP, Sacks FM, Bray GA, Vogt TM, Cutler JA, Windhauser MM, Lin PH, Karanja N. A clinical trial of the effects of dietary patterns on blood pressure. DASH Collaborative Research Group. *N Engl J Med.* 1997;336:1117–1124. Copyright © 1997 Massachusetts Medical Society. All rights reserved.

Typically, these diets are rich in plant foods (fruits, vegetables, breads, other forms of cereals, potatoes, beans, nuts, and seeds). Fruit is the typical daily dessert, and olive oil is the principal source of fat. Dairy products (principally cheese and yogurt), fish, and poultry are consumed in low to moderate amounts; zero to four eggs are consumed weekly; red meat is consumed in low amounts; and wine is consumed in low to moderate amounts, usually with meals. This diet is low in saturated fat ($\leq$ 7% to 8% of energy) but moderate to high in total fat, ranging from less than 25% to more than 40% of energy (10).

Despite the difficulties of characterizing a "Mediterranean-style" diet, interest in these diets is considerable because of their apparent health benefits, particularly a reduced risk of CHD. Results from observational studies suggest that consumption of a Mediterranean diet is associated with one of the lowest risks of CHD in the world. The Seven Countries Study, a landmark study initiated in the mid 1950s, was the first study that systematically examined the relationship between diet and risk of cardiovascular disease across geographically and culturally distinct populations (11). The countries were the United States, Finland, the Netherlands, Italy, Yugoslavia, Greece, and Japan. During the course of 10 years of follow-up, CHD mortality varied widely among these countries, with the highest age-adjusted incidence occurring in east Finland (68/1,000) and the United States (42/1,000), and the lowest in Greece (0/1,000) and Japan (7/1,000) (11).

Recent studies have used two score-based approaches to measure adherence to a Mediterranean diet among European and North American populations (12–14). Nine components similar to both the European and US score-based approaches are vegetables, legumes, fruits, nuts, whole grains, fish, monounsaturated fat–saturated fat ratio, alcohol, and meat. Using these score-based approaches, several prospective observational studies have documented that greater adherence with a Mediterranean diet is associated with lower mortality in both European and North American populations (14–16). In the European Prospective Investigation Into Cancer and Nutrition (EPIC) cohort, higher adherence to the Mediterranean diet by 2 units (according to the 9-point Mediterranean diet scale) was associated with a 27% lower mortality rate among subjects with prevalent CHD at enrollment (16).

Findings from the National Institutes of Health American Association of Retired Persons (NIH-AARP) Diet and Health study (14) suggest the inverse association between the Mediterranean diet and mortality is not limited to European populations or those at high risk for cardiovascular-related death. Among more than 380,000 retired women and men in the NIH-AARP Diet and Health study, both men and women with high adherence to a Mediterranean diet pattern had approximately 20% lower risk of all-cause mortality compared with those with low adherence ($P < .05$).

Few trials have tested the effects of the Mediterranean diet on weight and body composition (17). Of the three published trials, only the trial by McManus and colleagues (18) enrolled more than 50 participants and had a duration of more than 3 months. This trial randomly assigned overweight (body mass index [BMI] 26.5–46) men and women to follow a moderate-fat (35% of energy) Mediterranean diet or a low-fat (20% of energy) diet for 18 months; weight change was the primary outcome. Although attrition was high (40% after 18 months), adherence at 18 months was better in the moderate-fat group (54% or 27 of 50) compared with the low-fat group (20% or 10 of 51), ($P < .002$). In the moderate-fat group, there were mean decreases in body weight of 4.1 kg, BMI of 1.6, and waist circumference of 6.9 cm, compared with increases in the low-fat group of 2.9 kg, 1.4, and 2.6 cm, respectively (each $P \leq .001$). The moderate-fat diet group was continued for an additional year, and the mean weight loss after 30 months compared to baseline was 3.5 kg (n = 19; $P = .03$).

SUMMARY

In summary, the DASH and the Mediterranean diets are healthful dietary patterns with well-documented health benefits. Although the role of specific dietary patterns in controlling weight remains uncertain, it is reasonable to prescribe these diets, each of which should reduce the overall risk of chronic disease, particularly cardiovascular disease.

References

1. Appel LJ, Moore TJ, Obarzanek E, Vollmer WM, Svetkey LP, Sacks FM, Bray GA, Vogt TM, Cutler JA, Windhauser MM, Lin PH, Karanja N. A clinical trial of the effects of dietary patterns on blood pressure. DASH collaborative research group. *N Engl J Med*. 1997;336:1117–1124.

2. Obarzanek E, Proschan MA, Vollmer WM, Moore TJ, Sacks FM, Appel LJ, Svetkey LP, Most-Windhauser MM, Cutler JA. Individual blood pressure responses to changes in salt intake: results from the DASH-sodium trial. *Hypertension*. 2003;42: 459–467.

3. Fito M, Guxens M, Corella D, Sáez G, Estruch R, de la Torre R, Francés F, Cabezas C, López-Sabater Mdel C, Marrugat J, García-Arellano A, Arós F, Ruiz-Gutierrez V, Ros E, Salas-Salvadó J, Fiol M, Solá R, Covas MI; for the PREDIMED Study Investigators. Effect of a traditional Mediterranean diet on lipoprotein oxidation: a randomized controlled trial. *Arch Intern Med*. 2007;167:1195–1203.

4. Dietary Guidelines Advisory Committee. The Report of the Dietary Guidelines advisory committee on Dietary Guidelines for Americans, 2005. http://www.health. gov/DietaryGuidelines/dga2005/report. Accessed November 13, 2008.

5. Azadbakht L, Mirmiran P, Esmaillzadeh A, Azizi F. Better dietary adherence and weight maintenance achieved by a long-term moderate-fat diet. *Br J Nutr*. 2007;97: 399–404.

6. Karanja NM, Obarzanek E, Lin PH, McCullough ML, Phillips KM, Swain JF, Champagne CM, Hoben KP. Descriptive characteristics of the dietary patterns used in the Dietary Approaches to Stop Hypertension trial. DASH collaborative research group. *J Am Diet Assoc*. 1999;99(Suppl 8):S19–S27.

7. Hu FB, Willett WC. Optimal diets for prevention of coronary heart disease. *JAMA*. 2002;288:2569–2578.

8. Carey VJ, Bishop L, Charleston J, Conlin P, Erlinger T, Laranjo N, McCarron P, Miller E, Rosner B, Swain J, Sacks FM, Appel LJ. Rationale and design of the Optimal Macro-nutrient Intake Heart trial to prevent heart disease (OMNI-Heart). *Clin Trials*. 2005;2:529–537.

9. Appel LJ, Sacks FM, Carey VJ, Obarzanek E, Swain JF, Miller ER 3rd, Conlin PR, Erlinger TP, Rosner BA, Laranjo NM, Charleston J, McCarron P, Bishop LM; OmniHeart Collaborative Research Group. Effects of protein, monounsaturated fat, and carbohydrate intake on blood pressure and serum lipids: results of the OmniHeart randomized trial. *JAMA*. 2005;294:2455–2464.

10. Willett WC, Sacks F, Trichopoulou A, Drescher G, Ferro-Luzzi A, Helsing E, Trichopoulos D. Mediterranean diet pyramid: a cultural model for healthy eating. *Am J Clin Nutr*. 1995;61(Suppl 6):1402S–1406S.

11. Keys A. *Seven Countries: A Multivariate Analysis of Death and Coronary Heart Disease*. Cambridge, MA: Harvard University Press; 1980.

12. Fung TT, McCullough ML, Newby PK, Manson JE, Meigs JB, Rifai N, Willett WC, Hu FB. Diet-quality scores and plasma concentrations of markers of inflammation and endothelial dysfunction. *Am J Clin Nutr*. 2005;82:163–173.

13. Trichopoulou A, Costacou T, Bamia C, Trichopoulos D. Adherence to a Mediterranean diet and survival in a Greek population. *N Engl J Med*. 2003;348:2599–2608.

14. Mitrou PN, Kipnis V, Thiebaut AC, Reedy J, Subar AF, Wirfält E, Flood A, Mouw T, Hollenbeck AR, Leitzmann MF, Schatzkin A. Mediterranean dietary pattern and prediction of all-cause mortality in a US population: results from the NIH-AARP diet and health study. *Arch Intern Med.* 2007;167:2461–2468.

15. Trichopoulou A, Bamia C, Trichopoulos D. Mediterranean diet and survival among patients with coronary heart disease in Greece. *Arch Intern Med.* 2005;165:929–935.

16. Trichopoulou A, Orfanos P, Norat T, Bueno-de-Mesquita B, Ocké MC, Peeters PH, van der Schouw YT, Boeing H, Hoffmann K, Boffetta P, Nagel G, Masala G, Krogh V, Panico S, Tumino R, Vineis P, Bamia C, Naska A, Benetou V, Ferrari P, Slimani N, Pera G, Martinez-Garcia C, Navarro C, Rodriguez-Barranco M, Dorronsoro M, Spencer EA, Key TJ, Bingham S, Khaw KT, Kesse E, Clavel-Chapelon F, Boutron-Ruault MC, Berglund G, Wirfalt E, Hallmans G, Johansson I, Tjonneland A, Olsen A, Overvad K, Hundborg HH, Riboli E, Trichopoulos D. Modified Mediterranean diet and survival: EPIC-elderly prospective cohort study. *BMJ.* 2005;330:991.

17. Serra-Majem L, Roman B, Estruch R. Scientific evidence of interventions using the Mediterranean diet: a systematic review. *Nutr Rev.* 2006;64:S27–S47.

18. McManus K, Antinoro L, Sacks F. A randomized controlled trial of a moderate-fat, low-energy diet compared with a low fat, low-energy diet for weight loss in over-weight adults. *Int J Obes Relat Metab Disord.* 2001;25:1503–1511.

PART B: PRACTICAL APPLICATIONS

JUDITH WYLIE-ROSETT, EDD, RD, NICHOLA J. DAVIS, MD, MS, AND

CARMEN R. ISASI, MD, PHD

Many more clients need to lose weight than seek do it, but many overweight clients with associated risks such as cardiovascular disease, diabetes, and hypertension may seek out a dietetics professional for help in choosing more healthful foods to improve their medical condition. One question is whether the diet should address the cardiovascular disease with the possible added benefit of weight loss, or whether the diet should address weight loss first with the secondary expectation that weight loss will improve the cardiovascular disease. This chapter explores two diets that address cardiovascular disease and hypertension, but show signs of being successful weight-loss tools as well. Both the Mediterranean diet and the Dietary Approaches to Stop Hypertension (DASH) emphasize a plant-based approach with liberal servings of vegetables and fruits. However, the history of these approaches differs considerably.

Interest in the Mediterranean dietary pattern was based on observational data and subsequent clinical trials that demonstrated how cardiovascular morbidity and mortality could be reduced with a comprehensive dietary approach based on common foods in the Mediterranean (1). The term *Mediterranean diet* can describe the widely varying dietary patterns from at least 16 countries that border the Mediterranean Sea (2,3). Dietary traditions vary considerably between and within these countries. Differences in culture, ethnic background, religion, economy, and agricultural production result in considerable dietary variability. However, common elements include high consumption of fruits and vegetables; liberal use of legumes, nuts, and seeds; frequent intake of fish; use of olive oil in food preparation; and inclusion of grains in main dishes. Red wine is often associated with the Mediterranean diet, but consumption varies considerably based on religion and other factors.

Various scoring systems have been developed to evaluate dietary intake in relation to the Mediterranean dietary pattern (4,5) using these common elements. Some scores are based on being more or less than the average intake for the population (eg, based on American averages from the National Health and Nutrition Examination Survey). Scoring can also be based on a ratio of nutrients or food groups (eg, saturated to unsaturated fat ratio, or red meat to chicken/fish ratio). Mediterranean dietary scores based on being more or less than the average for a given population are highly correlated ($r = 0.75$) with the scores on the Alternative Healthy Eating Index (AHEI).

In contrast, the DASH clinical trial tested the effects of various dietary components, primarily increased fruit and vegetable and low-fat dairy intake, which were associated with reducing blood pressure (6). Clinical evidence from the DASH trial demonstrated significant reduction in blood pressure after 30 days of following the DASH dietary pattern. This reduction in blood pressure was particularly significant among subgroups of clients with stage 1 hypertension and African Americans. Although the initial DASH study was designed to test the efficacy of the dietary pattern while being weight stable, the subsequent PREMIER study demonstrated that the pattern had an additive effect in reducing blood pressure when combined with a weight-loss intervention (7,8). In clinical practice, this dietary strategy can be used to achieve modest blood pressure reduction in clients with borderline or stage 1 hypertension. Of particular interest, African Americans reduced blood pressure when following the DASH diet, and this approach is now being targeted to the dietary preferences of different cultural groups (eg, soul DASH cooking classes) (8). The DASH diet is so well-accepted that the National Institutes of Health have several publications regarding the clinical applications of the DASH diet, which includes menus and recipes to facilitate client adherence.

Table 4.1 (3) provides an overview of the food group recommendations from the DASH dietary pattern, the Mediterranean dietary pattern, and the 2005 MyPyramid (9) guidelines. These dietary patterns have considerable overlap, especially with regard to the emphasis on higher vegetable and fruit intake. Each dietary pattern has been evaluated with respect to health outcomes. Methods for evaluating the validity or predictive value of a dietary pattern is based on its relationship to current or future health parameters, such as life expectancy or the incidence of obesity, cardiovascular diseases, and some types of cancers (10,11). Dietary patterns and dietary indexes are also used to evaluate food consumption trends and to evaluate how well individuals and groups are achieving public health nutrition recommendations.

CASE STUDY 1

MG is a 47-year-old overweight man with hypertension and hyperlipidemia. He currently takes a diuretic and a beta blocker for his hypertension and a statin to reduce his

TABLE 4.1

DASH, Mediterranean, and MyPyramid Dietary Patterns: Recommendations by Food Groups

Food Group	DASH Recommendations	Mediterranean Diet Range for Average Daily Intake	MyPyramid Daily Recommendations
Vegetables	4–5 servings/d	6–9 oz	3–5 servings (1½–2½ cups)
Fruits	4-5 servings/d	5 oz–1 lb	2–4 servings (2 cups)
Nuts, seeds, and legumes	3–5 servings/wk	0.3–1 oz	
			Combined group
Red meat, poultry, and fish	Limit to ≤ 2 servings/d (6 oz total cooked weight)	1–7.5 oz meat	5–6 oz
Grains/fiber	6-8 servings/d (½ to⅓ as whole grains)	6–8.5 oz bread, 1–4 oz cereal	6–9 servings
Dairy	2–3 servings/d (low fat)	0.5–1 oz cheese 2.5–8 oz milk	2–3 servings
Fats and oils	2–3 tsp/d	Not available	Discretionary calories (for
Alcohol	Not specified	0.5–2 oz alcohol	solid fat, sugars, and alcohol):
Sweets/sugars	≤ 2 Tbsp sugars for 2,000 kcal/d plan (0 Tbsp for 1,600 kcal/d plan)	1–1.5 Tbsp	allotment is 130 kcal for 1,600 kcal/d level and 265 kcal for 2,000 kcal/d level

Source: Adapted by permission from Macmillan Publishers Ltd: *European Journal of Clinical Nutrition.* Karamanos B, Thanopoulou A, Angelico F, Assaad-Khalil S, Barbato A, Del Ben M, Dimitrijevic-Sreckovic V, Djordjevic P, Gallotti C, Katsilambros N, Migdalis I, Mrabet M, Petkova M, Roussi D, Tenconi MT. Nutritional habits in the Mediterranean Basin. The macronutrient composition of diet and its relation with the traditional Mediterranean diet. Multi-centre study of the Mediterranean Group for the Study of Diabetes (MGSD). *Eur J Clin Nutr.* 2002;56:983–991.

cholesterol. MG has a family history of coronary artery disease. His father had a heart attack at age 70, and his brother, who is 55, recently had a heart attack. Both were overweight with "large bellies." MG seeks advice to find out if losing weight and changing his diet can decrease his risk of having a heart attack. MG began to do research on his own and was overwhelmed by the number of different diets on the Internet. He started on his own to exercise, and he and his wife have been using more olive oil in their cooking. He has also tried to eat more fruits and vegetables, but he is frustrated because he has not lost any weight. See Box 4.1 for results of his laboratory tests and physical assessment. MG requests a registered dietitian (RD) referral to assist him in losing weight and prescribing a diet that may decrease his chances of having a heart attack.

MG's case demonstrates a client who is at risk for developing coronary artery disease. He has several risk factors: hypertension, hyperlipidemia, and a family history. Although his blood pressure and cholesterol seem to be moderately well controlled, MG may also have metabolic syndrome. He has impaired fasting glucose (> 110 mg/dL), borderline high triglycerides (150–200 mg/dL), low high-density lipoprotein (HDL) cholesterol, and hypertension. His waist measurement is not available, but metabolic syndrome is associated with a waist of more than 40 inches in men. In some cases, metabolic syndrome is associated with a waist measurement between 37 and 39 inches. Therefore, the goal of treating MG would be to reduce both his weight and his risk of coronary artery disease. The Mediterranean diet would be an ideal dietary plan for MG for two reasons: he has shown an interest in the kinds of foods that are central to this diet,

---

Box 4.1
Pertinent Laboratory and Physical Findings for Case Study 1

- Blood pressure: 126/82 mmHg
- Fasting blood glucose: 111 mg/dL
- Total cholesterol: 203 mg/dL
- HDL cholesterol: 43 mg/dL
- Triglycerides: 186 mg/dL
- LDL cholesterol: 134 mg/dL
- Weight: 187 pounds
- Height: 5 feet, 10 inches
- BMI: 26.8

---

and the diet itself has been demonstrated to reduce the rate of heart attacks in patients who are at high risk.

Counseling can be structured to address how his current intake relates to the Mediterranean dietary pattern. Understanding his frustration about not losing weight despite the changes he has already made, the RD can show him some of his errors, the biggest one being the liberal use of olive oil. Many patients seem to think that because olive oil has the connotation of being more healthful for the heart, it must also have fewer calories. MG is no different, and the RD begins by explaining the actual calorie content of all fats.

Both MG and the RD agree that the goal is to reduce calorie intake while considering the potential health benefits of a Mediterranean dietary pattern. The RD explains that in addition to fruit, vegetable, and olive oil intake, the Mediterranean diet also includes breads, pastas, fish, and nuts/seeds, many of which can add excess calories if portions are not controlled. Therefore, this dietary plan will need to be created carefully and MG must clearly understand the parameters. To make this plan workable and measurable, MG decides to limit his bread intake to one sandwich with two slices of whole-grain bread per day, measure his olive oil, and increase but vary his consumption of fruits and vegetables and fish. He agrees to keep food records and return to the RD the following week, and he understands that (*a*) this is probably the correct diet for him; (*b*) some modifications may have to be made; (*c*) the diet itself will help reduce his risk of coronary artery disease even if he does not lose weight; and (*d*) finally, he should not expect to lose weight quickly, although MG and the RD will work together to reach the best result possible.

CASE STUDY 2

LN is a 42-year-old African-American woman who was recently diagnosed with diabetes and hypertension. She was prescribed metformin, told to start monitoring her blood glucose before and after one meal each day, and advised to lose weight. LN is 5 feet, 3 inches in height and weighs 165 pounds (BMI 29.2). Her cousin, who also has

TABLE 4.2

My Pyramid 1,800-Calorie Meal Plan

Food Group	Amount
Grains[a]	6 ounces
Vegetables[b]	2.5 cups
Fruits	1.5 cups
Milk	3 cups
Meats and beans	5 ounces
Oils and discretionary calories	Aim for 5 tsp oils per day; limit your extras (extra fat and sugars) to 195 calories.

[a]Make Half Your Grains Whole: Aim for at least 3 ounces of whole grains a day.
[b]Vary Your Veggies: As weekly goals, aim for 3 cups dark-green vegetables, 2 cups orange vegetables, 3 cups dry beans and peas, 3 cups starchy vegetables, and 6½ cups other vegetables.
Adapted from MyPyramid Web site. http://www.mypyramid.gov. Accessed November 13, 2008.

diabetes, has teamed up with her to help. Originally LN focused on beginning to lose weight by using the MyPyramid Web site (http://www.mypyramid.gov) (9). LN received the 1,800-calorie meal plan listed in Table 4.2 after she entered her height and weight and indicated she was active for less than 30 minutes a day. On a follow-up physician visit 1 month later, LN had lost 2 pounds but her blood pressure remained high (150/85 mmHg) and her blood glucose remained moderately elevated 2 hours after her meal (150 mg/dL). LN and the physician both agreed that, although she had tried, this diet was not working.

LN remembered that her church had a "healthy soul" cooking program based on the DASH diet, and she decided to join it. There she learned to fine-tune some of the information she learned from MyPyramid, plus she could use foods that she was most comfortable with culturally.

At her next physician visit, LN's blood pressure is improved (135/82 mmHg) but her blood glucose diary still shows an elevation after her lunch meal, the meal she monitors. Before lunch her blood glucose is controlled, running between 90 and 110 mg/dL but 2 hours after lunch, her blood glucose ranges from 145 to 160 mg/dL. LN is very frustrated. She has started two different diets faithfully. Her lunch is simple: a sandwich using two slices of whole-wheat bread, a bowl of soup, and coffee with low-fat (2%) milk. Her usual breakfast is oatmeal with milk, juice, and coffee with low-fat milk. After starting the DASH diet, she noticed that her blood glucose had increased slightly after her meal. She was doing everything she was told, including eating more fruits and vegetables and drinking more fruit juices.

LN is an African-American woman, with stage 1 hypertension. The DASH diet would be an optimal diet for her to control her blood pressure *if* she did not have diabetes. The hallmark of the DASH diet is 9 to 11 servings of fruits and vegetables daily, which includes fruit juices. This can result in a substantial glycemic load in someone with diabetes, and can affect glycemic control. However, LN is comfortable with the idea of the DASH diet, she has a lot of support from her church, and this diet will help control her hypertension. Therefore, in counseling someone with diabetes who wants to follow the DASH diet, the RD should encourage her to choose lower carbohydrate fresh fruits rather than fruit juices. In addition, consumption of lower carbohydrate vegetables should be stressed.

It is also important to note that the DASH diet reduced blood pressure independent of weight loss. LN is overweight with diabetes and hypertension, and weight loss can have an additive effect on her blood pressure and help to reduce her blood glucose as well. Therefore, the dietary plan will need to also focus on achieving a negative energy balance.

It is helpful to consider how and why the Diabetes Food Pyramid (12) differs from MyPyramid and the DASH diet. The Diabetes Food Pyramid classifies starchy vegetables with other starches based on the carbohydrate content whereas MyPyramid (9) and the DASH diet group starchy and nonstarchy vegetables together. Consumption of nonstarchy vegetables is encouraged in both systems, but a nonpractitioner may not understand the nuances. The Diabetes Food Pyramid also may define portions differently to emphasize a standard amount of carbohydrate (15 g for the fruit and starch exchange groups). For LN, controlling postprandial blood glucose will probably be easier if she carefully monitors her carbohydrate intake. Monitoring her blood glucose before and after meals will help LN determine the glycemic effects of specific vegetables. A normal 2-hour postprandial blood glucose is ≤ 140 mg/dL, and it is important to evaluate whether the amount or type of carbohydrate intake is contributing to LN's elevated 2-hour blood glucose level (13).

LN is willing to monitor her blood glucose more often, but she wants to stay with her cousin in the church DASH diet program. To encourage weight loss, LN will also need to measure her intake of nuts and change from 2% milk to 1% or nonfat. After 2 months and two more meetings with the RD, LN has lost 5 pounds and her blood pressure and blood glucose are well controlled.

References

1. de Lorgeril M, Salen P, Martin JL, Monjaud I, Delaye J, Mamelle N. Mediterranean diet, traditional risk factors, and the rate of cardiovascular complications after myocardial infarction: final report of the Lyon Diet Heart Study. *Circulation*. 1999;99: 779–785.

2. Noah A, Truswell AS. There are many Mediterranean diets. *Asia Pac J Clin Nutr*. 2001;10:2–9.

3. Karamanos B, Thanopoulou A, Angelico F, Assaad-Khalil S, Barbato A, Del Ben M, Dimitrijevic-Sreckovic V, Djordjevic P, Gallotti C, Katsilambros N, Migdalis I, Mrabet M, Petkova M, Roussi D, Tenconi MT. Nutritional habits in the Mediterranean Basin. The macronutrient composition of diet and its relation with the traditional Mediterranean diet. Multi-centre study of the Mediterranean Group for the Study of Diabetes (MGSD). *Eur J Clin Nutr*. 2002;56:983–991.

4. Bach A, Serra-Majem L, Carrasco JL, Roman B, Ngo J, Bertomeu I, Obrador B. The use of indexes evaluating the adherence to the Mediterranean diet in epidemiological studies: a review. *Public Health Nutr*. 2006;9:132–146.

5. Trichopoulou A, Costacou T, Bamia C, Trichopoulos D. Adherence to a Mediterranean diet and survival in a Greek population. *N Engl J Med*. 2003;348:2599–2608.

6. Appel LJ, Moore TJ, Obarzanek E, Vollmer WM, Svetkey LP, Sacks FM, Bray GA, Vogt TM, Cutler JA, Windhauser MM, Lin PH, Karanja N. A clinical trial of the

effects of dietary patterns on blood pressure. DASH Collaborative Research Group. *N Engl J Med*. 1997;336:1117–1124.

7. Obarzanek E, Vollmer WM, Lin PH, Cooper LS, Young DR, Ard JD, Stevens VJ, Simons-Morton DG, Svetkey LP, Harsha DW, Elmer PJ, Appel LJ. Effects of individual components of multiple behavior changes: the PREMIER trial. *Am J Health Behav*. 2007;31:545–60.

8. Rankins J, Wortham J, Brown LL. Modifying soul food for the Dietary Approaches to Stop Hypertension diet (DASH) plan: implications for metabolic syndrome (DASH of Soul). *Ethn Dis*. 2007;17(3 Suppl 4):S4-7–12.

9. MyPyramid Web site. http://www.mypyramid.gov. Accessed November 12, 2008.

10. McCullough ML, Feskanich D, Stampfer MJ, Giovannucci EL, Rimm EB, Hu FB, Spiegelman D, Hunter DJ, Colditz GA, Willett WC. Diet quality and major chronic disease risk in men and women: moving toward improved dietary guidance. *Am J Clin Nutr*. 2002;76:1261–1271.

11. Fung TT, McCullough ML, Newby PK, Manson JE, Meigs JB, Rifai N, Willett WC, Hu FB. Diet-quality scores and plasma concentrations of markers of inflammation and endothelial dysfunction. *Am J Clin Nutr*. 2005;82:163–173.

12. Diabetes Food Pyramid. http://www.diabetes.org/nutrition-and-recipes/nutrition/foodpyramid.jsp. Accessed March 12, 2009.

13. Wylie-Rosett J, Albright AA, Apovian C, Clark NG, Delahanty L, Franz MJ, Hoogwerf B, Kulkarni K, Lichtenstein AH, Mayer-Davis E, Mooradian AD, Wheeler M. 2006–2007 American Diabetes Association nutrition recommendations: issues for practice translation. *J Am Diet Assoc*. 2007;107:1296–1304.

CHAPTER 5

DIET—LOW CARBOHYDRATE

PART A: OVERVIEW

FRANK B. HU, MD, PHD

The prevalence of obesity has increased dramatically in the United States despite a decreasing percentage of energy intake from fat. This has led to the hypothesis that compensatory increases in carbohydrate consumption as a result of fat reduction may be fueling the obesity epidemic (1). In recent years, low-carbohydrate diets, which have long been ignored or even dismissed by the nutrition community, have gained in popularity. Such diets typically recommend less than 10% to 30% of daily energy from carbohydrate (1). Dietary plans such as the Atkins diet minimize total carbohydrate consumption with no restriction on energy intake, whereas others such as Sugar Busters and Zone diets reduce carbohydrate intake and alter macronutrient composition. South Beach diet, a modified version of a low-carbohydrate diet, combines various strategies across different phases to modulate both quality and quantity of carbohydrates (2).

CLINICAL TRIAL EVIDENCE

Because of the increasing popularity of low-carbohydrate diets, several randomized controlled trials have been done to evaluate the efficacy of carbohydrate-restricted diets compared with fat-restricted diets on weight loss. A meta-analysis compared the effects on weight loss of ad libitum low-carbohydrate diets (allowing a maximum intake of 60 g of carbohydrates per day or ≤ 10% energy) vs low-fat (≤ 30% energy) energy-restricted diets (3). In total, five randomized controlled trials (N = 447) were summarized. These studies lasted 6 to 12 months. The meta-analysis found that after 6 months, participants randomly assigned to a low-carbohydrate diet had lost more weight than those randomly assigned to a low-fat diet (weighted mean difference 3.3 kg; 95% confidence interval [CI], –5.3 kg to –1.4 kg). However, after 12 months, this difference largely dissipated (weighted mean difference –1.0 kg; 95% CI, –3.5 kg to 1.5 kg). This meta-analysis also compared the effect of the two dietary patterns on cardiovascular disease risk factors and found that after 6 months, triglyceride and high-density lipoprotein (HDL) cholesterol level changes were more favorable in the low-carbohydrate diet group, but total cholesterol and low-density lipoprotein (LDL) cholesterol level changes were more favorable in the low-fat group. Overall, existing trials of low-carbohydrate/high-fat diets have shown greater short-term weight loss (within 6 months) than low-fat diets; however, most studies have been small and underpowered. Also, compliance to dietary interventions was poor and dropout rates were generally high.

Several recent trials on the effects of low carbohydrate diets vs other popular diets in weight control were much larger and lasted 1 to 2 years. Gardner et al (4) compared the effects of four popular diets—Atkins, Zone, Ornish (a very-low-fat diet), and LEARN (a moderately-low-fat diet)—on weight loss in a randomized trial of 311 free-living, over-weight/obese premenopausal women. Mean 12-month weight loss was 4.7 kg for the Atkins group, 1.6 kg for the Zone group, 2.6 kg for the LEARN group, and 2.2 kg for the Ornish group. At 12 months, the Atkins group had greater reductions in triglycerides, with only a small and nonsignificant increase in LDL cholesterol. Unlike other low-carbohydrate dietary intervention trials, this study had a relatively low dropout rate at 1 year (approximately 20%), although the degree of dietary adherence in all the groups was generally low.

In a 2-year trial, Shai et al (5) randomly assigned 322 moderately obese participants to one of three diets: low-fat, restricted-calorie; Mediterranean, restricted-calorie; or low-carbohydrate, nonrestricted-calorie. The mean weight loss was greatest for the low-carbohydrate group (4.7 kg), followed by the Mediterranean-diet group (4.4 kg) and the low-fat group (2.9 kg). The relative reduction in the ratio of total cholesterol to HDL cholesterol was greater in the low-carbohydrate group than the low-fat group (20% vs 12%; $P = .01$), whereas the greatest improvement in glycemic control was observed in the Mediterranean diet group. In this study, adherence to a study diet was very high (95.4% at 1 year and 84.6% at 2 years).

In a recent study, Sacks et al (6) randomly assigned 811 overweight adults to one of four hypocaloric diets with varying macronutrient compositions—the targeted percent-ages of energy from fat, protein, and carbohydrates, respectively, in the four diets were (a) 20%, 15%, and 65%; (b) 20%, 25%, and 55%; (c) 40%, 15%, and 45%; and (d) 40%, 25%, and 35%. At the end of 2-year intervention (primarily through dietary counseling), weight loss was similar across the four different diets (ranging from 2.9 to 3.6 kg). The amount of weight loss was primarily determined by the degree of adherence to the diets, regardless of macronutrient composition. These results are consistent with a 1-year study by Dansinger and colleagues (7), who found that diet compliance was a more im-portant factor in achieving greater weight loss than the type of popular diet used (Atkins, Ornish, Weight Watchers, and Zone diets).

Taken together, short-term studies (< 6 months) have in general demonstrated greater benefits of low carbohydrate diets on weight loss than low-fat diets. However, data from longer-term studies (1 to 2 years) are conflicting. This discrepancy may result from different population characteristics, different intervention methods (dietary coun-seling vs providing foods to the participants), and varying degree of adherence to the diets. Overall, current evidence suggests that more severe carbohydrate restriction may be moderately effective for weight loss.

POTENTIAL MECHANISMS

Malik and Hu (1) recently reviewed potential mechanisms for the greater efficacy of low-carbohydrate diets in weight loss compared with a conventional low-fat diet. Be-cause all low-carbohydrate diets are high in protein, much research has centered on pro-tein consumption and energy expenditure (eg, thermic effect of food, defined as the in-crease in energy expenditure above baseline after consumption of food, resting energy expenditure, and physical activity). Diets high in protein have been reported to induce a greater thermic effect than other diets because use of protein is energetically more costly. A systematic review of short-term studies found that, compared with low-fat diets, diets low in carbohydrates produced approximately 2.5 kg more weight loss after 12 weeks, with a 233 kcal/d greater energy deficit in the low-carbohydrate diets than low-fat diets (8). Neither macronutrient-specific differences in the availability of dietary energy nor changes in energy expenditure were able to explain the differences in weight loss. The most likely reason for the differential weight loss is a difference in energy intake between groups that was not apparent from diet records.

There is substantial evidence from short-term studies that higher protein diets increase satiety when compared with lower protein diets. This may enhance a participant's ability to "stick with" a hypocaloric diet over the long term. There is also some evidence that higher protein diets decrease subsequent energy intake at the next meal compared with lower protein diets, although the data are not consistent (8).

Ketogenesis has been suggested as an important component of the overall effects of a low-carbohydrate diet on weight loss. When dietary carbohydrate is restricted, glycogen stores are generally depleted within 48 hours, at which point fat oxidation increases (9). Fatty acids released into the blood can be partially oxidized to form acetoacetate, [beta]-hydroxybutyric acid, and acetone. These ketone bodies can be used by the brain and mitochondria-containing tissue as fuel. Ketosis is estimated to occur when carbohydrate intake is reduced to 50 g/d (9). It has been suggested that ketosis promotes weight loss by the excretion of energy through ketone bodies in urine, breath, and stool, although energy loss via urine cannot account for more than a few calories per day. Circulating ketone bodies might also be appetite-suppressing, mimicking the anorexia of starvation. However, none of weight-loss trials reviewed earlier have linked the amount of ketone bodies in urine and the degree of weight loss.

It has been suggested that early weight loss during carbohydrate restriction is primarily due to decrease in body water. Because each gram of glycogen is mobilized with approximately 2 g water, it is estimated that mobilization of total glycogen stores results in a weight loss of approximately 1 kg (10). Yang and Van Itallie (11) reported that loss of liver and muscle glycogen in the first 10 days of a low-carbohydrate diet resulted in a water loss of 1.9 kg, which could explain the early weight loss often seen in low-carbohydrate diets. In addition to water loss and the satiating effects of protein, limited food choice could also explain the spontaneous energy restriction seen in ad libitum low-carbohydrate diets. However, many foods are not permitted in low-carbohydrate diets, which might lead to decreased diet adherence in the long run. Two longer-term trials (5,7) have demonstrated that the degree of dietary adherence was a more important factor in achieving greater weight loss and reducing cardiovascular disease risk factors than macronutrient composition.

LONG-TERM EFFECTS ON CARDIOVASCULAR DISEASE

Current literature indicates that low-carbohydrate ad libitum dietary patterns are more effective in inducing weight loss in the short term (ie, 6 months), but little is known about their long-term influences on cardiovascular risk. Most carbohydrate-restricted diets tend to encourage increased consumption of animal products and therefore often contain high amounts of saturated fat and cholesterol. This may cause unfavorable changes in serum lipid concentrations and increase the risk of coronary heart disease (CHD). Some professional organizations, such as American Heart Association, have cautioned against the use of low-carbohydrate diets. Theoretically, chronic carbohydrate restriction might lead to nutritional inadequacy, osteoporosis, and kidney dysfunction, and could alter an individual's cancer risk and immune function through the restriction on fruit, vegetable, and fiber intake. On the other hand, low-carbohydrate/high-fat diets can be beneficial for cardiovascular disease risk provided that they are high in unsaturated fatty acids and limit saturated and *trans* fat.

Recently, my colleagues and I examined the relationship between low-carbohydrate diets and risk of CHD among 82,802 women in the Nurses' Health Study (12). During 20 years of follow-up, we documented 1,994 new cases of CHD. After multivariate adjustment, the relative risk of CHD comparing highest and lowest deciles of the low-carbohydrate-diet score (< 30% energy from carbohydrates) was 0.94 (95% CI, 0.76 to 1.18; *P* for trend = .19). The relative risk of CHD on the basis of a low-carbohydrate score characterized by a low intake of carbohydrates but high intakes of vegetable protein and vegetable fat was 0.70 (95% CI, 0.56 to 0.88; *P* for trend = .002). These findings suggest that diets lower in carbohydrates and higher in protein and fat are not associated with long-term risk of CHD in women. When vegetable sources of fat and protein are chosen, these diets may moderately reduce the risk of CHD.

In the Nurses' Health Study, most of the vegetable fat came from vegetable oil (soybean, corn, and canola oils), olive oil, mayonnaise, peanut butter, and nuts. Most of the vegetable protein came from whole-grain foods (dark bread and cold cereals), legumes (beans and peas), peanut butter, and nuts. Benefits of the plant-based low-carbohydrate diet on CHD are likely to stem from vegetable fat and protein as well as the reduced glycemic load (GL) in the dietary pattern. In several epidemiologic studies, a higher GL, a marker of refined carbohydrates in the diet, has been associated with long-term risk of type 2 diabetes and CHD (13). Thus, reducing dietary GL is considered a positive attribute of any low-carbohydrate diet. Refer to Chapter 3 for more information on GL.

CONCLUSION

Low-carbohydrate diets remain popular, but little is known about their long-term efficacy, safety, and ability to improve cardiovascular outcomes. Low-carbohydrate diets have promoted greater weight loss than low-fat diets in short-term clinical trials lasting no more than 1 year. However, the amount of weight loss is generally modest, and more severe restriction in carbohydrates may be required to achieve longer-term benefit. For any weight-loss diet, adherence to a dietary regimen may be more important than altering macronutrient compositions.

The long-term effects of low-carbohydrate diets on cardiovascular disease remain controversial. Recent data from the Nurses' Health Study suggest that diets lower in carbohydrates and higher in protein and fat were not associated with increased risk of CHD in women. In contrast, when vegetable sources of fat and protein were chosen, these diets were related to a reduced risk of CHD. These data support a potential benefit of a low-carbohydrate diet with an emphasis on plant sources of fat and protein in reducing

CHD risk. Randomized controlled trials are needed to test whether plant-based low-carbohydrate diets have the same or greater efficacy in achieving weight loss as compared with a conventional low-carbohydrate diet that is high in animal products.

References

1. Malik VS, Hu FB. Popular weight-loss diets: from evidence to practice. *Nat Clin Pract Cardiovasc Med*. 2007;4:34–41.

2. Agatston A. *The South Beach Diet: The Delicious, Doctor-Designed, Foolproof Plan for Fast and Healthy Weight Loss*. New York, NY: Macmillan; 2005.

3. Nordmann AJ, Nordmann A, Briel M, Keller U, Yancy WS Jr, Brehm BJ, Bucher HC. Effects of low-carbohydrate vs low-fat diets on weight loss and cardiovascular risk factors: a meta-analysis of randomized controlled trials. *Arch Intern Med*. 2006;166:285–293.

4. Gardner CD, Kiazand A, Alhassan S, Kim S, Stafford RS, Balise RR, Kraemer HC, King AC. Comparison of the Atkins, Zone, Ornish, and LEARN diets for change in weight and related risk factors among overweight premenopausal women: the A TO Z Weight Loss Study: a randomized trial. *JAMA*. 2007;297:969–977.

5. Shai I, Schwarzfuchs D, Henkin Y, Shahar DR, Witkow S, Greenberg I, Golan R, Fraser D, Bolotin A, Vardi H, Tangi-Rozental O, Zuk-Ramot R, Sarusi B, Brickner D, Schwartz Z, Sheiner E, Marko R, Katorza E, Thiery J, Fiedler GM, Blüher M, Stumvoll M, Stampfer MJ; Dietary Intervention Randomized Controlled Trial (DIRECT) Group. Weight loss with a low-carbohydrate, Mediterranean, or low-fat diet. *N Engl J Med*. 2008;359:229–241.

6. Sacks FM, Bray GA, Carey VJ, Smith SR, Ryan DH, Anton SD, McManus K, Champagne CM, Bishop LM, Laranjo N, Leboff MS, Rood JC, de Jonge L, Greenway FL, Loria CM, Obarzanek E, Williamson DA. Comparison of weight-loss diets with different compositions of fat, protein, and carbohydrates. *N Engl J Med*. 2009; 360:859–873.

7. Dansinger ML, Gleason JA, Griffith JL, Selker HP, Schaefer EJ. Comparison of the Atkins, Ornish, Weight Watchers, and Zone diets for weight loss and heart disease risk reduction: a randomized trial. *JAMA*. 2005;293:43–53.

8. Halton TL, Hu FB. The effects of high protein diets on thermogenesis, satiety and weight loss: a critical review. *J Am Coll Nutr*. 2004;23:373–385.

9. Adam-Perrot A, Clifton P, Brouns F. Low-carbohydrate diets: nutritional and physiological aspects. *Obes Rev*. 2006;7:49–58.

10. Denke MA. Metabolic effects of high-protein, low-carbohydrate diets. *Am J Cardiol*. 2001;88:59–61.

11. Yang MU, Van Itallie TB. Composition of weight lost during short-term weight reduction. Metabolic responses of obese subjects to starvation and low-calorie ketogenic and nonketogenic diets. *J Clin Invest*. 1976;58:722–730.

12. Halton TL, Willett WC, Liu S, Manson JE, Albert CM, Rexrode K, Hu FB. Low-carbohydrate-diet score and the risk of coronary heart disease in women. *N Engl J Med*. 2006;355:1991–2002.

13. Hu FB, Willett WC. Optimal diets for prevention of coronary heart disease. *JAMA*. 2002;288:2569–2578.

PART B: PRACTICAL APPLICATIONS

ANGELA MAKRIS, PHD, RD

INTRODUCTION

Among the most popular dietary alternatives for weight loss are low-carbohydrate, high-protein, high-fat diets. This dietary prescription can be achieved in a variety of ways, as evidenced by the numerous low-carbohydrate books on the market, each with a unique interpretation of optimal low-carbohydrate eating (eg, Atkins' *New Diet Revolution,* Protein Power, and the first phase of the South Beach diet). Although there is no universal definition for low-carbohydrate diets, they generally comprise fewer than 50 g carbohydrate per day or less than 10% of energy from carbohydrate (1) and consist of the following macronutrient distribution of energy intake: less than 10% carbohydrate, 25% to 35% protein, and 55% to 65% fat. Individuals are encouraged to consume controlled amounts of nutrient-dense carbohydrate-containing foods (ie, vegetables, fruits, and whole-grain products) and eliminate intake of carbohydrate-containing foods high in refined carbohydrate (ie, white bread, white rice, pasta, desserts, and chips). Although consumption of foods that do not contain carbohydrate (ie, meats, poultry, fish, and oils) is not restricted, the emphasis is on moderation, and some low-carbohydrate diets stress low-saturated fat intake.

Because of the high-fat and high-cholesterol nature of diets such as the Atkins diet that do not specify types of fat, there has been an understandable concern regarding potential adverse effects on cardiovascular disease risk; however, low-carbohydrate diets seem to be less harmful than anticipated in terms of traditional measures of cardiovascular disease risk, may be more efficacious than conventional approaches for short-term (< 6 months) weight loss, and are equally efficacious as more conventional weight-loss approaches up to 1 year (2–8). Given that low-carbohydrate diets are popular among the general public, do not seem to increase health risk in the short-term, and result in weight loss, registered dietitians (RDs) should be prepared to discuss this type of treatment with overweight and obese clients who show interest in trying this approach.

The following sections provide an overview of the various phases of the low-carbohydrate diet, clarify common misconceptions about the diet, and provide some practical suggestions related to a low-carbohydrate lifestyle, such as keeping track of carbohydrates, eating creatively, and dealing with potentially high-risk situations.

PHASES OF THE LOW-CARBOHYDRATE DIET: AN OVERVIEW

Phase I: Learning a New Way of Eating

No matter which low-carbohydrate approach is followed, the initial phase of the diet is the most restrictive. The purpose of the initial phase is to (*a*) jump start the weight loss process by decreasing carbohydrate intake, (*b*) heighten awareness of the carbohydrate content of various foods, and (*c*) establish a healthful foundation of eating in which nutrient-dense carbohydrates are featured rather than carbohydrates that have little nutritional value.

Phase II: Increasing Variety During Weight Loss

The purpose of the next phase is to support weight loss with greater flexibility in food choices. Carbohydrates (ie, primarily more vegetables, fruits, and eventually whole grains) are added back to the diet slowly to build upon the healthful foundation that was established during the first phase and help individuals maintain control of their eating while continuing to lose weight.

Phase III: Eating for Weight Maintenance

The purpose of the maintenance stage is to maintain a reduced body weight (see Chapter 10). Individuals entering this stage will consume a level of carbohydrate that supports weight maintenance. In other words, clients determine the maximum number of grams of carbohydrate they can consume to maintain their weight. By the time clients enter this phase of the diet, they should have a good idea of the type of carbohydrates they can safely incorporate into their diet (ie, foods that they can include in the diet without overeating) and maintain their weight.

UNDERSTANDING LOW-CARBOHYDRATE EATING

If asked to give an example of a carbohydrate, most people will list foods such as rice, pasta, bread, cereals, and potatoes. Although many will also name fruits, vegetables, and beverages, it is surprising how many people do not understand the variety of foods and beverages that actually contain carbohydrate. As such, it is probably a good idea in the beginning of weight-loss treatment to help clients understand what it means to eat a low-carbohydrate diet. The client who does not realize that he or she cannot reach for a bag of chips and soda or fruity yogurt, eat fried chicken or barbecue ribs with a cold beer, or a host of creamy entrees at a restaurant may be surprised by which foods have carbohydrate. Before clients commit to this way of eating, RDs may want to encourage them to keep a food record of the foods and beverages they eat and drink. Weekly food records are not only a good tool for self-monitoring, they also help clients develop a better understanding about sources of carbohydrate, especially those that are less obvious (such as gravies, sauces, and salad dressings) and quantities of carbohydrate in various foods and beverages. With this information, clients can avoid future frustration and make a more informed decision about whether this is an approach they are willing to follow.

RDs can use this opportunity to make sure clients know how to keep an accurate and complete food record (ie, time food was consumed, type and detailed description of food consumed, amount of carbohydrate per food or beverage, total carbohydrate intake at the end of the day). Whether or not a client decides to follow a low-carbohydrate diet, food record-keeping is an important skill to learn. Depending on the aptitude of the client, it may take several weeks to master record-keeping; therefore, for the first few weeks, the focus may be on completing detailed records and learning about sources of carbohydrate, rather than on carbohydrate counting.

Once clients understand how to complete food records, they can focus on counting carbohydrates and targeting a carbohydrate goal. Whether you are helping clients follow the Atkins or South Beach diet, it is important to clearly review the dietary guidelines of that approach (ie, which foods and beverages are and are not permitted, maximum amounts of carbohydrate per day during various phases of the diet, guidelines for eating food that contains fat and protein). In response to the recent popularity of these diets, many calorie-counting books and online sources, such as CalorieKing (http://www.calorieking.com), list the carbohydrate content of various foods. Clients should be encouraged to read food labels as often as possible because the carbohydrate content of some foods may vary depending on the manufacturer.

Although measuring food portions is time-consuming, clients should also be encouraged to use measuring utensils and a food scale to accurately determine the amount of carbohydrate consumed. Clients should weigh and measure foods in the short term (ie, at least the first 2 weeks) to become accustomed to actual portions because grams of carbohydrate are based on serving size. A benefit of the low-carbohydrate approach is that one only needs to count grams of carbohydrates, which means that clients do not need to weigh and measure all foods consumed (ie, one does not need to measure foods that do not contain carbohydrate). This makes the process of self-monitoring a little less burdensome. After reviewing the food records with the client, the RD should make brief comments about any patterns observed (eg, "I noticed that you have switched from using thousand island dressing to oil and vinegar on your salads") and make simple recommendations such as subtotaling carbohydrate intake throughout the day to stay on track.

ESTABLISHING A HEALTHFUL PATTERN OF EATING

Due to its restrictive nature in the initial stages, the low-carbohydrate approach can easily be viewed as an extreme and unnatural way of eating in the long term. Indeed, it would be rather difficult to maintain this way of eating over a long period of time; therefore, it is important to stress early in treatment that the first phase of this dietary approach is only a temporary period designed to initiate the process of consuming a low-carbohydrate diet. During this phase clients should establish a healthful pattern of eating that will become the basis of sustainable, long-term eating habits. The structured approach of the first phase will help clients focus on the fundamental feature of healthful eating according to this plan, consuming nutrient-dense carbohydrates while losing weight. RDs should explain that subsequent phases will slowly incorporate a larger variety of foods so that clients can learn to make healthful carbohydrate choices, choose foods they enjoy, and eat in a healthful way that is sustainable over the long term. The basic theme of any good nutritional approach is adaptability. Adding new carbohydrate-containing foods slowly and carefully will help clients learn good eating habits and be less prone to feeling hungry, irritated, and unhappy, which are feelings that may lead to overeating.

Because intake of foods that do not contain carbohydrates is not restricted, clients may wrongly believe that they can eat unlimited amounts of these foods. Although some of the books do not highly emphasize this point, the goal is to eat enough of these foods to feel satisfied but not stuffed. For example, in Dr. Atkins' *New Diet Revolution,* he states that although clients will not be counting calories on the Atkins' diet, calories do matter (9, p.143). He goes on to say that gaining weight results from eating more calories than are burned, so individuals should eat until satisfied and not gorge. Uncontrolled eating is generally not supported by any sound weight-control program.

Another misconception is that if restricting carbohydrate is good, eliminating carbohydrate altogether is better. In the early stages of the diet, low-carbohydrate approaches suggest that individuals consume most, if not all, of their carbohydrate in the form of vegetables. All RDs know that getting clients to eat their recommended amounts of vegetables each day is not an easy task. It is important to remind clients to get adequate amount of nutrients. Also, to prevent adverse symptoms related to electrolyte loss (eg, cramps), they should not eat less than the minimum amount of carbohydrate prescribed per day and they should drink adequate amounts of non-carbohydrate-containing fluids. Eating less than the recommended amount of carbohydrate per day offers no advantages in terms of weight loss.

To prevent constipation and dehydration, clients should drink at least eight 8-oz glasses of water per day (9, p.124). Low-carbohydrate plans generally allow diet sodas but alcohol is prohibited. Alcohol is not a source of nutritive carbohydrate and should not be consumed for a variety of reasons: (*a*) carbohydrate in alcoholic beverages takes the place of carbohydrate in nutritious foods; (*b*) it acts as alternate fuel source; (*c*) it decreases hydration; and (*d*) it decreases self-control.

THINKING "OUTSIDE OF THE BOX" DURING BREAKFAST, LUNCH, AND SNACKS

Eating a low-carbohydrate diet can be a challenge, especially in the beginning of the diet when there is less variety from which to choose. Dinner is less difficult because most dinners are planned around a protein source, but breakfast and lunch can be tricky due to time constraints and learned eating habits. Encourage your clients to be creative and to think beyond established mealtime "norms."

When you review your clients' food records, look for patterns in food selection. Ask clients how they feel about their food selections. Are they bored with their food choices? Boredom is a typical complaint among clients who follow low-carbohydrate diets. Therefore, it is important to take time to discuss methods of decreasing repetitiveness (ie, by altering the foods consumed or eating standard foods in different ways) and the advantages of increasing variety (ie, decreases monotony, improves nutrient intake).

Breakfast

Breakfast tends to be one of the most difficult meals for clients because common breakfast foods, such as cereals, waffles and pancakes with syrup, bagels, and muffins are

TABLE 5.1
Low-Carbohydrate and No-Carbohydrate Breakfast Options

Food	Serving Suggestions
Eggs	Eggs can be prepared in a variety of ways. Try omelets (with cheese, vegetables, meat, or a combination of all). Eggs can also be fried, poached, scrambled, boiled, or deviled.
Seafood and meat	Try shrimp, smoked salmon, tuna, or sardines. Serve with cream cheese and capers, cheddar cheese, mozzarella, and/or sliced vegetables like cucumber, tomato, or green pepper. A great example is smoked salmon wrapped around cream cheese.
Tofu	Tofu can be scrambled in olive oil or sesame oil with your favorite vegetables and herbs.
Nut butters	Celery topped with nut butters is a quick and easy start to the day.
Cheese	Try fresh mozzarella with tomato and avocado slices drizzled with olive oil and herbs.
Leftovers	Use the microwave to reheat leftovers from last night's dinner. Crustless quiche, zucchini pancakes, chicken drumsticks, tuna salad, or soup can be just as delicious at breakfast.

carbohydrate-laden; however, clients can be encouraged to choose foods conventionally eaten at other meals. Table 5.1 provides some examples of traditional and nontraditional foods that can be enjoyed for breakfast.

Lunch and Snacks

Given the time constraints at work and busy lifestyles, it can also be a challenge to put together a satisfying lunch. Brainstorm quick and easy lunch options with your clients. Salad topped with nuts, grilled chicken, steak strips, shrimp, or even pizza toppings can be a satisfying lunch. One can have soup with the salad to make the meal more complete. Many restaurants serve chicken, pork, fish, or shrimp, which can be grilled, broiled, or sautéed and served with sautéed or stir-fried vegetables. You can encourage clients to keep "quick-to-fix" foods on hand and freeze leftover foods in single-serving containers that can be easily carried in a lunch bag. Box 5.1 lists some food items that can be used to put together a quick and tasty lunch or snack.

DEALING WITH HIGH-RISK SITUATIONS

For many people, eating at restaurants, going on vacation, celebrating the holidays and other special occasions are opportunities to escape from everyday work and family responsibilities and relax or indulge in more pleasurable activities. Although eating should be an enjoyable activity, many people abandon healthful eating habits and excuse their behavior on special occasions. Individuals following a low-carbohydrate diet are at risk for selecting foods that are nutritionally inadequate and high in carbohydrate more often than nutrient-dense foods that are low in carbohydrate, and/or eat until they feel stuffed rather than stopping when they are satisfied. Clearly, these behaviors can jeopardize a client's long-term weight-control efforts. RDs can help their clients learn how to think about these special occasions a little differently and help them take control of the situation rather than allowing the situation to take control of them.

Box 5.1
Low-Carbohydrate and No-Carbohydrate Options for Lunches and Snacks

Nuts and seeds
- Sunflower seeds
- Pumpkin seeds
- Macadamia nuts, almonds, walnuts, hazelnuts, pecans
- Soy nuts or soy chips (relatively high in carbohydrate)

Fruits/Vegetables
- Avocado, guacamole
- Olives (plain or tuna stuffed)
- Frozen or roasted cherry tomatoes
- Raw vegetables from home or the salad bar
- Celery stuffed with cream cheese, nut butter, egg salad, or green salsa and cheese
- Salad greens in a bag
- Chef's salad, chicken caesar salad (no croutons)
- Frozen mixed vegetables, for soups, stir-fries, etc.
- Marinated artichoke hearts

Dairy
- Firm cheese
- String cheese
- Sour cream dip
- Cream cheese and feta dip

Meat, poultry, fish, eggs, tofu
- Canned tuna, salmon, sardines, mackerel, or chicken
- Lump crabmeat

- Precooked shrimp marinated in olive oil and herbs
- Homemade tuna or chicken salad
- Sliced turkey or chicken breast
- Turkey, romaine lettuce, and mayonnaise roll-up
- Smoked turkey wrapped around avocado
- Chicken wings or drumsticks
- Ham and cream cheese roll-up with an olive
- Cheeseburger without the bun
- Hard-boiled eggs
- Pre-marinated tofu
- Scrambled tofu with vegetables

Miscellaneous
- Soups and broths
- Bottled regular salad dressings
- Flavored vinegars
- Green salsa
- Spicy mustard
- Sugarless ketchup with horseradish
- Pork rinds (plain or with dip)
- Flavored gelatin made with artificial sweeteners and topped with whipped heavy cream

Eating Out

Given the variety of high-carbohydrate options offered at restaurants, eating out can be a challenge, but it can also be more manageable than clients may initially think. Clients can take charge of their meal before they go out to eat and while they are at the restaurant. They can call ahead of time to ask about low-carbohydrate choices and plan their meal before going to the restaurant. They may even want to eat a little something before they go out so they are not ravenous. The hungrier they are, the more tempted they will be by high-carbohydrate foods on the menu.

Restaurants are a service-oriented business and therefore inclined to cater to the customers' needs; clients can use this to their advantage and ask for what they want. Before the basket of warm bread comes to the table, clients can ask the server to *not* serve the bread (or chips or other high-carbohydrate "freebies"). They can also inquire whether a vegetable or olive tray can be served instead. RDs can point out to their clients the wording on menus that may indicate a method of preparation that uses flour, breading, fruit juice, or sugar—eg, terms such as breaded, deep fried, creamy, gravy, pastry, au gratin, southern style, escalloped/scalloped, or barbecued. Encourage clients to ask servers about the method of preparation. If the method of preparation is high in carbohydrate, they can ask whether the chef can modify the entrée to reduce the amount of carbohydrate. For example, a restaurant may broil or sauté a piece of fish rather than fry it in batter. Salad dressing, gravy, sauces, or spreads can be served "on the side." In many instances, high-carbohydrate foods can be replaced with lower carbohydrate items (eg, replace french fries with salad or broccoli). These are simple requests that most restaurants are happy to meet.

Vacations, Holidays, and Other Special Occasions

Although eating and drinking are part of vacations and celebrations, they should be kept in moderation. Ask your clients to share images (eg, good times, family traditions, stress, loneliness) and activities (eg, preparing for parties, baking, eating and drinking at parties) associated with vacations, holidays, or other special occasions. Although eating and drinking are often part of these celebrations, they are usually not the only activity. Encourage your clients to think of other opportunities to focus on during vacation (eg, sight-seeing, having more free time to exercise in a nicer climate and location, trying new activities and unique foods, having relaxed restaurant meals or sufficient time to prepare healthy meals). Similarly, help them think of holiday activities (eg, gift-giving, decorating, socializing, games, conversations, friendships, family time) that can make these times meaningful.

Discuss the advantages and disadvantages of incorporating or abandoning healthful eating and activity during these situations. For example, healthful eating and activity may help clients feel light, energetic, in control, and attractive, whereas temporarily letting go of healthful pursuits may involve less planning but make the client feel like she or he is doing nothing, out of control, or regaining weight/heavy. Work closely with the client to identify strategies for handling special occasions. Work through one or two potentially difficult situations and problem-solve these issues.

A FINAL NOTE

As with any change, modifying eating habits can be challenging. In an environment in which high-carbohydrate foods (particularly highly refined carbohydrates) are readily available, limiting carbohydrate intake can initially be difficult. However, this dietary approach has several benefits. By limiting the customary array of less-healthful carbohydrate foods, individuals are obliged to explore a larger variety of fruits and vegetables that they may increasingly appreciate over time. This approach also allows individuals to enjoy tasty protein-rich foods and does not restrict the use of a variety of fats, which can also be very pleasing to the palate. In addition, for those who do not like to count calories, this approach limits counting to only foods that contain carbohydrate, making the important process of self-monitoring easier. If participants have faithfully followed the phases of the low-carbohydrate diet, they should have a new and more healthful pattern of eating by the time they reach the maintenance phase.

References

1. Freedman MR, King J, Kennedy E. Popular diets: a scientific review. *Obes Res.* 2001;9(1 suppl):1S–40S.

2. Foster GD, Wyatt, HR, Hill JO, McGuckin BG, Brill C, Mohammed S, Szapary PO, Rader DJ, Edman JS, Klein S. A randomized trial of a low-carbohydrate diet for obesity. *N Engl J Med.* 2003,348:2082–2090.

3. Brehm BJ, Seeley RJ, Daniels SR, D'Allesio DA. A randomized trial comparing a very low-carbohydrate diet and a calorie-restricted low-fat diet on body weight and cardiovascular risk factors in healthy women. *J Clin Endocrin Metab.* 2003;88: 1617–1623.

4. Samaha FF, Iqbal N, Seshadri P, Chicano KL, Daily DA, McGrory J, Williams T, Williams M, Gracely EJ, Stern L. A low-carbohydrate as compared with a low-fat diet in severe obesity. *N Engl J Med.* 2003,348:2074–2081.

5. Stern L, Iqbal N, Seshadri P, Chicano KL, Daily DA, McGrory J, Williams M, Gracely EJ, Samaha FF. The effects of low-carbohydrate versus conventional weight loss diets in severely obese adults: one-year follow-up of a randomized trial. *Ann Intern Med.* 2004;140:778–785.

6. Yancy WS, Olsen MK, Guyton JR, Bakst RP, Westman EC. A low-carbohydrate, ketogenic diet versus a low-fat diet to treat obesity and hyperlipidemia. *Ann Intern Med.* 2004;140:769–777.

7. Dansinger ML, Gleason JA, Griffith JL, Selker HP, Schaefer EJ. Comparison of the Atkins, Ornish, Weight Watchers, and Zone diets for weight loss and heart disease risk reduction: a randomized trial. *JAMA.* 2005;293:43–53.

8. Gardner CD, Kiazand A, Alhassan S, Kim S, Stafford RS, Balise RR, Kraemer HC, King AC. Comparison of the Atkins, Zone, Ornish, and LEARN diets for change in weight and related risk factors among overweight premenopausal women: the A TO Z Weight Loss Study: a randomized trial. *JAMA.* 2007;297:969–977.

9. Atkins RC. *Dr. Atkins' New Diet Revolution.* New York, NY: Harper Collins; 2002.

CHAPTER 6

PHYSICAL ACTIVITY AND WEIGHT MANAGEMENT

PART A: OVERVIEW

JOHN M. JAKICIC, PHD

INTRODUCTION

There has been a consistent increase in the prevalence of overweight and obesity in the United States over the past few decades (1). Moreover, individuals trying to maintain weight loss are frequently unsuccessful. Body-weight regulation is influenced by the balance between energy intake and energy expenditure. In the most basic context, body weight will remain stable when energy intake equals energy expenditure, with weight loss occurring when energy expenditure exceeds energy intake and weight gain occurring when energy intake exceeds energy expenditure. Physical activity may be the most variable component of total energy expenditure (2), suggesting that physical activity may be an important intervention to influence weight loss and prevent weight gain.

THE EFFECT OF PHYSICAL ACTIVITY ON PRIMARY PREVENTION OF WEIGHT GAIN

A potential strategy to combat the obesity epidemic is to not only focus interventions on weight loss, but to also develop effective strategies to prevent weight gain. Results from numerous studies point to an important role of physical activity in the prevention of weight gain. For example, cross-sectional evidence indicates that individuals who are more active have a lower body weight than less-active individuals (3). Results from the Pound of Prevention Study also demonstrated that physical activity was predictive of less weight gain over a 3-year period (4), with additional long-term prospective studies supporting the effectiveness of physical activity in the primary prevention of weight gain (5–13).

Whereas increasing physical activity seems to be an important component of weight gain prevention, it may also be important to focus on reducing sedentary behaviors. Ball et al (14) reported that young women who gained 5% or more of their initial body weight over a 4-year period reported more time sitting compared with those who did not gain weight. Data from the Nurses' Health Study also demonstrated that across a 6-year period, the risk of becoming obese increased with increased time spent watching television, and the risk of becoming obese decreased with increased time spent walking (15). Thus, focusing interventions on increasing physical activity and decreasing sedentary behaviors may prove to be effective at preventing weight gain and the development of obesity.

THE EFFECT OF PHYSICAL ACTIVITY ON WEIGHT LOSS

Physical activity is a common component of behavioral intervention for weight loss. However, physical activity alone may have only a modest effect on weight loss. A review of the literature demonstrated that physical activity resulted in weight loss of approximately 1 to 2 kg (16). This magnitude of weight loss seems to be consistent with the conclusions of clinical guidelines developed by the Expert Panel on the Identification, Evaluation, and Treatment of Overweight and Obesity in Adults (17), which reported that physical activity resulted in 2.4 kg of weight loss. However, the magnitude of weight loss may be dependent on the duration of moderate-to-vigorous physical activity that is done as well as the diet that is consumed, and studies have shown modest to significant weight losses with a range of 180 to 270 minutes per week of exercise (18–20).

The magnitude of weight loss achieved from physical activity seems to be less than what can be achieved through reductions in dietary intake. This was confirmed in a study conducted by Wood et al (21), who reported weight loss at 12 months from physical activity to be 4.0 kg vs a weight loss of 7.2 kg achieved through a reduction in energy intake. However, when added to an energy-restricted diet, physical activity can have an additive effect compared with what can be achieved through either diet or physical activity alone. For example, in a study by Wing et al, weight losses achieved at 6 months through diet alone, physical activity alone, and the combination of diet plus physical activity were 9.1 kg, 2.1 kg, and 10.3 kg, respectively (22), and this pattern has been confirmed by other investigators (23).

There is an increasing interest in the effects of resistance exercise on body weight regulation. However, resistance exercise seems to have a modest effect on body weight, typically resulting in less than 1 kg decrease (24). This lack of an effect of resistance exercise on body weight may be a result of the reduction in body fat being countered by a concurrent increase in fat-free mass. Therefore, assessment of body composition rather than body weight may be necessary to best understand the effect of resistance exercise on body weight regulation. Resistance exercise may also result in additional benefits for overweight and obese adults, such as improving muscular strength, which can result in improvements in physical function (25).

THE ROLE OF PHYSICAL ACTIVITY IN THE MAINTENANCE OF WEIGHT LOSS

Although the scientific evidence seems to support that physical activity has a modest effect on weight loss, there is growing evidence to support the role of physical activity in the maintenance of weight loss and the prevention of weight regain. More importantly, the scientific evidence also supports the belief that relative high doses of physical activity may be required to sustain long-term weight loss. For example, self-report data from the National Weight Control Registry have demonstrated that individuals sustaining weight loss of 13.6 kg (30 lb) or more expend 2,800 kcal per week through physical activity, which is the equivalent of 5 to 6 hours of walking per week (26). In a follow-up to the initial report, McGuire et al (27) reported that individuals in the National Weight Control Registry who gained weight after 1 year also reported greater decreases in energy expenditure compared with individuals who maintained their weight loss. Additional prospective studies further support the importance of physical activity for the prevention of weight regain. For example, Leser et al (28) reported a significant inverse correlation ($r = -0.53$; $P = .005$) between physical activity and weight change at a 3-year follow-up, and Schoeller et al (29) reported that 80 minutes per day of moderate-intensity physical activity was required to sustain weight loss long-term.

Evidence from clinical trials supports the need for relatively high levels of physical activity to sustain long-term weight loss. In two independently conducted studies (30,31), Jakicic et al have demonstrated that physical activity equivalent to 250 to 300 minutes per week was required to sustain weight loss of 10% or more for a period of 12 to 18 months. These findings are supported by research by Jeffery et al (32) and are consistent with recommendations of the American College of Sports Medicine (33), the Institute of Medicine (34), the International Association for the Study of Obesity (IASO) (35), and the 2005 US Dietary Guidelines for Americans (36). In sum, the scientific evidence supports the need for 60 to 90 minutes of physical activity per day to sustain long-term weight loss.

FITNESS VS FATNESS

In recent years there has been an increasing interest in the debate about whether physical activity improves health-related outcomes independent of its effect on body weight. If this hypothesis is accurate, focusing on increasing physical activity in the context of modest or no actual change in body weight would still result in substantial improvements in health. The majority of the research in this area has focused on cardiorespiratory fitness rather than on physical activity per se. To date, a considerable amount of research has supported that an improvement in cardiorespiratory fitness can improve health outcomes independent of body weight. These independent effects of fitness on health-related outcomes have been demonstrated for both women (37) and men (38–40). A more recent study has also reported that higher levels of cardiorespiratory fitness result in lower all-cause mortality in individuals with type 2 diabetes independent of body weight (41). Moreover, Wing et al (42) reported that both fitness and fatness affect cardiovascular disease risk factors in individuals with type 2 diabetes, potentially high-lighting the importance of increasing fitness and decreasing weight.

Although these studies emphasize the importance of sufficient physical activity to improve cardiorespiratory fitness in overweight and obese adults, these results do not suggest that weight loss should be ignored, especially in the most severe obese individuals. For example, many of these studies had limited numbers of subjects with a body mass index (BMI) more than 35, which limits the generalizability of these findings to individuals classified as overweight (BMI 25–29.9) and individuals with Class 1 obesity (BMI 30–34.9). Moreover, Wing et al (42) reported that only 2.4% of subjects who were classified as Class 3 obese were also in the highest classifications for fitness, suggesting that it may be difficult to sufficiently increase fitness in this population group. Therefore, it may be important to focus on both improving cardiorespiratory fitness along with re-ducing body weight in overweight and obese adults to maximize the improvements in health-related outcomes.

SUMMARY

The consensus public health recommendation for physical activity is to participate in at least 30 minutes of moderate-intensity activity on most days of the week (43), which is commonly interpreted as at least 150 minutes of physical activity per week. This level of physical activity has been shown to improve health-related outcomes associated with nu-merous chronic diseases and prevent or delay onset of these conditions. However, this level of physical activity may not be sufficient for optimal body weight control. This is confirmed in numerous recommendations and position stands (33–35). More recently, the 2005 US Dietary Guidelines have recommended 60 minutes of physical activity per day to prevent weight gain and 60 to 90 minutes per day to maintain weight loss and to prevent weight regain (36). Thus, interventions should target this amount of physical ac-tivity and help individuals progressively increase to these levels to maximize the effect on body weight.

References

1. Ogden CL, Carroll MD, Curtin LR, McDowell MA, Tabak CJ, Flegal KM. Preva-lence of overweight and obesity in the United States, 1999–2004. *JAMA*. 2006;295: 1549–1555.

2. Ravussin E, Bogardus C. Relationship of genetics, age, and physical fitness to daily energy expenditure and fuel utilization. *Am J Clin Nutr*. 1989;49:968–975.

3. Lee IM, Paffenbarger R. Associations of light, moderate, and vigorous intensity physical activity with longevity: the Harvard Alumni Health Study. *Am J Epi-demiol*. 2000;151:293–299.

4. Sherwood NE, Jeffery RW, French SA, Hannan PJ, Murray DM. Predictors of weight gain in the Pound of Prevention study. *Int J Obes*. 2000;24:395–403.

5. Balkau B, Vierron E, Vernay M, Born C, Arondel D, Petrella A, Ducimetiere P; D.E.S.I.R. Study Group. The impact of 3-year changes in lifestyle habits on meta-

bolic syndrome parameters: the D.E.S.I.R. study. *Eur J Cardiovasc Prev Rehabil*. 2006;13:334–340.

6. Berk DR, Hubert HB, Fries JF. Associations of changes in exercise level with subsequent disability among seniors: a 16-year longitudinal study. *J Gerontol A Biol Sci Med Sci*. 2006;1:97–102.

7. Droyvold WB, Holmen J, Midthjell K, Lydersen S. BMI change and leisure time physical activity (LTPA): an 11-y follow-up study in apparently healthy men aged 20–69 y with normal weight at baseline. *Int J Obes*. 2004;28:410–417.

8. Kyle UG, Genton L, Gremion G, Slosman DO, Pichard C. Aging, physical activity and height-normalized body composition parameters. *Clin Nutr*. 2004;23:79–88.

9. Kyle UG, Melzer K, Kayser B, Picard-Kossovsky M, Gremion G, Pichard C. Eight-year longitudinal changes in body composition in healthy Swiss adults. *J Am Coll Nutr*. 2006;25:493–501.

10. Murray LA, Reilly JJ, Choudhry M, Durnin JVGA. A longitudinal study of changes in body composition and basal metabolism in physically active elderly men. *Eur J Appl Physiol*. 1996;72:215–218.

11. Schroeder ET, Hawkins SA, Hyslop D, Vallejo AF, Jensky NE, Wiswell RA. Longitudinal change in coronary heart disease risk factors in older runners. *Age Aging*. 2007;36:57–62.

12. Wang BWE, Ramey DR, Schettler JD, Hubert HB, Fries JF. Postponed development of disability in elderly runners: a 13-year longitudinal study. *Arch Intern Med*. 2002;162:2285–2294.

13. Williams PT, Wood PD. The effects of changing exercise levels on weight and age-related weight gain. *Int J Obes*. 2006;30:543–551.

14. Ball K, Brown W, Crawford D. Who does not gain weight? Prevalence and predictors of weight maintenance in young women. *Int J Obes*. 2002;26:1570–1578.

15. Hu FB, Li TY, Colditz GA, Willett WC, Manson JE. Television watching and other sedentary behaviors in relation to risk of obesity and type 2 diabetes mellitus in women. *JAMA*. 2003;289:1785–1791.

16. Wing RR. Physical activity in the treatment of the adulthood overweight and obesity: current evidence and research issues. *Med Sci Sports Exerc*. 1999;31(Suppl 11):S547–S552.

17. National Institutes of Health. Clinical Guidelines on the Identification, Evaluation, and Treatment of Overweight and Obesity in Adults: the Evidence Report. *Obes Res*. 1998;6(Suppl 2):51S–209S.

18. Irwin ML, Tasui Y, Ulrich CM, Bowen D, Rudolph RE, Schwartz RS, Yukawa M, Aiello E, Potter JD, McTiernan A. Effect of exercise on total and intra-abdominal body fat in postmenopausal women: a randomized controlled trial. *JAMA*. 2003;289:323–330.

19. Nakamura Y, Tanaka K, Yabushita N, Sakai T, Shigematsu R. Effects of exercise frequency on functional fitness in older adult women. *Arch Gerontol Geriatr*. 2007;44:163–173.

20. Skrinar GS, Huxley NA, Hutchinson DS, Menninger E, Glew P. The role of a fitness intervention on people with serious psychiatric disabilities. *Psychiatr Rehabil J*. 2005;29:122–127.

21. Wood PD, Stefanick ML, Dreon DM, Frey-Hewitt B, Garay SC, Williams PT, Superko HR, Fortmann SP, Albers JJ, Vranizan KM, et al. Changes in plasma lipids

and lipoproteins in overweight men during weight loss through dieting as compared with exercise. *N Engl J Med*. 1988;319:1173–1179.

22. Wing RR, Venditti EM, Jakicic JM, Polley BA, Lang W. Lifestyle intervention in overweight individuals with a family history of diabetes. *Diabetes Care*. 1998;21:350–359.

23. Hagan RD, Upton SJ, Wong L, Whittam J. The effects of aerobic conditioning and/or calorie restriction in overweight men and women. *Med Sci Sports Exerc*. 1986;18:87–94.

24. Donnelly JE, Jakicic JM, Pronk NP, Kirk EP, Jacobsen DJ, Washburn R. Is resistance exercise effective for weight management? *Evidence Based Prevent Med*. 2004;1:21–29.

25. Jakicic JM. Physical activity considerations for the treatment and prevention of obesity. *Am J Clin Nutr*. 2005;82(Suppl 1):226S–229S.

26. Klem ML, Wing RR, McGuire MT, Seagle HM, Hill JO. A descriptive study of individuals successful at long-term maintenance of substantial weight loss. *Am J Clin Nutr*. 1997;66:239–246.

27. McGuire MT, Wing RR, Klem ML, Lang W, Hill JO. What predicts weight regain in a group of successful weight losers? *J Consult Clin Psychol*. 1999;67:177–185.

28. Leser MS, Yanovski SZ, Yanovski JA. A low-fat intake and greater activity level are associated with lower weight regain 3 years after completing a very-low-calorie diet. *J Am Diet Assoc*. 2002;102:1252–1256.

29. Schoeller DA, Shay K, Kushner RF. How much physical activity is needed to minimize weight gain in previously obese women. *Am J Clin Nutr*. 1997;66:551–556.

30. Jakicic JM, Marcus BH, Gallagher KI, Napolitano M, Lang W. Effect of exercise duration and intensity on weight loss in overweight, sedentary women. A randomized trial. *JAMA*. 2003;290:1323–1330.

31. Jakicic JM, Winters C, Lang W, Wing RR. Effects of intermittent exercise and use of home exercise equipment on adherence, weight loss, and fitness in overweight women: a randomized trial. *JAMA*. 1999;282:1554–1560.

32. Jeffery RW, Wing RR, Sherwood NE, Tate DF. Physical activity and weight loss: does prescribing higher physical activity goals improve outcome? *Am J Clin Nutr*. 2003;78:684–689.

33. Jakicic JM, Clark K, Coleman E, Donnelly JE, Foreyt J, Melanson E, Volek J, Volpe SL; American College of Sports Medicine. American College of Sports Medicine position stand: appropriate intervention strategies for weight loss and prevention of weight regain for adults. *Med Sci Sports Exerc*. 2001;33:2145–2156.

34. Institute of Medicine. *Dietary Reference Intakes for Energy, Carbohydrates, Fiber, Fat, Protein and Amino Acids (Macronutrients)*. Washington, DC: National Academies Press; 2002.

35. Saris WH, Blair SN, van Baak MA, Eaton SB, Davies PS, Di Pietro L, Fogelholm M, Rissanen A, Schoeller D, Swinburn B, Tremblay A, Westerterp KR, Wyatt H. How much physical activity is enough to prevent unhealthy weight gain? Outcome of the IASO 1st Stock Conference and consensus statement. *Obes Rev*. 2003;4:101–114.

36. US Department of Health and Human Services and US Department of Agriculture. *Dietary Guidelines for Americans*. 2005. http://www.healthierus.gov/dietary guidelines. Accessed November 14, 2008.

37. Barlow CE, Gibbons LW, Blair SN. Physical activity, mortality, and obesity. *Int J Obes*. 1995;19(suppl):S41–S44.

38. Lee S, Kuk JL, Davidson LE, Hudson R, Kilpatrick K, Graham TE, Ross R. Exercise without weight loss is an effective strategy for obesity reduction in obese individuals with and without type 2 diabetes. *J Appl Physiol*. 2005;99:1220–1225.

39. Wei M, Kampert J, Barlow CE, Nichaman MZ, Gibbons LW, Paffenbarger RS Jr, Blair SN. Relationship between low cardiorespiratory fitness and mortality in normal-weight, overweight, and obese men. *JAMA*. 1999;282:1547–1553.

40. Farrell SW, Braun L, Barlow CE, Cheng YJ, Blair SN. The relation of body mass index, cardiorespiratory fitness, and all-cause mortality in women. *Obes Res*. 2002;10:417–423.

41. Church TS, LaMonte MJ, Barlow CE, Blair SN. Cardiorespiratory fitness and body mass index as predictors of cardiovascular disease mortality among men with diabetes. *Arch Intern Med*. 2005;165:2114–2120.

42. Wing RR, Jakicic J, Neiberg R, Lang W, Blair SN, Cooper L, Hill JO, Johnson KC, Lewis CE; LOOK AHEAD Research Group. Fitness, fatness, and cardiovascular risk factors in type 2 diabetes: Look AHEAD Study. *Med Sci Sports Exerc*. 2007;39:2107–2116.

43. Pate RR, Pratt M, Blair SN, Haskell WL, Macera CA, Bouchard C, Buchner D, Ettinger W, Heath GW, King AC, et al. Physical activity and public health: a recommendation from the Centers for Disease and Prevention and the American College of Sports Medicine. *JAMA*. 1995;273:402–407.

PART B: PRACTICAL APPLICATIONS

RUTH ANN CARPENTER, MS, RD

INTRODUCTION

In the past, many clinicians, including registered dietitians (RDs), were trained to refer clients to exercise physiologists or other exercise specialists for exercise counseling. Although this remains a good practice in some instances, the convergence of several new developments in health promotion has made it important, if not imperative, for all health professionals working with overweight and obese clients to provide physical activity guidance. As described in the Overview section of this chapter, recent research has shown that moderate amounts of physical activity provide substantial health benefits, regardless of weight status. The body of evidence and the ensuing public health recommendations expand the options that health professionals can use to promote physical activity.

In addition, the increasing prevalence of obesity suggests that it will take a concerted effort from all health professionals—physicians, RDs, dietetic technicians registered (DTRs), exercise physiologists, nurses, health educators, and others—to help stem this disturbing trend. Research is leading to evidenced-based physical activity interventions that can be delivered by non-exercise professionals. Studies at the Cooper Institute and Brown University have shown that a lifestyle approach to physical activity is just as effective, and is more cost-effective, than a structured exercise program in improving physical fitness, physical activity, and many cardiovascular risk factors (1,2).

Given these recent developments and the fact that physical activity is essential for long-term weight management, the time is right for RDs and other health professionals to provide physical activity guidance as part of a comprehensive approach to treating overweight and obese clients. This section will (*a*) provide examples of how to help clients implement public health recommendations for physical activity; (*b*) review methods for physical activity assessment; and (*c*) address several exercise-related topics that are unique to the obese client.

PUBLIC HEALTH GUIDELINES

In October 2008, the Department of Health and Human Services published the first-ever Physical Activity Guidelines for Americans (3). These guidelines are the main source of information about the amount, intensity, and types of physical activity needed to attain health benefits for Americans. The Physical Activity Guidelines for Americans complement the Dietary Guidelines for Americans that RDs know intimately and use regularly in their practices. Together, these two documents provide evidence-based recommendations to promote good health and reduce the risk of chronic diseases, including overweight and obesity.

The bottom line is that the harder, longer, and more frequently a person exercises, the more health benefits they accrue and the more calories they burn. Although increasing energy expenditure is a primary focus for physical activity's role in weight management, regular moderate-intensity physical activity also provides substantial health benefits, regardless of weight loss.

Physical Activity Guidelines for Adults

The Physical Activity Guidelines (3) provide specific recommendations for children, adolescents, adults, older adults, and special populations (such as women during pregnancy and the postpartum period, adults with disabilities, and people with chronic medical conditions). The focus of this chapter will be on the recommendations for adults. They are as follows:

- Avoid inactivity.
- For health benefits, do:
  - At least 150 minutes a week of moderate-intensity, or
  - At least 75 minutes a week of vigorous-intensity, or
  - A combination of moderate- and vigorous-intensity physical activities to equal these amounts (eg, 60 minutes of moderate-intensity *plus* 45 minutes of vigorous-intensity activities per week).

- For additional health benefits, increase physical activity to 300 minutes of moderate-intensity or 150 minutes of vigorous-intensity per week.
- For weight-management benefits, reduce energy intake and gradually increase physical activity level to at least 150 minutes of moderate-intensity or 75 minutes of vigorous-intensity physical activity per week. Many adults will need to do much more than 150 minutes of moderate-intensity activity per week to lose weight or keep it off. Some will need to do 300 minutes or more of moderate-intensity physical activity per week to effectively manage their weight.
- Activity should be done in bouts of at least 10 minutes and it should be spread across numerous days of the week. That is, it is not recommended that an entire week's worth of activity be done on the weekend.
- Muscle-strengthening activities (eg, weight training, resistance bands, calisthenics) for all major muscle groups should be done at least 2 days per week.

Physical Activity Guidelines for Older Adults

For older adults, the physical activity recommendations are essentially the same as for other adults (3). Additional considerations include the following:

- If older adults have chronic conditions, they should discuss with their physician whether regular physical activity is safe.
- If they cannot do the 150 minutes of moderate-intensity activity because of chronic medical conditions, older adults should be as physically active as their abilities and health conditions allow.
- Older adults should do exercises, such as tai chi, that improve their balance.

PHYSICAL ACTIVITY: HOW HARD?

Although any amount of physical activity is beneficial, the current recommendations emphasize activity that is at least moderate in intensity. Exercise physiologists classify this as any activity that requires 3 to 6 metabolic equivalents (METS) of energy expenditure, or 3 to 6 times more than resting intensity. This is equivalent to walking 1 mile in 15 to 20 minutes, a brisk walk for most individuals.

Walking is not the only moderate-intensity physical activity. Box 6.1 lists many other activity ideas. Notice that many of these do not require a gym membership or special exercise equipment.

Does this mean that overweight clients should not exercise at more vigorous levels? Not necessarily. A major advantage of vigorous activity is that it burns calories at a higher rate than moderate-intensity activities do. In fact, the public health physical activity recommendations were recently clarified (3) to reinforce to clinicians and the public that vigorous activities, such as those listed in Box 6.1, are appropriate.

However, many weight-management clients are inactive and have low fitness levels. This makes it difficult to do vigorous activities for very long or without significant risk of injury or burnout. In addition, many vigorous activities require special equipment or instruction (eg, aerobics classes, weight-training). Also, engaging in vigorous activity

Box 6.1
Selected Moderate- and Vigorous-intensity Activities

Moderate-intensity Activities	Vigorous-intensity Activities
• Walking briskly	• Jogging and running
• Gardening	• Walking up stairs
• Golfing (without a cart)	• Jumping rope
• Bicycling, less than 10 mph	• Calisthenics
• Raking leaves	• Aerobic dance
• Washing and waxing a car	• Tennis (doubles)
• Vigorous vacuuming	• Circuit weight-training
• Hiking	• Competitive sports (soccer, basketball, hockey)
• Dancing	• Swimming laps
• Tai chi	• Tennis (singles)
• Softball	• Heavy gardening

would require some overweight clients to obtain a physician's clearance. Therefore, it is best to help participants to simply start moving and building up to doing at least moderate-intensity activities. In time, as their fitness level improves and their exercise interests expand, you can encourage them to increase the intensity and duration of activity. For clients who are capable of and interested in vigorous activity at the beginning of treatment, consider recommending a certified personal trainer, fitness center, or exercise physiologist who can help with their fitness and exercise training goals. Another option is for RDs to obtain certification in personal training or other exercise credentialing (4).

PHYSICAL ACTIVITY: HOW OFTEN?

The Physical Activity Guidelines for Americans (3) indicate that people should spread their 150 minutes of moderate-intensity or 75 minutes of vigorous-intensity physical activity throughout the week. This allows flexibility to help clients meet this physical activity goal. The main point is that clients should embrace the important concept that to get health benefits, especially weight-management benefits, physical activity must be regular and sustained.

PHYSICAL ACTIVITY: HOW LONG?

For most people, overweight or not, exercising at a moderate intensity for 150 to 300 minutes (or more) per week seems daunting. That is why it is important to inform clients that they do not need to complete all their daily physical activity in one exercise session. Research now shows that people can obtain similar health and fitness benefits by either accumulating physical activity throughout the day or by exercising in one single exercise session. One study demonstrated that obese women who did four 10-minute bouts of activity throughout the day, 5 days per week, did more minutes of moderate activity—and lost more weight—than women who were instructed to do one 40-minute bout of exercise, 5 days per week (5). The bottom line is that you should help clients identify ways to include physical activities in their daily routine. Some clients will be able to do one long bout of physical activity each day. Others will need ideas to do enough short (10 minutes or more) bouts of activity to reach the weekly goal of at least 150 to 300 minutes of moderate-intensity activity.

LIFESTYLE PHYSICAL ACTIVITY

The new public health recommendations for physical activity remove barriers (eg, lack of time, don't like to sweat, don't like sports) to being more active. Still, clients may need an RD's help to find individualized, creative ways to introduce more physical activity into their lifestyle. One way to do this is to ask clients to identify how they can take normally sedentary activities and add activity to them. For example, one client started using used a cordless telephone and walked up and down the corridor outside his office as he was making business calls. Likewise, a woman started walking around her daughter's soccer practice field instead of sitting on the sidelines talking with the other moms. Yet another client used a home exercise bike while watching the evening news to burn a few calories and relieve stress. Also, encourage clients to replace sedentary activities with more active pursuits. One client started bicycling to work instead of driving several times per week. A volunteer at the local animal shelter asked to be switched from the receptionist's desk to walking the dogs.

Building small bouts of activity into a daily routine is one part of lifestyle physical activity. Another important aspect of lifestyle physical activity is the development of life-management skills that are necessary to make physical activity a regular part of daily living. These cognitive and behavioral skills enable clients to make behavior change relevant to their particular lifestyle and help them cope with the many challenges of becoming more active. Teaching clients these strategies is nothing new to RDs. For example, Table 6.1 compares how different cognitive and behavior-change skills can be applied to both diet and physical activity.

As stated earlier, increased physical activity may contribute modestly to weight loss, but being active is especially important to prevent weight regain after weight loss. Teaching these lifestyle-management skills helps build the skills to maintain physical activity for a lifetime.

STEPS TO PROVIDING
PHYSICAL ACTIVITY GUIDANCE

To provide physical activity guidance to for overweight and obese clients, RDs will need to assess readiness for physical activity. Then, treatment guidelines can be adapted to the client's interests, abilities, and readiness to change.

TABLE 6.1
Applications of Lifestyle Skills to Change Dietary and Physical Activity Behaviors

Lifestyle Skill	Dietary Application	Physical Activity Application
Self-monitoring	• Food records	• Physical activity behavior logs • Periodic fitness assessments • Step counters
Goal-setting	• Reduced energy intake • Balanced diet	• Increased energy expenditure • Step counters
Reward setting	• Tied to healthful eating goals	• Tied to physical activity goals
Social support	• People to help with healthful shopping and cooking tasks • People to encourage healthful eating habits	• People with whom to exercise and to help with life activities so client can have time to be active
Stimulus control	• Removing empty-calorie items from counters, cupboards, and refrigerators	• Keeping walking shoes at office, in car, in travel bag
Cognitive restructuring	• All foods can fit (eliminating all-or-none thinking)	• Any activity is better than no activity
Increasing healthy opportunities	• Finding restaurants that offer heart-healthy options • Try new low-fat food • Take healthful cooking classes	• Finding parks, recreation centers, trails, activity clubs in local community • Putting home exercise equipment in conspicuous place
Relapse prevention	• Planning ahead for high-calorie or unusual eating situations • Positive-thinking strategies to get back on track after a lapse • Cognitive skills to cope with urges to eat unhealthful foods	• Planning ahead for disruptions to activity plans (time constraints, weather, injury, etc) • Positive thinking strategies to get back on track after a lapse • Cognitive skills to cope with urges to skip doing physical activity

Assessment

Three types of assessments can be useful in helping overweight and obese clients prepare physical activity plans. One is the assessment of a client's current physical fitness status. Traditional exercise interventions use measured fitness level as the base on which a structured exercise prescription is developed. The lifestyle approach suggested earlier does not require a baseline fitness assessment. Still, periodic fitness assessments can provide useful feedback to the client and the clinician about the effects of an increase in physical activity level. Fitness assessment tests are normally administered by trained clinicians, exercise physiologists, or other experts and, as such, are beyond the scope of this section. If the client is interested in obtaining this information, refer him or her to a qualified exercise professional, such as a certified personal trainer or exercise physiologist. Two assessments that should be administered to all clients are an exercise preparticipation screening and an assessment of motivational readiness to become more physically active.

Physical Activity Readiness Questionnaire (PAR-Q)

The Physical Activity Readiness Questionnaire (PAR-Q) is one way to discern who should get a physician's clearance to exercise (6). To download the PAR-Q form, go to the Canadian Society for Exercise Physiology Web site (http://www.csep.ca) and click the Publications link on the left navigation bar.

The PAR-Q is very specific about the steps that should be taken before starting an exercise program. It is best to administer the PAR-Q during a client's initial visit. If, after completing the PAR-Q, it seems safe for the client to start exercising, proceed with the motivational readiness assessment process. However, if the client's answers to the questions on the PAR-Q indicate that he or she should see a physician, then delay discussing physical activity until the client obtains written medical clearance to start exercising.

If the screening protocol recommends the client seek a physician's clearance before beginning activity but the client is not able or willing to see a doctor, refrain from discussing physical activity changes. Address the benefits of physical activity, but do not start working with the client to devise a specific physical activity plan.

Assessing Motivational Readiness

An individual may be physically ready to start moving more, but this does not mean that he or she will start. Motivational readiness plays a big role in a person's willingness to listen to messages about physical activity and to start becoming more active. Behavior change is a complex process, but the transtheoretical, or stages of change (SOC), model provides a useful tool for clinicians to be more effective in their physical activity guidance. The SOC model posits that people move through different stages in the process of adopting a new health behavior (7). People move through the stages by applying different behavioral and cognitive skills. Table 6.2 lists the five stages of readiness, typical characteristics of people in each physical activity readiness stage, and appropriate goals and actions for counseling clients in each stage.

The counselor's goal should be to help a client move from one stage to the next. For example, it may be inappropriate to tell a person in the precontemplation stage that he or she should start exercising. They are simply not ready to change. Instead, the goal should be to get a precontemplator to start thinking about being more active (ie, to move to the contemplation stage). Be prepared to help the client understand the many benefits of physical activity, dispel myths about exercise (eg, that it has to be done all at once, it has to be vigorous to get benefits, it has to be done at a gym, it requires special equipment or instruction), and help the client identify personal exercise barriers. These actions are likely to help the client take the next step (ie, thinking about being more active) in the journey to reaching the maintenance stage. Remember, different clients are going to be in different stages. Tailor your guidance to each client's motivational readiness. A "one size fits all" physical activity recommendation will not help most clients.

Simply listening to what a client says about physical activity can often be very revealing. "I don't exercise now and I don't see what good it is going to do me" is something a precontemplator might say. A person in the preparation stage might say, "I bought a new pair of walking shoes and I am going to starting exercise on Monday." The comment "I've been doing at least 30 minutes of moderate exercise at least 5 days a week for the last 3 months, but I am getting bored," might be something you would hear from a person in the action stage.

Figure 6.1 (8) shows another way to determine a person's stage of readiness to become more physically active. This simple flow diagram is easy to administer. Be sure that clients fully comprehend the first box. Some people do not give themselves enough credit for the smaller (eg, 10-minute or more) bouts of moderate activity (eg, walking the

TABLE 6.2

Characteristics, Goals, and Actions for Different Stages of Readiness to Change Physical Activity Level

Stage of Readiness	Characteristics of Stage	Stage-Appropriate Goal and Actions
Precontemplation	• Not thinking about being more active • Doesn't recognize personal benefits to being active; may have tried and failed in the past • Has lots of barriers (real and perceived) • Very low exercise self-efficacy (ie, self-confidence)	*Goal: Move to Contemplation* 1. Discuss the benefits of regular physical activity (ie, weight management, CHD risk reduction, reduced stress, bone health, diabetes risk reduction). 2. Identify the client's personal barriers. 3. Educate about moderate-intensity activity and accumulating physical activity. 4. Encourage client to think about physical activity, not necessarily do more activity.
Contemplation	• Thinking about being more active but not doing anything • Knows some benefits but has many barriers • Doesn't know how to get started	*Goal: Move to Preparation* 1. Numbers 1 through 3 in Precontemplation plus have client: (*a*) commit to doing a few 2-minute walks each week, gradually building up to several per day; (*b*) begin to address major barriers. 2. Identify how client can turn sedentary activities into more active ones (eg, walking at the park while children have soccer practice).
Preparation	• Intending to become more active in the near future, or doing some physical activity but not enough to meet public health guidelines • Can get started but can't stay with it • More benefits but still have a lot of barriers	*Goal: Move to Action* 1. All of the Precontemplation and Contemplation goals plus help client: (*a*) set short- and long-term goals and rewards; (*b*) recruit support; (*c*) track thoughts about activity or actual activity (ie, minutes, steps, distance). 2. Also congratulate client on doing something.
Action	• Meeting activity goal in public health guidelines but for fewer than 6 months • Most use of cognitive and behavioral skills (ie, goal-setting, self-monitoring, social support) • At the greatest risk of relapse • Knows or has experienced some physical activity benefits	*Goal: Move to Maintenance* 1. All of the goals in the preceding stages plus help client: (*a*) plan for lapses and high-risk situations; (*b*) identify physical activity resources in their community; (*c*) try new activities; (*d*) track their activity (steps, minutes, distance); (*e*) set new short-term and long-term goals. 2. Also praise client's progress and commitment.
Maintenance	• Meeting activity goal in public health guidelines for more than 6 months • Very high exercise self-efficacy • Has realized many physical activity benefits • Physical activity is a personal value	*Goal: Stay in Maintenance* 1. All of the goals in the preceding stages plus have client: (*a*) cite keys for personal success; (*b*) encourage client to help others become more active; (*c*) identify alternative physical activities; (*d*) determine whether client is ready to add other or more vigorous activities to program.

Abbreviation: CHD, coronary heart disease.

dog, walking from the subway to the office, raking leaves) that they get throughout the day. At the same time, many people have a tendency to overestimate their activity level.

Neither the professional nor the client should expect a linear progression through the stages of change. Behavior change is often a process of two steps forward, one step back. In other words, lapses are to be expected. Advise clients that lapses are part of the learning process. On the positive side, if clients experience lapses during treatment, help them to (*a*) identify what triggered the lapse and how to deal with the trigger in the future and (*b*) develop cognitive skills to accept a lapse as a temporary setback and use positive-thinking skills to prevent the lapse from leading to a total collapse of efforts to adopt

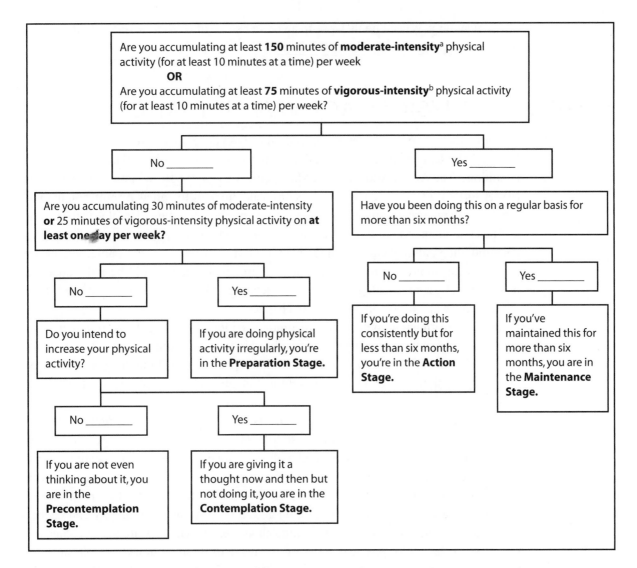

[a]Moderate-intensity physical activities are equal in effort to a brisk walk (walking 1 mile in 15 to 20 minutes) and increase your heart rate or breathing rate slightly. Activities of moderate intensity are: slow bicycling, dancing, gardening and yard work, golfing without a cart, hiking, raking leaves, vacuuming carpet, washing and waxing a car.
[b]Vigorous-intensity physical activities are harder than brisk walking and increase your heart rate or breathing rate a lot. Activities of vigorous intensity include: jogging, running, basketball, soccer, walking up stairs, fast bicycling, shoveling snow, and other activities of similar intensity.

FIGURE 6.1   Readiness to change.

Adapted with permission from Blair SN, Dunn AL, Marcus BH, Carpenter RA, Jaret P. *Active Living Every Day*. Champaign, IL: Human Kinetics; 2001:9,77,116

physical activity. When clients lapse to an earlier stage of readiness, return to the strategies that helped them move forward initially.

PROVIDING PHYSICAL ACTIVITY GUIDANCE

Recently, the American Dietetic Association (ADA) developed a set of practice guidelines to help RDs enhance the standard of care for several nutrition-related diseases and conditions. The ADA's Adult Weight Management Evidence-Based Practice Guidelines (9) set forth a set of evidence-based recommendations in the areas of nutrition assessment and treatment, weight-management interventions (including diet, physical activity, and behavioral interventions), weight-loss medications, and bariatric surgery. The ADA's corresponding Adult Weight Management Toolkit (10) provides companion resources and tools for implementing the guidelines. A treatment plan should be individualized based on a client's risk category, extent of dietary and lifestyle changes that need to be made, and the client's readiness to make changes.

Per the treatment guidelines, the recommended length of weight-loss treatment is at least 6 months. After an initial visit, it is feasible to plan multiple visits, 2 to 4 weeks apart during the 6 months, with periodic follow-up as needed. Table 6.3 shows the recommended actions and practical counseling strategies related to physical activity for a hypothetical client.

Depending on whether it is an initial visit or follow-up visit, a typical weight-management counseling session may last 20 to 60 minutes. This is a limited amount of time to cover the many tasks associated with assessment, diagnosis, intervention, monitoring, and evaluation in nutrition, physical activity, and behavior. Plus, clinicians who do not specialize in exercise may not be as comfortable talking about exercise issues. Likewise, many clients tend to be more interested in learning about dietary approaches to weight reduction than they are in learning about exercise (ie, they are in early stages of readiness to change for physical activity). Be aware of these roadblocks to physical activity intervention and work to help your overweight clients improve their physical activity behaviors as well as their eating habits.

CASE STUDY: MEET DORA

Dora is 47-year-old woman living in central Ohio with three children (ages 20, 15, and 12 years), her husband, who drives a delivery truck for a national overnight shipping company, and two large dogs. Dora works part time (3 days per week) as an accounting clerk at a local newspaper publisher near her home. A good portion of her day is spent shuttling her two youngest children to school and sports activities. She also volunteers 2 days per month at a local nursing home.

Dora is 64 inches tall and weighs 190 pounds (BMI = 33). Her weight history indicates a gradual increase in weight since high school, when she weighed 140 pounds. She started gaining weight after her pregnancies—approximately 10 to 12 additional pounds with each child. At times she had lost 10 to 15 pounds on various fad diets, but she always gained the weight back plus more.

TABLE 6.3

Physical Activity Recommendations for Medical Nutrition Therapy for Adult Weight Management

Encounter	Interval Between Visits	Physical Activity Recommendations	Practical Application
1	Within 30 days of referral	• Assess client's readiness to learn. • Assess physical activity pattern (attitude about physical activity, personal history, knowledge about physical activity). • Mutually establish short- and long-term goals for physical activity.	• If not previously cleared for exercise, administer PAR-Q. • Ask about client's personal barriers and potential benefits to being more active. • Administer "Readiness to Change" flowsheet. • Set goals according to client's readiness stage.[a] • Educate about physical activity's role in weight loss and especially in maintenance of weight loss.
2, 3, and 4	2–4 weeks	• Assess client's adherence to and comprehension of physical activity. Compare to expected outcomes and goals. • Reinforce or modify life skills strategies.[c] • Reinforce or modify mutual short- and long-term goals for physical activity.	• Review physical activity logs.[b] • Help client use problem-solving mindset to address one or two physical activity barriers. • Re-administer "Readiness to Change" flowsheet every 4 weeks. • Set goals according to client's readiness stage.[a] • Reinforce role of physical activity in weight loss and prevention of weight regain.
5 and 6	4–6 weeks	• Assess client's adherence to and comprehension of physical activity. Compare to expected outcomes and goals. • Reinforce or modify life skills strategies.[c] • Reinforce or modify mutual short- and long-term goals for physical activity. • Discuss lapse and relapse prevention.	• Review physical activity logs.[b] • Help client use problem-solving mindset to address one or two physical activity barriers. • Re-administer "Readiness to Change" flowsheet. • Set goals according to client's readiness stage.[a] • Reinforce role of physical activity in weight loss and prevention of weight regain. • Have client make plans for coping with high-risk situations (eg, holidays, vacations, travel, family emergencies, bad weather).

Abbreviation: PAR-Q, Physical Activity Readiness Questionnaire.
[a]See Table 6.2.
[b]Logging thoughts about physical activity is a good self-monitoring skill for people who have not yet begun to be more active.
[c]See Table 6.1.

Dora has borderline hypertension and normal fasting glucose and triglyceride levels. Lipitor has brought her blood cholesterol levels into an acceptable range. She is not using any other medication on a regular basis.

Dora comes to you on the advice of a friend who is a client. Your nutrition assessment indicates that she eats excessive fat and sugar calories, mostly from snack foods. Jellybeans are a "stress food" for her. Her fruit intake is inadequate, but she does "pretty well" in the other food groups. She has indicated that she is very ready to start eating better. As for physical activity, she loved tap and jazz dance as a child but did not do any organized activities as an adolescent or young adult. She has tried aerobics classes but found them too strenuous and inconvenient.

As she has gotten older, Dora's knees have begun to hurt more, especially while climbing hills and stairs. Her doctor has told her that the pain is probably the beginning of arthritis and that physical activity and weight loss would likely improve her symptoms. Dora likes being outside except when it is really cold or wet, which in central Ohio is a substantial part of the year.

The following are some questions to consider:

- Does Dora need to see a physician before you start working with her on her physical activity?
- Which stage of readiness to change is Dora in?
- What seem to be her barriers to physical activity?
- What benefits might she gain from being active?

Using the principles described in this chapter, here are clinical guidelines for providing physical activity guidance to Dora during a 6-month weight-management program.

Encounter 1: March 1

Assessment

- Not previously cleared for exercise.
- Not capable or interested in doing vigorous activities; willing to try moderate-intensity activities.
- Cleared, using PAR-Q instrument, for moderate-intensity activities.
- Barriers to activity: time, family responsibilities, doesn't like to sweat, uncomfortable wearing exercise clothes.
- Perceived personal benefits: weight loss.
- Stage of readiness to change physical activity: contemplation.
- Enjoyed dance as a child but was not active as an adolescent or young adult; aerobics classes were too strenuous; enjoys walking in neighborhood; doesn't like cold weather; knows exercise is important.

Intervention

- Educate about physical activity's role in weight loss and especially in maintenance of weight loss.
- Educate on the personally relevant benefits of moderate-intensity physical activity, especially weight management, stress management, energy enhancement, and cardiovascular disease risk reduction.
- Educate on accumulation of activity throughout the day.
- Short-term goal (next 2 weeks): keep a log of thoughts about physical activity and actual physical activity; do one brisk 2-minute walk per day for 10 of the next 14 days.

- Long-term goal (in 5 months): accumulate at least 150 minutes of moderate-intensity activity per week.

Encounter 2: March 15

Assessment

- Log indicated increased number of thoughts about physical activity in second week; did not log activity time.
- Achieved goal for 2-minute walks on 5 days; has a hard time remembering to think about being more active.
- Family responsibilities often upset her physical activity plans.
- Purchased comfortable walking shoes.

Intervention

- Dora brainstormed ways to fit physical activity into family time (walk around soccer field, go dancing with husband on "date night," walk the dog after dinner).
- Reinforced role of physical activity in weight loss and prevention of weight regain.
- Short-term goal(s) (next 2 weeks): keep a log of thoughts about physical activity and actual physical activity; do one brisk 2-minute walk per day for 10 of the next 14 days; do at least one activity with family that is active.
- Long-term goal (in 5 months): accumulate at least 150 minutes of moderate-intensity activity per week.

Encounter 3: March 30

Assessment

- Continuing to increase number of thoughts about physical activity; logged activity for 2 weeks.
- Achieved goal for 2-minute walks on 10 days; family walked to church together one day (15 minutes each way); walked around ball field during son's game for 10 minutes.
- Knees hurt during walk to church.
- Feels more confident about ability to fit in short bouts of activity; wants to do more.
- Administration of "Readiness to Change" flowsheet shows Dora is still in contemplation stage.

Intervention

- Discussed need to be more gradual in increasing activity to prevent pain and injury.
- Encouraged Dora to identify sedentary activities that she does and ways to make them more active.

- Short-term goal(s) (next 4 weeks): keep a log of thoughts about physical activity and actual physical activity; do two brisk 5-minute walks per day for at least 5 days each week; turn one sedentary activity into an opportunity for activity.
- Long-term goal (in 5 months): accumulate at least 150 minutes of moderate-intensity activity per week.

Encounter 4: May 1

Assessment

- Logged activity for 3 of 4 weeks; accumulated more than 30 minutes on 5 days during this period!
- Achieved goal for 5-minute walks (two per day) for 4 weeks; walked instead of drove to neighbor's for monthly bridge game; continued walking at soccer games for 15 minutes twice per week (found two other mothers to walk with her); walks dogs for 10 to 15 minutes several times per week.
- Has a hard time fitting in walks on days that she works at the newspaper publisher.
- Beginning to feel less tired when walking and has a little more energy, but getting a little bored with walking.
- Administration of "Readiness to Change" flowsheet shows Dora has moved to preparation stage.

Intervention

- Encouraged Dora to increase number of 5-minute walks; point out how close she is to reaching long-term goal of at least 150 minutes per week; encouraged her to find new activities or people with whom to do activities.
- Short-term goal(s) (next 4 weeks): keep a log of physical activity; do two brisk 10-minute walks per day for at least 5 days per week; walk to part-time job (20 minutes) at least 2 days per week.
- Long-term goal (in 5 months): accumulate at least 150 minutes of moderate-intensity activity per week.

Encounter 5: June 1

Assessment

- Logged activity for first 2 weeks only; stress at work, lost logging sheets, and end of school year activities prevented logging.
- Unsure what, if any, goals she met since last visit; she did think about being active and fit in some walks; did not walk to job.
- Feeling "stressed out," having a hard time making time for herself.
- Very discouraged and ready to give up.

- Administration of "Readiness to Change" flowsheet shows Dora has lapsed back to contemplation stage.

Intervention

- Praised her for doing what she could under the circumstances.
- Discussed the inevitability of lapses; described importance of positive thinking to prevent a lapse from becoming a relapse; encouraged Dora to analyze what contributed to the lapse and to learn from it.
- Emphasized the importance of physical activity in managing stress.
- Introduced the step counter as a simple method for logging activity; demonstrated its use.
- Short-term goal(s) (next 6 weeks): keep a log of steps taken each day; increase average daily number of steps by 200 to 500 steps each week after first week; build back up to doing at least two brisk 10-minute walks per day for at least 5 days per week; walk to part-time job (20 minutes) at least 2 days per week; find ways to be active with family.
- Long-term goal (in 5 months): accumulate at least 150 minutes of moderate-intensity activity per week; do strength-building exercises on 2 days per week.

Encounter 6: July 15

Assessment

- Loved step counter! Averaged 6,300 steps the first week; increased 500+ daily steps per week so she is now averaging nearly 10,000 steps per day.
- Administration of "Readiness to Change" flowsheet shows Dora has progressed to the action stage.
- Feeling more confident after recovering from her lapse; not as stressed out.
- Blood pressure has decreased and her knees do not hurt as much.

Intervention

- Praised her for reaching her long-term goal.
- Reviewed the strategies that worked best for her. Reminded her that she will need to keep using these strategies to maintain her activity level.
- Reminded her about the long-term benefits of physical activity regardless of weight loss and the importance of activity for long-term weight management.
- Encouraged her to increase daily activity time gradually to 60 minutes or to begin to include more vigorous activities by trying new activities.
- Made plans for maintaining activity level when weather turns cold and icy (get comfortable, safe boots to wear so she can still walk to work, check ads for used treadmills or stationary bikes, walk at shopping mall, learn to cross-country ski).

- Short-term goal(s) (next 4 weeks): increase activity time by 10 minutes to 40 minutes per day; go dancing with husband at least three times per month; find new physical activities to enjoy.
- Long-term goal (in 6 months): accumulate at least 45 to 60 minutes of moderate-intensity activity 5 or more days per week; do strength-building exercises 2 days per week.

SPECIAL TOPICS IN PHYSICAL ACTIVITY FOR WEIGHT MANAGEMENT

In trying to be better equipped to provide physical activity guidance to overweight clients, clinicians often have questions about the role of strength training in weight management. In addition, many clinicians want help with physical activity issues that are of particular concern for severely obese clients. We conclude this chapter by addressing these two important topics.

The Role of Strength Training in Weight Management

This chapter has focused primarily on moderate-intensity lifestyle activities as the preferred type of physical activity for clients who are overweight or obese. Moderate-intensity activities (*a*) can provide weight management and health benefits; (*b*) can remove the barrier of getting a medical clearance before exercising for many clients; (*c*) do not require special equipment or instruction and can be incorporated into many daily routines; and (*d*) are appropriate for those who are not physically fit enough to start with vigorous activities. Still, it is important to recognize the role that strength or resistance training (considered a vigorous activity) can have in promoting health and maintaining weight.

First, as individuals lose weight, they often lose muscle tissue. Because muscle is very metabolically active—ie, it burns a lot of calories all day—muscle loss can lead to a decrease in total daily energy expenditure and, hence, difficulty in preventing weight regain. Any physical activity will help to attenuate this loss, but strength training may be the most effective exercise for minimizing muscle loss. Second, new studies suggest that resistance training may have health benefits independent of total physical activity level (11). Third, strength training can improve an individual's ability to perform daily tasks such as carrying groceries, climbing stairs, getting up from a sofa or chair, and general mobility. Finally, strength training can tone muscles, which may help reduce the appearance of sagging skin that some overweight individuals experience after losing weight.

From a practical perspective, strength-building activities are a great complement to aerobic activity. In fact, the new Physical Activity Guidelines for Americans state, "Adults should also do muscle-strengthening activities that are moderate or high intensity and involve all major muscle groups on two or more days a week" (3).

Most obese clients are not ready to do strength training activities at the beginning of treatment. However, as clients gain more fitness and more confidence in their ability to be active, clinicians can recommend strength training as another important component of a healthful lifestyle. There are many tools that can help clients improve their strength and fitness, including resistance bands, hand weights, calisthenics (ie, using own body weight as resistance), weight machines, and free weights. Each of these methods requires some instruction. Some equipment comes with directions for use. In the absence of specialized training in this area, it best to refer your clients to certified personal trainers or to exercise physiologists for strength training instruction.

Issues for the Severely Obese

Although being physically active is healthful for people of every weight, severely obese clients may have special concerns. Orthopedic problems, body image issues, health risk factors, balance problems, and chafing can be roadblocks to physical activity for many obese clients. Some obese clients may want to wait until they have lost weight before they start increasing their activity. Be mindful not to ignore the topic of physical activity with these individuals, however. Instead, use the strategies outlined in Table 6.2 for precontemplators and contemplators.

For severely obese clients who do want to begin doing some activity, the following are suggestions for coping with some of the common problems they may face. Also, many of the resources listed in Box 6.2 are specifically relevant to this population.

- Orthopedic or balance problems: non–weight-bearing activities, such as water exercise classes, chair aerobics, and recumbent stationary cycling, are good options.
- Body image issues: suggest videos/DVDs they use at home (see Box 6.2); seek out exercise facilities/instructors who are sensitive to clients with severe obesity.
- Health risk factors: Use the assessment guidelines in this chapter to evaluate the need to seek medical clearance before increasing physical activity level; periodically check risk-factor status to determine whether adjustments to medication are needed.
- Chafing: encourage very gradual increase in activity; tight clothing will minimize chafing better than loose clothing; areas that rub should be kept as dry as possible (talcum or baby powder can help); or a lubricant, such as bag balm, petroleum jelly, or another lubricating gel, can be used.

When working with severely obese clients, it is important to remember that although they may have some issues that require special consideration, you should treat them as you would any overweight client—that is, match your recommendations to their readiness to change, their physical activity interests, and their abilities.

FINAL NOTE

Remember, even if your clients do not lose any weight after increasing their physical activity level, they are likely to be healthier than when they started. The following are a few final preparations that you can make to be ready to provide physical activity guidance to your overweight clients.

- Complete the PAR-Q form yourself so that you are familiar with it and know when a referral to a physician is necessary. (The form can be downloaded from http://www. csep.ca.)

Box 6.2
Additional Resources[a]

Books

Jonas S, Konner L. Just *the Weigh You Are: How to Be Fit and Healthy Whatever Your Size*. New York, NY: Houghton Mifflin Company; 1998.

Lyons P, Burgard D. *Great Shape: The First Fitness Guide for Large Women*. Palo Alto, CA: Bull Publishing Company; 1990.

Marcus BH, Forsyth LH. *Motivating People to Be Physically Active*. Champaign, IL: Human Kinetics; 2003.

Pappas Baun M. *Fantastic Water Workouts*, 2nd ed. Champaign, IL: Human Kinetics; 2007.

Prochaska JO, Norcross JC, DiClemente CC. *Changing for Good*. New York, NY: Avon Books: 1994.

Sullivan J. *Size Wise: A Catalog of More Than 1000 Resources for Living With Confidence and Comfort at Any Size*. New York, NY: Avon Books; 1997.

Pamphlet

National Institutes of Diabetes and Digestive and Kidney Diseases. *Active at Any Size*. October 2006. NIH pub 04-4352. http://win.niddk.nih.gov/publications/active.htm. Accessed November 14, 2008.

Videos

Yoga for Round Bodies: Three 30-minute classes using traditional yoga poses adapted for large bodies. Available through online bookstores.

Chair Dancing: Videos designed to improve muscle tone, flexibility, and cardiovascular endurance without putting stress on knees, back, hips, or feet. 800/551-4386 or http://www.chairdancing.com.

Step Counter Distributors

Accusplit: 800/935-1996 or http://www.accusplit.com

Walk4Life: 888-422-1806 or http://walk4life.com

Organizations and Programs

Council on Size and Weight Discrimination: 914/679-1209 or http://www.cswd.org.

National Association to Advance Fat Acceptance: 916/558-6880 or http://www.naafa.org.

Weight-control Information Network: 877/946-4627 or http://win.niddk.nih.gov/index.htm.

Web Sites

Choose to Move: A 12-week program from the American Heart Association designed to help women begin a personalized physical activity program. http://www.choosetomove.org.

Healthy Living with Bliss: Includes information and resources related to fitness activities for large and very large people. http://www.KellyBliss.com.

Start! A Web site from the American Heart Association that focuses on getting individuals and organizations to start moving through walking. htpp://www.americanheart.org/start

StrongWomen: This interactive Web site includes three specialized fitness programs, health information, recipes, and tips for empowering women. http://www.strongwomen.com.

[a]Parts of this resource list were adapted from National Institutes of Diabetes and Digestive and Kidney Diseases *Active at Any Size*, NIH Publication No. 04-4352, October 2006. These resources are included for information only and do not imply endorsement by the authors.

- Use the "Readiness to Change" flowsheet (Figure 6.1) to assess your readiness to change your own physical activity level.
- Develop a referral list of exercise physiologists or certified personal trainers who are capable of working with overweight clients who want to do more vigorous exercise.

References

1. Dunn AL, Garcia ME, Kohl HW 3rd, Blair SN. Comparison of lifestyle and structured interventions to increase physical activity and cardiorespiratory fitness: a randomized trial. *JAMA*. 1999;281:327–334.

2. Sevick MA, Dunn AL, Morrow MS, Marcus BH, Chen GJ, Blair SN. Cost-effectiveness of lifestyle and structured exercise interventions in sedentary adults: results of Project ACTIVE. *Am J Prev Med*. 2000;19:1–8.

3. *2008 Physical Activity Guidelines for Americans*. Washington, DC: Department of Health and Human Services; 2008. ODPHP Publication no. U0036.

4. Carpenter RA. Going the extra mile to obtain fitness certifications. *Weight Management Dietetic Practice Group Newsletter*. 2007;4(4).

5. Jakicic JM, Wing RR, Butler BA, Robertson RJ. Prescribing exercise in multiple short bouts versus one continuous bout: effects on adherence, cardiorespiratory fitness, and weight loss in overweight women. *Int J Obes Relat Metab Disord*. 1995;19:893–901.

6. Physical Activity Readiness Questionnaire (PAR-Q). Canadian Society of Exercise Physiology Web site. http://www.csep.ca/forms.asp. Accessed November 14, 2008.

7. Prochaska JO, Norcross JC, DiClemente CC. *Changing for Good: A Revolutionary Six-Stage Program for Overcoming Bad Habits and Moving Your Life Positively Forward*. New York, NY: Avon Books; 1994.

8. Blair SN, Dunn AL, Marcus BH, Carpenter RA, Jaret P. *Active Living Every Day*. Champaign, IL: Human Kinetics; 2001.

9. American Dietetic Association. Adult Weight Management Evidence Based Nutrition Practice Guideline. http://www.adaevidencelibrary.com/topic.cfm?cat=2798. Accessed November 14, 2008.

10. American Dietetic Association. Adult Weight Management Toolkit. 2007. http://www.adaevidencelibrary.com. Accessed November 14, 2008.

11. Tanasescu M, Leitzmann MF, Rimm EB, Willett WC, Stampfer MJ, Hu FB. Exercise type and intensity in relation to coronary heart disease in men. *JAMA*. 2002;288:1994–2000.

Acknowledgment: The author would like to thank William J. Wilkinson, MD, for reading an earlier draft of this manuscript.

CHAPTER 7

BEHAVIOR MODIFICATION

PART A: OVERVIEW

JOHN P. FOREYT, PHD

All of us who counsel obese patients have heard the familiar mantra of intervention: diet, physical activity, and behavior modification. The diet and physical activity interventions are reviewed in Chapters 2 through 6. This chapter focuses on the behavior part of the triad. What exactly is behavior modification? What is the scientific evidence for its efficacy? What about *behavior therapy, behavioral treatment, cognitive-behavior therapy*, and *lifestyle modification*? Do these terms all refer to the same principles and techniques, or is there something different about each of them?

First, let's be clear about the terms. On a practical, clinical level the terms *behavior modification, behavior therapy, behavioral treatment, cognitive-behavior therapy*, and *lifestyle modification* are all fairly synonymous. Technically, they differ slightly. For example, *behavior modification* refers to strategies developed through research on animals and humans based on learning theories. When applied to humans in a treatment setting, it becomes *behavior therapy*. *Lifestyle modification* refers specifically to strategies for achieving a healthful diet and exercise. But today all these terms are typically used interchangeably in the obesity field to refer to a combination of strategies to help make it easier for obese individuals to do what they want to do—ie, lose weight and maintain their losses.

From a historical perspective, behavior modification was originally based on learning theories, both classical and operant conditioning (1). Becoming obese was seen as the result of undesirable behaviors that needed modifying, ie, overeating and underexercising (2,3). Learning theorists speculated that these unhealthful behaviors could easily be corrected by applying classical and operant conditioning strategies. Several interesting research papers, many of them published in the 1960s and 1970s, imply that these conditioning approaches were effective and would be the solution to cure obesity (4,5). Although of interest to students of behavior theory, these historical behavior interventions typically were of short duration, with small numbers of oftentimes highly selected participants. We hopefully have learned a lot since those early studies. Today, we recognize that obesity may result from more than bad habits. Genetic, metabolic, hormonal, cultural, and psychological factors can play a role in development of obesity and make it more difficult for some individuals to lose much weight. For those individuals, focusing on the health benefits of improving their diets and physical activity, rather than on weight loss, seems to make more sense.

Today, behavior modification for managing obesity means teaching clients specific skills to make it easier for them to modify their diet and improve their physical activity to lose and maintain a more healthful weight. Behavior modification strategies focus on clients' current behaviors. It is not psychotherapy. It is not focused on how they were raised or their relationships with their parents during childhood. Behavior modification focuses on the here and now, with an emphasis on improving current dietary and physical activity patterns. It is based on problem-solving and goal-setting. It involves small changes that are thought to be more easily made and have a better chance of being maintained than large ones that typically do not last.

STANDARD BEHAVIOR MODIFICATION

Today, standard behavior modification almost always involves a package—several strategies tailored to a client's specific needs. The individual strategies include goal-setting, self-monitoring, stimulus control, cognitive restructuring, stress management, social support, and relapse prevention (6,7).

Goal-setting

Goal-setting involves helping clients make specific and realistic plans for changing their behaviors. The primary goal for most clients in behavioral weight-loss programs is to lose 1 to 2 pounds (0.5 to 1.0 kg) per week. Clients are prescribed diets of approximately 1,200 kcal/d for women and 1,500 kcal/d for men. Physical activity of approximately 30 minutes per day for 5 days per week is recommended (8).

Unfortunately, many obese clients begin their weight-loss program with unrealistic goals. For example, Foster and colleagues (9) reported that obese individuals commonly expect to lose 25% to 32% of their body weight. Even informing clients about their probable weight losses had little effect on their unrealistically high expectations (10). Such unreasonable and unachievable expectations can lead some clients to dismiss the likely benefits of a modest, realistic weight loss, leading to poor morale and poor maintenance, and high attrition rates in treatment programs.

A goal of 10% weight loss over 24 weeks is reasonable for most obese clients. Goals need to be quantifiable. Rather than a goal of "I'll do better next week," clients are asked to set specific objectives, such as "I will walk for 30 minutes on Monday, Wednesday, and Friday at 8:00 AM." Goals should also be time-limited, usually a week or two, and realistic, but somewhat challenging. Achieving realistic goals provides feelings of accomplishment, which can be reinforcing for clients (11).

Self-monitoring

Self-monitoring refers to the systematic observation, recording, and feedback of specific target behaviors. At a minimum, clients are asked to record their food, physical activity, and weight. Often, clients also are asked to record additional behaviors, such as time of day they eat and exercise, their mood states, and other factors that might influence their intake or physical activity. The recording is frequently used by registered dietitians (RDs) to assess how their clients are doing, to identify potential problems that need addressing, and to make suggestions for change. However, self-monitoring has another even more important role. That role is to increase clients' awareness of their eating, physical activity, and weight. The act of observing and recording one's behaviors will often have the effect of changing those behaviors in the desired direction (12–14).

In addition to observing and recording key behaviors, the third element, that of feedback, should not be overlooked. The feedback can be provided by the RD, but ideally should come from the clients themselves. It may include the client looking up the calories consumed from the food record, the number of minutes walked, the steps on the pedometer, or the calories expended. Yes, clients underreport their intake on food records by approximately one third (15,16) and overreport their physical activity by a half or so (17). It does not matter. Remember, the most important goal of self-monitoring is to increase clients' awareness of their eating, physical activity, and weight. For example, daily self-weighing has been shown to be associated with less weight regain in individuals who were trying to maintain weight loss (18). Weighing on a regular schedule provides consistent feedback about how a client's diet and physical activity are affecting positive changes. If RDs incorporate only one behavioral strategy into their client interventions, research suggests that it should be self-monitoring.

Stimulus Control

Stimulus control involves managing the cues associated with overeating and underexercising (19). For the RD, it typically involves helping clients change their daily environment to make it easier to eat more healthfully and be more physically active. Examples include encouraging clients to remove high-fat foods from their homes, change the way they drive home if they have trouble passing the local fast-food restaurant, lay out their exercise clothes before they go to bed, or turn off the computer or television when they are eating. Stimulus control strategies work best when individuals identify their own cues for eating and figure out their own strategies for changing them, rather than having the RD provide the answers.

Cognitive Restructuring

Cognitive restructuring helps clients improve their unhealthful beliefs about their ability to make healthful lifestyle changes (20,21). Clients can be asked to self-monitor their thoughts that may be making it difficult to achieve their goals and replace them with more realistic ones. The client might be asked to repeat a positive affirmation several times a day. The assumption is that clients can more effectively change their behaviors by changing unhealthful thoughts. Although sometimes helpful, cognitive restructuring is supported by less evidence than some of the other behavior modification strategies, such as self-monitoring.

Stress Management

Overeating can be a coping mechanism for stress and negative emotions. One study reported that individuals reporting the highest emotion- and stress-related eating on a questionnaire were 13.38 times more likely to be overweight or obese as compared with individuals scoring the lowest on those factors (22). RDs can teach clients several strategies, including increased physical activity, meditation, and progressive relaxation, when stress interferes with program goals.

Social Support

Social support is an important component of behavioral interventions, although the evidence for its long-term effectiveness is mixed (23,24). Support from groups such as Weight Watchers or Take Off Pounds Sensibly (TOPS) may provide motivation to help clients make changes ("If they can do it, so can I"). Families, close friends, coworkers, and counselors can serve as potential sources of support for the client attempting to make positive changes. Unfortunately, some potential sources of support, such as spouses, can also serve as saboteurs and undermine the behavior modification process. Picking the right sources of support can make the difference between success and failure.

Relapse Prevention

Relapse prevention strategies emphasize that lapses are normal, to be expected, and a natural part of attempts to lose and maintain weight (25). RDs can help clients anticipate the situations in which lapses may occur, such as holidays, vacations, and eating away from home, and help them plan behavioral strategies to cope with the events. The behavioral goal is to prevent the lapses from becoming relapses. Unfortunately, research studies have not strongly supported the role of relapse prevention strategies in helping with long-term maintenance (26).

STRUCTURE OF STANDARD BEHAVIOR MODIFICATION PROGRAMS

The structure of standard behavior modification programs has evolved over the past few decades. Typically, clients are asked to attend 60- to 90-minute weekly group meetings led by an RD or other health care professional. The standard intervention has increased from 8 to 24 weekly group sessions (26). Group sizes typically range from 8 to 15 participants. The standard program also can be taught by an RD in individual client sessions.

Both group and individual approaches have advantages and disadvantages. The major advantages of group sessions are that larger numbers of clients can be seen at once by an RD and the group can be a source of support for participants. The disadvantage is that there is less time to tailor programs for each client. Individual sessions provide more time for tailoring, but fewer clients can be seen and support from fellow participants is lacking. Overall, group sessions are preferable. Lifestyle interventions are best delivered by a multidisciplinary team of health care professionals, including RDs, behavioral specialists, and personal trainers/exercise physiologists (27). Physicians also serve as team members and tend to focus on the client's medical management. Today, because of busy schedules and time pressures, the Internet and other technological approaches increasingly are being used to present standard behavioral programs (28).

RESULTS OF BEHAVIOR MODIFICATION INTERVENTIONS

Individual behavior modification strategies typically have not been researched. For example, there are few intervention programs that test only cognitive restructuring, or only stress management, or only social support for obesity management. Rather, the research has tested a combination of behavioral strategies for achieving weight loss. Published reviews have clearly documented the beneficial effects of the combination of diet, physical activity, and behavior modification (26). Randomized clinical trials, considered the gold standard in research, show that this combination, usually delivered in weekly group sessions of approximately 16 to 24 weeks, leads to mean weight losses of 5% to 10% (5 to 10 kg) (26). Mean weight losses of 5% to 10% typically result in positive changes in blood pressure, blood glucose, blood lipids, insulin sensitivity, endothelial function, and psychological well-being, and reduced thrombosis and inflammatory markers (26,29).

Long-term maintenance of initial losses has been less successful. A review that summarized the results of 21 studies that included 25 behavioral intervention groups with follow-ups of 2 years or more showed that few obese patients succeed at maintaining losses of 10 kg or more over the long term (26). However, studies showing long-term weight-loss outcomes of 5% were more encouraging. Since 2000, eight studies (out of 15) have reported mean weight loss outcomes of 5% or more at 2 years (26). These interventions typically involved an intensive weight-maintenance program that included monthly or bimonthly meetings during the entire 2 years. The attrition rate at 2 years was a mean of 39%, suggesting that the results may be somewhat lower than reported (individuals who gained their weight back are less likely to return for follow-up assessments). The bottom line, however, suggests that with extended follow-up intervention programs, some individuals are able to maintain modest but clinically significant losses of 5% to 10% for at least 2 years.

It is important to consider what might have happened to these individuals without intervention. Obese individuals gain approximately 0.6 kg per year (30). Also, looking only at mean weight losses hides that fact that some individuals have long-term success. For example, one study reported that approximately 20% of their patients maintained losses of 5 kg or more for 4 years or more (31). Although not everyone succeeds in long-term maintenance, many do very well.

EXAMPLES OF SUCCESSFUL BEHAVIOR MODIFICATION INTERVENTIONS

Diabetes Prevention Program

The Diabetes Prevention Program (DPP) is an outstanding example demonstrating the implementation of a behavioral intervention for preventing or delaying the onset of type 2 diabetes in overweight and obese individuals at risk for its development (32). The researchers randomly assigned 3,234 nondiabetic overweight and obese adults at risk for the disease to placebo, metformin, or a lifestyle-modification program, with a goal of 7% weight loss and 150 minutes of physical activity per week for all participants. The lifestyle-modification participants received a 16-week curriculum covering diet, physical activity, and behavior modification. The curriculum was taught by case managers on a one-to-one basis during the first 24 weeks. Subsequent individual sessions, usually monthly, and group sessions were added to reinforce the behavior changes.

Mean weight loss in the lifestyle-modification group was 6.7 kg after 1 year, compared with mean weight losses of 2.7 kg and 0.4 kg in the metformin and placebo groups, respectively. At 4 years, the lifestyle group had maintained losses of 3.5 kg, compared with 1.3 kg and 0.2 kg in the metformin and placebo groups, respectively. Most striking, compared with the placebo group, the lifestyle-modification intervention reduced the incidence of diabetes by 58% whereas incidence in the metformin intervention group was reduced by 31% (32). The lifestyle-modification intervention was significantly more effective than metformin. The study clearly demonstrated the efficacy of a lifestyle intervention for improving long-term health benefits.

Look AHEAD (Action for Health in Diabetes)

The Look AHEAD (Action for Health in Diabetes) study is a second example showing the efficacy of behavior modification (33). Look AHEAD is a multicenter, randomized controlled trial designed to determine whether modest weight losses reduce cardiovascular morbidity and mortality in overweight and obese individuals with type 2 diabetes. The researchers randomly assigned 5,145 adults with diabetes to either a lifestyle-modification intervention or a usual-care group. The intervention goals included a 7% weight loss and 175 minutes of physical activity per week. Individuals assigned to the lifestyle-modification intervention attended 24 treatment sessions during the first 6 months. The study combined both group and individual sessions. Between 6 and 12 months, participants attended three sessions per month. The behavior modification protocol included food and physical activity self-monitoring, eating at regular times, limiting times and places of eating, cognitive restructuring, and relapse prevention. Participants who struggled to meet study goals were offered special interventions from an intervention "toolbox" (34).

Results at 1 year exceeded study goals. Participants assigned to the lifestyle-modification group lost a mean of 8.6% of their initial weight compared with 0.7% in the usual-care group (33). The significant weight loss was associated with improved diabetes control and cardiovascular risk factors and reduced medication needs in the lifestyle-modification group compared with the usual-care group. The study is currently ongoing, and continued intervention and follow-up will determine whether these changes are maintained. Look AHEAD is the first randomized controlled trial to assess whether a behavioral intervention aimed at weight reduction will reduce cardiovascular morbidity and mortality. Both DPP (32) and Look AHEAD (33) demonstrate that RDs can successfully intervene to implement a behavior modification intervention to induce weight loss, which is associated with considerable health benefits.

THE FUTURE OF BEHAVIOR MODIFICATION

Research studies with long-term follow-up typically show a pattern in which individuals regain lost weight. One hope for long-term maintenance seems to be extended interventions. Unfortunately, this is not the answer for all people. Extended intervention is too labor-intensive and expensive to be very practical for all but a few individuals. Motivation wanes and attrition increases after initial interventions. The seemingly inevitable weight regain is probably the result of psychological, physiological, and environmental factors making it extremely difficult to maintain initial losses.

Research strategies that have attempted to improve maintenance but to date have not seemed to be appreciably effective long-term include peer group meetings, relapse-prevention training, supervised group exercise, the use of personal trainers, and using monetary incentives for either weight loss or exercise (26). Research has shown some positive evidence for improving maintenance with strategies such as extending intervention beyond 6 months with weekly or biweekly sessions, and providing multicomponent interventions with ongoing client-counselor contact in person or via telephone or mail. Other strategies that have shown some promise include the use of no-cost meal replacements, home-based exercise programs aimed at achieving high levels of physical activity, the use of home exercise equipment, and pharmacotherapy (26).

The greatest challenge for RDs and other health care professionals is to improve behavioral strategies for the long-term management of obesity. For effective management, obesity, like type 2 diabetes and hypertension, requires intensive programs of ongoing care. Registered dietitians, trained in behavior modification, seem to be the ideal case managers.

References

1. Ullmann LP, Krasner L, eds. *Case Studies in Behavior Modification.* New York, NY: Holt, Rinehart and Winston; 1965.

2. Ferster CB, Nurnberger JI, Levitt E. The control of eating. *J Mathetics.* 1962;1: 87–109.

3. Stuart RB. Behavioral control of overeating. *Behav Res Ther.* 1967;5:357–365.

4. Foreyt JP, ed. *Behavioral Treatments of Obesity.* New York, NY: Pergamon Press; 1977.

5. Walen S, Hauserman NM, Lavin PJ. *Clinical Guide to Behavior Therapy.* Baltimore, MD: Williams & Wilkins; 1977.

6. Foreyt JP, Poston WSC. What is the role of cognitive behavior therapy in patient management? *Obes Res.* 1998;6(suppl):18S–22S.

7. Berkel LA, Poston WSC, Reeves RS, Foreyt JP. Behavioral interventions for obesity. *J Am Diet Assoc.* 2005;105(suppl):S35–S43.

8. Foreyt JP, Pendleton VR. Management of obesity. *Primary Care Rep.* 2000;6:19–30.

9. Foster GD, Wadden TA, Vogt RA, Brewer G. What is a reasonable weight loss? Patients' expectations and evaluations of obesity treatment outcomes. *J Consult Clin Psychol.* 1997;65:79–85.

10. Wadden TA, Womble LG, Sarwer DB, Berkowitz RI, Clark VL, Foster GD. Great expectations: "I'm losing 25% of my weight no matter what you say." *J Consult Clin Psychol.* 2003;71:1084–1087.

11. Bandura A, Simon KM. The role of proximal intentions in self-regulation of refractory behavior. *Cognit Ther Res.* 1977;1:177–193.

12. Foreyt JP, Goodrick GK. Factors common to successful therapy of the obese patient. *Med Sci Sports Exerc.* 1991;23:292–297.

13. Wadden TA, Letizia KA. Predictors of attrition and weight loss in patients treated by moderate and severe caloric restriction. In: Wadden TA, Van Itallie TB, eds. *Treatment of the Seriously Obese Patient.* New York, NY: Guilford Press;1992:383–410.

14. Baker RC, Kirschenbaum DS. Self-monitoring may be necessary for successful weight control. *Behav Ther.* 1993;24:377–394.

15. de Vries JH, Zock PL, Mensink RP, Kaan MB. Underestimation of energy intake by 3-d records compared with energy intake to maintain body weight in 269 nonobese adults. *Am J Clin Nutr.* 1994;60:855–860.

16. Tooze JA, Subar AF, Thompson FE, Troiano R, Schatzkin A, Kipnis V. Psychosocial predictors of energy underreporting in a large doubly labeled water study. *Am J Clin Nutr.* 2004;79:795–804.

17. Lichtman SW, Piscarka K, Berman ER, Pestone M, Dowling H, Offenbacher E, Weisel H, Heshka S, Matthews DE, Heymsfield SB. Discrepancy between self-reported and actual caloric intake and exercise in obese subjects. *N Engl J Med.* 1992;327:1893–1898.

18. Wing RR, Tate DF, Gorin AA, Raynor HA, Fava JL. A self-regulation program for maintenance of weight loss. *N Engl J Med.* 2006;355:1563–1571.

19. McReynolds WT, Paulsen, BK. Stimulus control as the behavioral basis of weight loss procedures. In: Williams BJ, Martin S, Foreyt JP, eds. *Obesity: Behavioral Approaches to Dietary Management.* New York, NY: Brunner/Mazel; 1976:43–64.

20. Foreyt JP, Rathjen DP, eds. *Cognitive Behavior Therapy: Research and Application.* New York, NY: Plenum Press; 1978.

21. Dobson KS, ed. *Handbook of Cognitive-Behavioral Therapies.* New York, NY: Guilford Press; 2001.

22. Ozier AD, Kendrick OW, Leeper JD, Knol LL, Perko M, Burnham J. Overweight and obesity are associated with emotion- and stress-related eating as measured by the Eating and Appraisal Due to Emotions and Stress Questionnaire. *J Am Diet Assoc.* 2008;108:49–56.

23. Wing RR, Jeffery RW. Benefits of recruiting participants with friends and increasing social support for weight loss and maintenance. *J Consult Clin Psychol.* 1999;66:132–138.

24. Milsom VA, Perri MG, Rejeski WJ. Guided group support and the long-term management of obesity. In: Latner JD, Wilson GT, eds. *Self-Help for Obesity and Binge Eating.* New York, NY: Guilford; 2006:205–222.

25. Marlatt GA, Gordon JR, eds. *Relapse Prevention.* New York, NY: Guilford; 1985.

26. Perri MG, Foreyt JP, Anton SD. Preventing weight regain after weight loss. In: Bray GA. Bouchard. C, eds. *Handbook of Obesity.* 2nd ed. New York, NY: Marcel Dekker; 2008:249–268.

27. Melanson KJ, McInnis KJ, Rippe JM. Modern management of obesity: the value of a multidisciplinary approach. In: Foreyt JP, Poston WSC, McInnis KJ, Rippe JM, eds. *Lifestyle Obesity Management.* Malden, MA: Blackwell; 2003:1–33.

28. Tyler C, Johnston CA, Foreyt JP. Lifestyle management of obesity. *Am J Lifestyle Med.* 2007;1:423–429.

29. Aronne LJ, Brown WV, Isoldi KK. Cardiovascular disease in obesity: a review of related risk factors and risk-reduction strategies. *J Clin Lipid.* 2007;1:575–582.

30. Shah M, Hannan PJ, Jeffery RW. Secular trends in body mass index in the adult population of three communities from the upper mid-western part of the USA: the Minnesota Heart Health Program. *Int J Obes Relat Metab Disord.* 1991;15: 499–503.

31. Kramer FM, Jeffery RW, Forster JL, Snell, MK. Long-term follow-up of behavioral treatment for obesity: patterns of weight regain among men and women. *Int J Obes Relat Metab Disord.* 1989;13:123–126.

32. Diabetes Prevention Program Research Group. Reduction in the incidence of type 2 diabetes with lifestyle intervention or metformin. *N Engl J Med.* 2002;346: 393–403.

33. The Look AHEAD Research Group. Reduction in weight and cardiovascular disease risk factors in individuals with type 2 diabetes: one-year results of the Look AHEAD trial. *Diabetes Care.* 2007;30:1374–1383.

34. The Look AHEAD Research Group. The Look AHEAD study: a description of the lifestyle intervention and the evidence supporting it. *Obesity.* 2006;14:737–752.

PART B: PRACTICAL APPLICATIONS

MOLLY GEE, MED, RD, AND REBECCA REEVES, DRPH, RD

Evidence-based practice is the gold standard of any medical treatment, disease prevention program, or health promotion (1,2). This sets registered dietitians (RDs) apart from others in weight management. The American Dietetic Association (ADA) Evidence Analysis Library (EAL) Adult Weight Management Guideline concludes (2, p.77):

A comprehensive weight management program should make maximum use of multiple strategies for behavior therapy (eg, self monitoring, stress management, stimulus control, problem solving, contingency management, cognitive restructuring, and social support). Behavior therapy in addition to diet and physical activity leads to additional weight loss. Continued behavioral interventions may be necessary to prevent a return to baseline weight.

Nutrition counseling, including behavior modification strategies, is an integral part of ADA's Nutrition Care Process (NCP), which consists of four interrelated steps: nutrition assessment, nutrition diagnosis, nutrition intervention, and nutrition monitoring and evaluation (3,4). This process is defined as "a systematic problem-solving method that dietetics professionals use to critically think and make decisions to address nutrition related problems and provide safe and effective quality nutrition care" (3). Step 3 of the NCP, nutrition intervention, identifies behavior-modification strategies as key tools for behavior change.

This chapter takes a practical look at the *what, where, when,* and *how* issues related to our application of these strategies or interventions. In the first part of this chapter,

John Foreyt, PhD, answered the "*what*" with a comprehensive description of the behavior-modification techniques plus a review of recent randomized clinical trials using behavior-modification strategies.

Behavior-modification strategies focus on restructuring a client's environment to reduce habits or actions thought to contribute to inappropriate behaviors. For example, graphic food commercials on television have motivated many clients to get up and "shop" in the refrigerator or pantry. Food records can provide startling insight into cues that trigger inappropriate eating behavior and lack of physical activity. "All-or-nothing thinking"—ie, a client believes he or she must follow the diet "perfectly"—often sabotages a weight-loss plan. Using reframing or cognitive restructuring and goal-setting, the RD provides a reality check to help the client stay on course. Self-monitoring, goal-setting, stimulus control, problem-solving, stress management, cognitive restructuring, and social support are the most common techniques to achieve behavior change (4–6).

Where should behavior modification strategies be used? RDs work in a variety of practice settings, from acute clinical care to disease prevention and health promotion. Inpatient or outpatient clinics, community centers, public health clinics, research intervention protocols, corporate programs, private practice, and schools are just some of the places where behavior change will be prescribed. One-on-one or group settings can be equally effective. Groups can become a primary source of social support for clients, and some medical and commercial weight-management programs structure weekly meetings for that reason. The Look AHEAD study (discussed in Part A of this chapter) structured the intervention arm with a combination of both group and individual sessions.

Practitioners should tailor any strategy based on their personal counseling philosophy or style and the assessment of the client. The following series of case studies are used to illustrate the *when* and *how* of applying some behavior-modification strategies.

CASE STUDY: MRS. GARCIA

Mrs. Garcia is a 54-year-old Hispanic female who was referred to a registered dietitian (RD) by her primary care physician for weight loss as treatment for her diagnosis of type 2 diabetes and arthritis in her hips and knees. She is married with two adult sons, works full time in retail, and attends nursing school in the evenings. She is the primary caregiver for her aging parents.

Initial Visit

Mrs. Garcia weighs 222.6 pounds, and her height is 5 feet, 2.5 inches (BMI = 40.1). Her blood pressure is 129/76 mmHg, and her hemoglobin A1C is 8.5%.

This client has a long history of dieting with the typical pattern of losing weight and regaining the weight as old habits resurface. She has tried all the latest popular diets, including Atkins, Weight Watchers, Jenny Craig, and more. She is frustrated with herself about her weight going up and down on the scale. Physical activity is not a priority because she does not have time.

Setting Priorities and Goals

When asked about what she wants to accomplish with the diet instruction, Mrs. Garcia says that she is concerned about her health, especially since her diagnosis of diabetes. She has difficulty moving around and knows that the extra weight does not help matters. She and the RD discuss how her life will be different after losing weight and keeping it off. It is clear that she wants to be healthy to enjoy life with her husband and her future grandchildren.

Of course, she wants to lose 82 pounds in 4 months but cannot remember the last time she weighed 140 pounds. After talking out loud, she comes to the realization she would have to lose 5 pounds each week to meet her goal. Reality has spoken to her, and she revises her goal to losing 2 pounds per week.

Diet Recall, Diet Prescription, and Self-monitoring

Mrs. Garcia eats most of her meals away from home because of her erratic work schedule. When asked about what she usually orders, she says that she tries to order sensibly but knows that she probably eats too much because she gets "so hungry." The RD asks her how much and how often she eats on an average day. She is not at all sure and remembers keeping food records when she was going to Weight Watchers. During that time she counted points and found that it controlled how much she ate and she lost weight. The RD asks Mrs. Garcia what she thinks about trying food records again. After some discussion, she seems excited to get back in control by keeping food records and looking up calories for her food choices.

Mrs. Garcia says that she does very well on approximately 1,400 calories a day. She and the RD set a range between 1,400 and 1,600 kcal/d. She is not receptive to incorporating physical activity at this time.

Mrs. Garcia's weight on the scale fluctuates throughout the day. In fact, she weighs herself several times a day and is never happy. The RD and Mrs. Garcia talk about the importance of keeping track of her weight and negotiate how often and when she will monitor her weight. It upsets her to get on the scale every day, and she decides that weighing once per week on Wednesday morning would be the best for her.

Summary

Mrs. Garcia confirms her goals for the upcoming weeks of keeping food records, staying within 1,400 and 1,600 calories, and weighing only once per week on Wednesday morning. The RD gives her food records, measuring cups and spoons, a food scale, and a calorie pamphlet. A follow-up appointment in 2 weeks is scheduled.

Follow-up Visit

At her follow-up, Mrs. Garcia weighs 221.6 pounds. Her blood pressure is 130/77 mmHg.

Cognitive Restructuring

Mrs. Garcia is disappointed that she only lost 1 pound. She feels like she will never lose reach her goal weight and will be fat the rest of her life. She feels like she failed *again*. She describes her last 2 weeks as really stressful and crazy, and she felt out of control.

Mrs. Garcia's father had a medical emergency last week that required 48 hours in the emergency department, which challenged her schedule. Fortunately, he is doing okay. She has had no extra time for herself because of all her work and other family responsibilities. She has slept very little and eaten whatever is available.

After talking about all of the things that had happened, the RD reminds Mrs. Garcia that she was able to lose 1 pound. She acknowledges that she "really did pretty well considering how crazy things were going."

Goal-setting

Mrs. Garcia asks the RD what she thought about her goal of losing 2 pounds per week. The RD asks her how she felt about it in light of all drama that is happening with her family. After talking about the added responsibilities she will have, Mrs. Garcia revises her goal to losing 1 pound per week.

Stimulus Control and Problem-solving to Manage Stress

Mrs. Garcia does not have control of her eating when under stress. When she was in the hospital with her father, she ate foods she did not even like. This was really obvious to her when she attempted to keep some food records. Although this was a specific stressor episode, she identifies that any type of stress triggers her to overeat. How often she uses "stress" as an excuse to eat is a surprise to her. She indicates that she wants to find ways to deal with stress other than with food. The RD and Mrs. Garcia do some quick problem-solving to come up with some options to manage her stress. Taking a bubble bath, calling a friend, journaling, and taking a walk are some ideas that appeal to her. She decides that taking a 5- to 10-minute walk when life becomes too much is doable. She will record these walks on her food records.

Self-reward

By keeping food records, Mrs. Garcia realizes the large amount of calories in meals she eats at fast-food restaurants at lunchtime. Recently she has been bringing some low-calorie frozen meals to the office for lunch to save calories and money. The RD asks her what she is going to do with that money she saved. This change in behavior is considerable and needs to be reinforced. They talk about what Mrs. Garcia likes and what would be a good reward. Initially, she rejects the idea of rewarding herself for doing what she should be doing to lose weight. However, the calculation of the savings of $100 per month on fast-food lunches multiplied by 5 months is a real motivator about the reality of buying an MP3 player and music for herself.

Summary

Mrs. Garcia confirms that she is still going to stay within the prescribed range of 1,400 to 1,600 calories per day, and self-monitor by keeping food records and weighing herself every Wednesday to keep track of her progress.

A follow-up appointment in 2 weeks is scheduled.

CASE STUDY 2: MR. JONES

Mr. Jones is a 34-year-old white divorced male who was referred by his primary care physician for weight loss as treatment for his diagnosis of hypertension and prediabetes. His father died of a heart attack at age 57, and his 45-year-old sister has diabetes.

He works for the county as a corrections officer and reports to work at 5:00 AM Monday through Friday. He rarely eats breakfast because he is in a hurry to get to work. He does not enjoy cooking for himself and eats out at least four times per week for lunch and dinner. Fast foods are the typical choice for meals.

Initial Visit

At his first visit, Mr. Jones weighs 215 pounds. He is 5 feet, 7 inches tall (BMI = 33.7). His blood pressure is 150/92 mmHg with medication. His blood glucose level is 105 mg/dL.

Mr. Jones has never really been serious about losing weight. Once, he tried Weight Watchers. Most of the time, he tries to "cut back" his portions. As a corrections officer, he spends a great deal of time outdoors with the inmates. He does enjoy walking approximately 30 minutes per day, 5 days a week at the local high school track.

Setting Priorities and Goals

When asked about how he wants to spend our time together, Mr. Jones says that he wants to look better and be healthier. He and the RD then discuss what looking better and being healthier would look like for him. He wants to lose 50 pounds.

It has been more than 10 years since Mr. Jones weighed 165 pounds. However, he wants to lose the weight as quickly as possible—ie, in 3 or 4 months. Losing 50 pounds in 4 months translates to losing more than 3 pounds per week. He is motivated about that kind of weight loss and sets that as his goal.

Diet Recall, Diet Prescription, and Self-monitoring

Being single, Mr. Jones eats out at most meals. He knows that the calories can add up and has caused his weight gain over the years. He is very fond of burgers with fries and Mexican and Italian food. He remembers keeping food journals when he attended a weight-loss program at his church. He says he actually lost weight and felt good about writing things down. He does not have any problems keeping food records (self-monitoring).

Mr. Jones follows a 1,100-calorie diet, but is hungry all the time. Obviously, feeling hungry is not a good strategy for weight loss. Mr. Jones and the RD set a target goal of 1,600 calories. He has a recent copy of a calorie-counting book, which includes food from popular restaurants. The RD and Mr. Jones discuss the importance of a regular eating schedule, with meals or snacks at least every 5 hours.

Mr. Jones has a reliable home scale and weighs himself every morning. He will chart his daily weight to self-monitor his progress.

Summary

Mr. Jones confirms his goals for the upcoming weeks of following a 1,600-calorie plan, keeping food records, and charting his weight daily. The RD provides food records, daily weight graph, measuring cups and spoons, and a food scale. A follow-up appointment in 2 weeks is scheduled.

CONCLUSION

There is no magic in behavior-modification strategies. RDs use these strategies in combination with client-centered counseling for the best outcomes. It is very satisfying to collaborate with a client on behavior change that results in weight loss. However, we cannot control a client's readiness to change or willingness to change. We can provide some tools as simple as a food and activity diary to help clients become aware of what they are doing. We can provide the steps of the problem-solving model. We can teach progressive relaxation in an effort to help clients manage stressors that are bound to occur. We can teach them about identifying negative self-talk and strategies to disrupt and reframe self-talk. We can provide accountability and support. We cannot lose the weight for them, but we can teach skills and strategies.

"Give a man a fish and you feed him for a day. Teach a man to fish and you feed him for a lifetime."—a Chinese proverb

References

1. American Dietetic Association. Evidence Analysis Library. http://www.adaevidencelibrary.com. Accessed November 14, 2008.
2. National Heart, Lung, and Blood Institute. *The Practical Guide: Identification, Evaluation and Treatment of Overweight and Obesity in Adults.* October 2000. NIH publication 00-4084. http://www.nhlbi.nih./gov/guidelines/obesity/prctgd_c.pdf. Accessed June 2, 2009.
3. Lacey K, Pritchett E. Nutrition care process and model: ADA adopts road map to quality care and outcomes management. *J Am Diet Assoc.* 2003;103:1061–1072.

4. *International Dietetics & Nutrition Terminology (IDNT) Reference Manual: Standardized Language for the Nutrition Care Process.* Chicago, IL: American Dietetic Association; 2008.

5. Berkel AL, Poston WS, Reeves RS, Foreyt JP. Behavioral interventions for obesity. *J Am Diet Assoc.* 2005;105(suppl):S35–S43.

6. Melanson KJ. Dietary considerations for obesity treatment. *Am J Lifestyle Med.* 2007;1:433–436.

CHAPTER 8

MEDICATION

PART A: OVERVIEW

DONNA H. RYAN, MD, AND GEORGE A. BRAY, MD

PRINCIPLES FOR USING OBESITY MEDICATIONS

The rationale for the use of medications in the management of obesity is that medications can help more individuals achieve clinically meaningful weight loss, when they are making lifestyle changes to reduce energy intake and increase energy expenditure through physical activity. Medications are adjuncts to lifestyle change. Compared with lifestyle changes alone, currently available medications have been shown to produce greater weight loss, and the chances of achieving 5% to 10% loss are at least twice as good. Several key points are essential background to understanding the role of medications as adjuncts to dieting.

First, because every medication has associated side effects and risks, there is no way to justify their use for cosmetic weight loss. The individual's health risk must justify the use of obesity medication. The *Clinical Guidelines on the Identification, Evaluation, and Treatment of Overweight and Obesity in Adults: The Evidence Report* (1) states that medications may be indicated for individuals with a BMI of 30 or more, or for BMI of 27 or more with a comorbid condition. Individuals with hypertension, diabetes, dyslipidemia, metabolic syndrome, or another obesity-related disorder might qualify as a candidate for medication with a BMI of 27 or more.

Second, medications for obesity are not panaceas and should always be used as part of a comprehensive weight-loss program with an effective weight-maintenance plan to follow. The operant concept is that available obesity medications, in and of themselves, produce modest weight loss, but they can help reinforce behavioral approaches to weight loss and weight loss maintenance. Therefore, it is important to use the medication's mechanism of action in a dieting approach that maximizes effectiveness. For example, sibutramine promotes satiety and weight loss that is greatest when the medication is used with a sensible diet of three portion-controlled meals and two snacks. Orlistat blocks intestinal fat absorption and should be prescribed with a diet that is approximately 30% or less of energy as fat, with avoidance of high-fat foods at meals and snacks.

Third, not all people will respond to all medications; approximately one fourth of individuals who are prescribed medications will not have the expected response. Because medications should not be continued if the patient is not responding, it is helpful to have an idea after the first month of treatment about ultimate response. The rule of thumb is that a loss of 4 pounds (1.8 kg) in the first 4 weeks generally predicts at least 5% weight loss at 6 months of therapy.

Fourth, obesity medications do not cure obesity. Like medications for hypertension, they will help reduce weight to a certain level and then, as long as they are continued, help maintain that weight. The currently available medications typically are associated with a weight-loss plateau after approximately 6 months, and if medications are stopped, weight regain will occur. If medications are started, it should be with a commitment to continue for at least 1 year.

Fifth, medications will work only if used. Individuals who achieve weight loss with medications will likely experience weight regain if medications are stopped. Most physicians who manage patients with medications will advise that medications be restarted if more than 5 pounds (2.3 kg) of weight is regained.

REALITIES OF PRESCRIBING FOR OBESITY

Although evidence supports the benefits of weight-loss medications in increasing the likelihood of achieving clinically meaningful weight loss, there are still considerable barriers to prescribing for obesity. Because of these barriers, obesity medications are prescribed in only a fraction of the people who are eligible, according to the Clinical Guidelines (1). The reasons for this are many. First, it is unusual for insurers to reimburse for treatments for obesity, especially medications. Second, drugs approved by the US Food and Drug Administration (FDA) on the market today are associated with only modest weight loss (4%–5% better than placebo), although this can be greater when combined with lifestyle approaches. Physicians and patients may not appreciate the benefits of modest weight loss, especially when the patient must pay out-of-pocket for the medications. Third, physicians who manage obese patients, especially those who prescribe medications, tend to be stigmatized by their peers. This is due to the stigma associated with obesity itself, and the residual stigma associated with the use and abuse of amphetamine and amphetamine derivatives for weight loss in the last century. Physicians are reluctant to be known as obesity medication prescribers because patients may seek them out for recreational drugs.

Thus, the realities of prescribing for obesity are that the current pharmacopoeia and prescribing landscape leave us with unmet needs. Health care providers need medications that are safe, effective, and reasonably tolerable. The health care system must develop ways to reimburse for treating obesity, and for reimbursing for obesity pharmacotherapy. There is some promise in the investment by virtually all pharmaceutical companies to develop medications for obesity management and to try novel approaches to medicating. We believe that in the future we will approach obesity like we treat hypertension, using several medications at tolerable doses to aid in attaining clinically meaningful weight loss.

BENEFITS OF MODEST WEIGHT LOSS

Loss of 5% to 10% of body weight by obese individuals can translate into improvement in glycemic control, blood pressure and hypertension control, lipid profile, and improvements in symptoms of sleep apnea, arthritis, and other comorbid conditions (1). Furthermore, modest weight loss can translate into reduction in morbidity. Weight loss of 7% from baseline produced a 58% reduction in risk for developing type 2 diabetes over 2 to 5 years in the Diabetes Prevention Program (DPP) in individuals with impaired glucose tolerance (2). Health care professionals must encourage individuals to set achievable weight-loss goals and help them recognize the health benefits of achieving those goals. Medications can help more patients achieve clinically meaningful weight loss, and that is how they should be used—as adjuncts to lifestyle modification.

AVAILABLE MEDICATIONS
FOR OBESITY MANAGEMENT

We recently reviewed the literature on drug treatment (3). There are only two drugs approved by the FDA for long-term obesity management: sibutramine (Meridia [Abbott US; http://www.abbott.us]; sold as Reductil in other countries) and orlistat (sold by prescription as Xenical [Roche; http://www.roche.com]) and over-the-counter as Alli [GlaxoSmithKline; http://www.gsk.com]). Phentermine and diethylpropion are still widely prescribed because they are inexpensive and somewhat stimulatory, but those drugs have approval only for short-term obesity management (usually interpreted to mean use up to 12 weeks). Table 8.1 (3–6) compares the drugs with an obesity indication currently used in the United States.

Sibutramine

We recently reviewed the literature on sibutramine (4). This medication was first tested as a potential antidepressant but did not show efficacy. However, weight loss was observed in the obese and normal-weight volunteers and the drug was developed for obesity management. Marketed as Meridia in the United States and Reductil in other countries, sibutramine entered the market in March 1998. It generally costs approximately $100 for 1 month's supply.

Sibutramine is a beta-phenethylamine with a cyclobutyl group on the side chain. It inhibits the reuptake of serotonin, norepinephrine, and, to a lesser extent, dopamine. Sibutramine produces weight loss by a dual mechanism of action. It promotes satiety, which is the primary mechanism for the weight-loss effect. The drug also has a small effect to increase energy expenditure by blocking the reduction in metabolic rate that accompanies weight loss. One key to successful use of sibutramine is to prescribe it with an appropriate dietary approach. Because sibutramine promotes satiety (it does not produce anorexia), it works best in a program that enforces regular portion-controlled meals.

There are several published meta-analyses (5,7–9) of the weight-loss effects of sibutramine and its effects on blood pressure and other risk factors. One meta analysis of sibutramine (7), with findings that are typical for all published reports, found a mean difference between placebo and drug-treated groups of 4.5 kg weight loss (95% confidence interval [CI], 3.62–5.29 kg) at 12 months. However, only five studies met the predefined criteria for inclusion in the meta-analysis. A second report (8) shows 12-month weight

TABLE 8.1

Drugs with Indication for Obesity Management Used in the United States

	Diethylpropion	**Phentermine**	**Sibutramine**	**Orlistat**
Trade name	Tenuate	Adipex-P, Ionamin	Meridia	Xenical (Rx); Alli (OTC)
Year of approval	1959	1959	1997	1999 for Xenical; 2007 for Alli
Controlled substance class	IV	IV	IV	Not scheduled; OTC
Dose	25 mg 3 times/d (or 75 mg every morning)	37.5 mg every morning (Adipex-P); 30 mg or 15 mg once daily before breakfast (Ionamin)	5, 10, or 15 mg in the morning	120 mg 3 times/d (Rx); 60 mg 3 times/d (OTC)
Mechanism	Noradrenergic; loss of appetite	Noradrenergic; loss of appetite	Serotonin and norepinephrine reuptake inhibitor; promotes satiety	Pancreatic lipase inhibitor; blocks fat absorption
Approved for long-term use?	No	No	Yes	Yes
Average weight loss efficacy, drug alone	4%–6%	4%–6%	4%–6%	4%–6%
Weight loss efficacy with appropriate lifestyle	No data	No data	Up to 16% with strong behavioral approach (4,5)	For Xenical, up to 8% with behavioral approach (3,6)
Safety issues	Increased blood pressure possible; small abuse potential	Increased blood pressure possible; small abuse potential	Increased blood pressure possible	No safety issues; vitamin supplement recommended
Tolerability	Insomnia, stimulation	Insomnia, stimulation	Dry mouth	GI side effects, anal leakage
Advantages	Low cost, patient acceptance	Low cost, patient acceptance	Supported by clinical trials	Safe; supported by clinical trials
Disadvantages	Inadequate data (no long-term studies) to support use for more than a few months	Inadequate data (no long-term studies) to support use for more than a few months	Blood pressure must be monitored; cost	Tolerability, cost

Manufacturer information: Tenuate, Aventis Pharmaceuticals, http://www.sanofi-aventis.com; Adipex-P, Gate Pharmaceuticals, http://www.gatepharma.com; Ionamin, Celltech Pharmaceuticals, http://www.celltechgroup.com; Meridia, Abbott US, http://www.abbott.us; Xenical, Roche, http://www.roche.com; Alli, GlaxoSmithKline, http://www.gsk.com.
Abbreviations: Rx, prescription; OTC, over-the-counter; GI, gastrointestinal.
Source: Data on efficacy with appropriate lifestyle are from references 3–6.

change difference between sibutramine and placebo of -4.18 kg (95% CI, -5.14 to -3.21 kg). These meta-analyses, despite limitations of small numbers of studies, reinforce the concept that independent of the behavioral intervention, weight loss with sibutramine is modest.

There are three key factors in the efficacy of sibutramine (4). First, weight loss is dose-related. The usual starting dosage is 10 mg, but the drug may be increased to 15 mg (or decreased to 5 mg if there are adverse effects). An advantage is sibutramine's once-a-day dosing. Second, the amount of initial weight loss is related to the intensity of the behavioral intervention. Highly structured, portion-controlled schemes produce the most weight loss. Third, sibutramine is very effective during weight-loss maintenance. Placebo-controlled studies (5,9) demonstrate successful weight-loss maintenance with sibutramine for up to 2 years.

In general, clinical trials with sibutramine inform us that approximately three quarters of patients treated with 15 mg/day sibutramine will achieve more than 5% weight loss, and 80% of those will maintain that loss for 2 years if they continue taking the drug. Approximately 5% of patients will not tolerate the drug because of adverse effects on blood pressure and pulse. Some patients (usually approximately 25%) are nonresponders (4).

In clinical trials, sibutramine, like other sympathomimetic agents, produced a small increase in mean heart rate and mean blood pressure (4,7,8,10,11). However, the blood pressure response is variable. A subset (approximately 5% of patients) seem to be sensitive to the blood pressure effects and cannot tolerate sibutramine. Some people may need to discontinue sibutramine because of blood pressure elevations into the hypertensive range. Other adverse effects, including dry mouth, insomnia, and asthenia, are similar to those of other noradrenergic drugs. Sibutramine is not associated with valvular heart disease, primary pulmonary hypertension, or substance abuse.

Sibutramine should be used with caution in individuals with cardiovascular disease and those taking selective serotonin reuptake inhibitors. It should not be used within 2 weeks of taking monoamine oxidase inhibitors and should not be used with other noradrenergic agents.

Orlistat

Orlistat, reviewed by us recently (4), is available by prescription (Xenical) in a dosage of 120 mg three times a day before meals and over-the-counter as Alli at a lower dosage of 60 mg. Both types are taken three times daily before meals. Alli is sold for approximately $60 for 90 capsules (1 month's supply) whereas Xenical is sold for $100 to $200 per month.

These medications block the enzymatic action of pancreatic lipase, thereby inhibiting the digestion of dietary fat and reducing the amount of calories absorbed. Orlistat (tetrahydrolipstatin) is a potent inhibitor of lipase activity that decreases intestinal triglyceride hydrolysis in a dose-dependent manner. In clinical trials (3,6,8), it also has a dose-dependent effect on fat absorption and weight loss. After a high-fat meal, steatorrheal diarrhea is expected when using this medication, but gastrointestinal events in practice are mild to moderate, resolve spontaneously, and are usually limited to no more than one or two episodes per patient. Deficiency of fat-soluble vitamins can occur, and vitamin supplementation, usually with a daily multivitamin, is recommended. In general, individuals tolerate the drug very well, especially if they receive advance patient education.

⟶ Orlistat works best when given with a diet that has approximately 30% fat content, so patient counseling is important. If a high-fat meal or snack is consumed, gastrointestinal distress can result. For a very-low-fat meal, orlistat is not going to produce a caloric deficit, and individuals on a low-fat diet will not lose weight on orlistat.

Orlistat is effective in producing and sustaining modest weight loss (3). Data from clinical trials suggest that approximately 70% of patients will achieve more than 5% weight loss, and at 2 years 70% of them will have maintained that loss. Clinical trials have documented orlistat use for up to 4 years; one of the studies targeted diabetes prevention (6).

Several meta-analyses of orlistat have been published (7,8,12). By pooling six studies, Haddock and associates (12) estimated the weight loss in patients treated with orlistat as –7.1 kg (range –4.0 to –10.3 kg) compared with –5.02 kg (range –3.0 to –6.1 kg) for the placebo-treated groups. In another meta-analysis by Li et al (5), the overall mean difference between drug-treated and placebo-treated groups after 12 months of therapy in 22 studies was –2.70 kg (95% CI, –3.79 to –1.61 kg). Another meta-analysis (8) examined the effects in eight 1-year studies on weight loss at 1 and 2 years and on the various laboratory and clinical responses. (Only one of the eight studies involved patients with diabetes.) The overall effect of orlistat on weight loss at 12 months using the weighted mean difference between orlistat and placebo was –3.01 kg (95% CI, –3.48 to –2.54 kg) (8). After 24 months, the overall effect of orlistat on weight loss was –3.26 kg (95% CI, –4.15 to –2.37 kg).

One advantage to orlistat is its beneficial effect on low-density lipoprotein (LDL) cholesterol. Because orlistat blocks fat absorption, the LDL reduction is about twice that seen with weight loss alone (3).

Phentermine and Diethylpropion

Phentermine and diethylpropion are classified by the US Drug Enforcement Agency (DEA) as schedule IV drugs; however, some state regulatory systems classify phentermine as a schedule II drug. This regulatory classification requiring scheduling for sibutramine indicates the government's belief that these drugs have the potential for abuse, although this potential seems to be very low. These drugs are only approved for a "few weeks" of use, which is usually interpreted as up to 12 weeks.

We recently reviewed these agents (3). Weight loss with phentermine and diethylpropion persists for the duration of treatment, suggesting that tolerance to these drugs does not develop. If tolerance developed, the drugs would lose their effectiveness or increased amounts of drug would be required for individuals to maintain weight loss. Phentermine and diethylpropion are no longer protected by patents and are therefore inexpensive—generally approximately $30 for a 1-month supply. Phentermine is not available in Europe. A review in the *New England Journal of Medicine* (13) recommends obtaining written informed consent if phentermine is prescribed for longer than 12 weeks because there are not sufficient published reports on the long-term use of phentermine.

The only published studies of these medications involve small numbers of individuals treated for a short duration. Because of the lack of long-term studies and the lack of sufficient safety data, we do not recommend the routine use of these agents. One 36-week study (14) using phentermine showed that intermittent use of phentermine (1 month on, 1 month off) is just as effective in producing weight loss as continuous therapy. This approach is occasionally useful.

The adverse effect profiles for sympathomimetic drugs are similar. They produce insomnia, dry mouth, asthenia, and constipation. Sympathomimetic drugs can also increase blood pressure.

Off-label Prescribing

Weight loss has been reported with several medications that we reviewed earlier (3), including bupropion (an approved antidepressant and smoking cessation aid), venlafaxine (an antidepressant with structural similarity to sibutramine), topiramate (an anticonvulsant also used for migraine prophylaxis), metformin (an antidiabetic), exenatide (an incretin mimetic used in diabetes), and pramlintide (an amylin analog used in diabetes). We discourage off-label prescribing for obesity. However, because many antidepressants produce weight gain, bupropion or venlafaxine may be good choices for the obese patient with diabetes. Clinical trials of topiramate as an anti-obesity agent were undertaken, but the drug was not pursued as a single agent because of tolerability issues; topiramate is sedating and causes cognitive slowing at dosages that produce significant weight loss. Because of this, we do not advocate use of topiramate. Metformin, exenatide, and pramlintide may be good choices in obese individuals with diabetes because of the added benefit of weight loss with these drugs, whereas most antidiabetic agents produce weight gain.

SPECIAL ISSUES IN DIABETES

In regard to individuals with diabetes, diabetic control improves with weight reduction, and hypoglycemia becomes a possibility for those people, especially if they are on insulin or sulfonylurea medications. Some individuals may develop increased hunger due to hypoglycemia, and weight loss may slow or stop. Physicians must remember to monitor glucose carefully and reduce or stop diabetes medications as weight loss occurs. In our clinic, we halve or discontinue insulin and sulfonylureas at the start of the weight-loss program. The Look AHEAD (Action for Health in Diabetes) study (15) randomly assigned more than 5,000 participants with diabetes to either a control group or a weight-loss intervention. The intervention group achieved an average of nearly 9% weight loss in more than 2,500 individuals with diabetes, in part by careful attention to medication management during weight loss and a portion-control diet. That study should be noted by every clinician who cares for patients with diabetes because of its demonstration of the powerful effect of weight loss in achieving lipid and glycemic targets. It is a strong statement promoting a weight-centric approach to diabetes management.

FUTURE DIRECTIONS IN OBESITY PHARMACOTHERAPY

Interest in developing new drugs for obesity is high, not only because of the high rates of obesity but also because of advances in understanding the biology of energy balance regulation. Several trends are emerging. First, the identification of "druggable targets" in the brain and periphery has produced several new agents that are in development. Second, combination therapies are emerging.

A major disappointment has been with compounds directed at the endocannabinoid system, a complex endogenous system that affects many different metabolic pathways, including physical and emotional reactions to stress and appetite. Rimonabant, one of the drugs in this category, failed to obtain FDA approval and was withdrawn from the market abroad in 2008. Rimonabant acts to inhibit CB-1 receptors, which are found primarily in the brain in areas related to feeding, on fat cells, and in the gastrointestinal tract; inactivation of these receptors serves to "dampen" the desire for palatable food. Studies indicate a statistically significant improvement in lipids and a dose-dependent decrease in waist circumference and well as more efficacious weight loss than with diet and physical activity alone (16). However, adverse effects include depressed moods and sometimes severe and increased risk for suicide. Thus, rimonabant was withdrawn from use and, in fact, investigation of all drugs in the CB-1 antagonist class have been stopped.

There are many other drugs in the pipeline: New antagonists of neuro-peptide-Y (NPY), peptide-YY (PYY), oxyntomodulin, amylin, and glucagon-like peptide-1 (GLP-1) are being used for their abilities to reduce food intake. Because the 5-hydroxytryptamine$_{2b}$ (5 HT) receptor is implicated in valvulopathy, agonists for $5HT_{2c}$ and $5HT_6$ are in development. Cetilistat (17), a lipase inhibitor, seems to have a more favorable side effect profile and similar efficacy to orlistat. Tesofensine (18), a reuptake inhibitor of norepinephrine, dopamine, and serotonin, is being studied and has shown dose-related weight loss, albeit with dose-related side effects on blood pressure and heart rate.

Several companies have combinations in development, and the ones that are farthest along are combinations of topiramate-phentermine, bupropion-naltrexone and bupropion-zonisamide. The concept with combination therapy is to maximize efficacy by additive effects (or more) and to minimize adverse effects by using lower dosages. Some older compounds may return to use as part of a combination and, in particular, leptin and NPY antagonists may have a new role as part of a combination.

Overall, the future of obesity pharmacotherapy seems to be evolving similar to the historical development of effective drug strategies for hypertension. We predict that new drugs will eventually make it to market, based on advances in understanding the biology of energy balance. The approach will be to use weight-loss drugs in combinations, keeping individual doses low to avoid adverse effects and tolerability issues but achieving greater efficacy by targeting multiple mechanisms. Another trend that we predict is the emergence of greater emphasis on weight management as a pathway to better diabetes control, so the weight-gain or weight-loss impact of antidiabetic agents is likely to come under greater scrutiny.

References

1. National Institutes of Health, National Heart, Lung, and Blood Institute. Clinical Guidelines on the Identification, Evaluation, and Treatment of Overweight and Obesity in Adults: the evidence report. *Obes Res.* 1998;6(Suppl 2):51S–209S.
2. Knowler WC, Barrett-Connor E, Fowler SE, Hamman RF, Lachin JM, Walker EA, Nathan DM, Diabetes Prevention Program Research Group. Reduction in the incidence of type 2 diabetes with lifestyle intervention or metformin. *N Engl J Med.* 2002;346:393–403.
3. Bray GA, Ryan DH. Drug treatment of the overweight patient. *Gastroenterology.* 2007;132:2239–2252

4. Ryan DH. The role of sibutramine in the clinical management of obesity. In: Medeiros-Neto G, Halpern A, Bouchard C, eds. *Progress in Obesity Research: 9.* Montrouge, France: John Libbey Eurotext; 2003:1051–1057.4.

5. Apfelbaum M, Vague P, Ziegler O, Hanotin C, Thomas F, Leutenegger E. Long-term maintenance of weight loss after a very-low-calorie diet: a randomized blinded trial of the efficacy and tolerability of sibutramine. *Am J Med.* 1999;106: 179–184.

6. Torgerson JS, Hauptman J, Boldrin MN, Sjostrom L. Xenical in the prevention of diabetes in obese subjects (XENDOS) study: a randomized study of orlistat as an adjunct to lifestyle changes for the prevention of type 2 diabetes in obese patients. *Diabetes Care.* 2004;27:155–161.

7. Li Z, Maglione M, Tu W, Mojica W, Arterburn D, Shugarman LR, Hilton L, Suttorp M, Solomon V, Shekelle PG, Morton SC. Meta-analysis: pharmacologic treatment of obesity. *Ann Intern Med.* 2005;142:532–546.

8. Avenell A, Brown TJ, McGee MA, Campbell MK, Grant AM, Broom J, Jung RT, Smith WC. What interventions should we add to weight reducing diets in adults with obesity? A systematic review of randomized controlled trials of adding drug therapy, exercise, behaviour therapy or combinations of these interventions. *J Hum Nutr Diet.* 2004;17:293–316.

9. James WPT, Astrup A, Finer N, Hilsted J, Kopelman P, Rossner S, Saris WHM, van Gaal L, for the STORM study group. Effect of sibutramine on weight maintenance after weight loss: a randomized trial. *Lancet.* 2000;356:2119–2125.

10. Kim SH, Lee YM, Jee SH, Nam CM. Effect of sibutramine on weight loss and blood pressure: a meta-analysis of controlled trials. *Obes Res.* 2003;11:1116–1123.

11. Bettor R, Serra R, Fabris R, Pagano C, Federspil G. Effect of sibutramine on weight management and metabolic control in type 2 diabetes: a meta-analysis of clinical studies. *Diabetes Care.* 2005;28:942–949.

12. Haddock CK, Poston WS, Dill PL, Foreyt JP, Ericsson M. Pharmacotherapy for obesity: a quantitative analysis of four decades of published randomized clinical trials. *Int J Obes Relat Metab Disord.* 2002;26:262–273.

13. Yanovski SZ, Yanovski JA. Drugs in obesity. *N Engl J Med.* 2002;346:591–602.

14. Munro J, MacCuish A. Comparison of continuous and intermittent anorectic therapy in obesity. *BMJ.* 1968;1:352–354.

15. The Look AHEAD Research Group. Reduction in weight and cardiovascular disease risk factors in individuals with type 2 diabetes. One year results of the Look AHEAD Trial. *Diabetes Care.* 2007;30:1374–1383.

16. Sheen AJ. CB1 receptor blockade and its impact on cardiometabolic risk factors: overview of the RIO programme with rimonabant. *J Neuroendocrinol.* 2008;20 (suppl 1): S139–S146.

17. Kopelman P, Bryson A, Hickling R, Rissanen A, Rossner S, Toubro S, Valensi P. Cetilistat (ATL-962), a novel lipase inhibitor: a 12-week randomized, placebo-controlled study of weight reduction in obese patients. *Int J Obes.* 2007;31:494–499.

18. Astrup A, Madsbad S, Breum L, Jensen TJ, Kroustrup JP, Larsen TM. Effect of tesofensine on bodyweight loss, body composition, and quality of life in obese patients: a randomized, double-blind, placebo-controlled trial. *Lancet.* 2008;372: 1906–1913.

PART B: PRACTICAL APPLICATIONS

CATHY A. NONAS, MS, RD, CDE

CASE STUDY: PART 1—JANE CONSIDERS THE USE OF MEDICATIONS

Jane is one of those people who has so much experience with diets that she could write a perfectly balanced 1,200-calorie diet for anyone who had asked her for one. Her problem is the she cannot follow her own advice. She is 46 years old with a BMI of 32. She has two children, a husband, and an executive position in an advertising firm. She has a gym membership, which she uses three times each week on good weeks.

During the initial visit, Jane brings food records without being asked, and then she proceeds to tell the registered dietitian (RD) exactly what she (Jane) has been doing wrong. This leaves the RD with little to say. But Jane has reasons for coming to see the RD: her serum cholesterol has increased and her blood pressure is prehypertensive, so her physician has told her she must lose weight. She has not seen an RD in the past decade and wondered whether an RD would have a different perspective. She has a friend who had good results with this particular RD.

The RD is a little taken aback because Jane has tried just about everything the RD could suggest: low-carbohydrate, low-fat, low-glycemic, meal replacements, vegetarian, Weight Watchers, Jenny Craig, Optifast, and Health Management Resources, to name a few, and she had done well with all of them, even, in some cases, keeping her weight off for long periods of time. Now Jane is having trouble returning to any one of those diets for more than a few days.

Jane takes no prescription medication, although her physician had recommended a statin for her cholesterol. At this point, the RD asks Jane if she has ever considered weight-loss medication. "No," she replies, "the idea scares me."

There are many biases against medication for weight control. For example, there is a long history of addiction. In the 1960s, amphetamines were prescribed for short-term weight loss, with the unrealistic expectation that a "head start" would magically help the individual continue to lose weight after the amphetamines were stopped. As we now know, this was not the case. First, sympathomimetic stimulants such as amphetamines can cause severe cardiovascular adverse effects ranging from tachycardia to death; second, they are addictive; and third, short-term medication use for weight loss is ineffective for long-term weight loss (1).

All medications, including weight-loss medications, have side effects. The difference, however, is that obesity is not universally considered a disease (eg, most health insurers do not reimburse for treatment), and, people still consider obesity a behavioral problem only. Adverse effects for a "non-disease" are a bigger concern for both prescribers and patients. Furthermore, the history of weight-loss medication has not been positive. Not only have there been concerns about amphetamines, but there was the well-known fen/phen debacle. The popular medication fenfluramine (Pondimin) and its dextroisomer, dexfenfluramine (Redux) caused a dangerous valvulopathy in some individuals and was ultimately taken off the market (2). This made both prescribers and patients very wary about weight-loss medications.

The other problem with medications that result in weight loss is that there are very few whose original purpose was weight loss. Medications that result in weight loss can be divided into three categories: (*a*) those that are approved by the US Food and Drug Administration (FDA) for the specific purpose of weight loss, such as sibutramine (Meridia [Abbott US; http://www.abbott.us]) and orlistat (sold by prescription as Xenical [Roche; http://www.roche.com] and over-the-counter as Alli [GlaxoSmith Kline; http://www.gsk.com]); (*b*) those that are approved for another purpose but affect weight as well, such as topiramate (Topamax [Ortho-McNeil, USA; http://www.ortho-mcneil.com/ortho-mcneil] or dextroamphetamine (Adderall [Shire, USA; http://www.shire.com]) for attention deficit disorder; and (*c*) those that are "recreational" drugs that are not approved for any disease and are taken for pleasure with a side effect of weight loss (eg, crack cocaine).

It is interesting that the approved drugs for weight loss are not regarded in the same way as other medications that are FDA-approved. For example, if a statin was efficacious for lowering cholesterol, and was generally safe but with an adverse effect on the liver in some people, the physician would take liver enzyme tests at specific periods to ensure that there were no side effects. If there were an adverse effect, the statin would likely be stopped. Likewise, if the statin worked and there were no adverse effects for that patient, the physician would not consider stopping the statin when the serum cholesterol fell to normal range. If the statin were stopped, the serum cholesterol would likely return to its original elevated level. The same thing happens with weight-loss medication: although the FDA has approved three medications for long-term use (sibutramine, orlistat by prescription, and lower-dose orlistat over-the-counter), many clinicians believe they should stop weight-loss medication after a time, and when it is stopped they are surprised that weight regain occurs and consider the medication to be ineffective.

Finally, current FDA-approved weight-loss medications result in only a modest weight loss. This is actually not surprising. The body is not built to sustain weight loss. Humans have evolved to defend against famines, and the body works hard to defend its weight. Energy expenditure decreases when food is unobtainable, and adipose tissue increases when food is readily available. It is, therefore, reasonable to consider that to sustain life during periods of famine, more than one system evolved to guard the body. When a hazardous signal such as weight loss is transmitted, the body signals for backup. When a medication successfully targets a signal in the brain to reduce appetite, another signal may try to restore the weight status quo. Even so, it is important to remember that this modest effect of weight-loss medications often produces a 5% to 10% weight loss, an amount that makes a substantial difference in the health profile (3).

The positive health consequences of a 5% to 10% weight loss are one reason why the FDA will approve a medication that may only have a "modest" effect. If that medication can result in more people losing 5% or 10% over a rigorous intervention of diet alone, and if more of those people can maintain that 5% to 10% weight loss *and* the medication is deemed safe, then the FDA will approve the drug. On the other hand, the modest weight loss is one reason why medication for weight loss is not as popular as it might be. The modest weight loss is countered by the expense of the medication (rarely insurance-reimbursable), and by its side effects profile, which, no matter how benign, is often deemed not worth the effort for such modest outcomes. In different studies by Foster et al and Fabricatore et al (4–6), both physicians and patients were asked what their dream/ideal weight losses were. Both groups replied that more that 30% of body weight would be ideal, even though that kind of weight loss is usually limited to successful bariatric surgeries. When asked what was acceptable, patients said 25% while physicians answered that 14% weight loss was acceptable. Clearly, these answers are substantially more than what is practical and what is clinically significant. Thus, one of the cruxes of medication use for weight loss: the outcomes are too modest for both the physicians and the clients, no matter how impressive the data are for health improvements.

Jane's RD lets her know that the weight-loss effect from medication will be modest, but the current approved medications have been used for years and the health profiles are very good. The RD also explains that medication may help Jane be more consistent with her diet plan. After all, no medication works as well without the supportive behavioral changes. Jane is ready to make some behavioral changes; she is just having trouble doing it consistently.

Jane is still leery, particularly because she wanted to lose 20% of her weight and is not sure that it is worth the risk of adverse effects to lose only 5% to 10%. Both Jane and her RD are well aware of the literature on successful diets, so Jane decides to first try a well-balanced plan for 1,200 calories.

At her follow-up visit 1 week later, Jane has lost 2 pounds. But as a seasoned dieter, she also knows that this is a diuresis period and she expected to lose at least 5 pounds in her first week. Two pounds is discouraging. She decides to discuss weight-loss medication with her physician.

FDA APPROVAL

For a medication to cause weight loss, it must do one of three things: (*a*) reduce appetite; (*b*) stop absorption of some calories; or (*c*) increase metabolism. Medications that have been approved for weight loss thus far affect the first two, but no medication has been created to safely increase metabolism.

The FDA approves weight-loss medications if studies show that, by using the medication along with intensive diet therapy, more subjects can safely reach and maintain a 5% to 10% weight loss than with intensive diet therapy and placebo. This is an important point. Studies 40 to 50 years ago did not use intensive diet therapy as part of the placebo protocol and therefore the effect of the drug in those studies was larger. Studies today are more sophisticated, and FDA approval is more rigorous. The intensity of the diet therapy makes the comparison between medication and placebo look modest. But that is exactly the point: the medication must help more people reach a clinically significant weight loss compared with rigorous diet therapy alone, and it must do so safely. If the medication does this, then it stands to reason that it should be approved by the FDA and welcomed by all who treat obesity and overweight.

The idea that a weight-loss medication should be more efficacious than diet alone works in reverse as well—no medication works as well alone as it will with diet and behavior change (see Table 1.4 in Chapter 1). Therefore, RDs have become an integral and consistent part of any guideline for prescriptive treatment. This is also why it is incumbent upon RDs to understand the actions of various medications for weight loss to more effectively counsel their clients.

SCHEDULING

Medications are scheduled by the FDA in terms of abuse potential. Amphetamines are schedule II or III, which means they have a highly addictive quality. Most FDA-approved weight-loss medications currently prescribed have a lower abuse potential and are therefore schedule IV (see Table 8.1), or, in the case of orlistat, are not scheduled at all (7). These drugs also have a more benign side effect profile. The FDA approves medications for short-term and long-term use. For example, phentermine, one of the best-selling medications for weight loss, is approved for short-term use (no more than 12 weeks). Deemed a nonamphetamine amphetamine (schedule IV for low-abuse potential), phentermine is generic and therefore less expensive. It is approved for short-term use because there are no long-term studies. Orlistat (Xenical) and sibutramine (Meridia) are prescription medications approved for long-term use because they have outcome studies to support more than 2 years of use. As the maintenance of weight loss becomes integral to treatment paradigms, long-term effects of medications become important criteria for success. In clinical trials in which subjects after weight loss are randomly assigned to either placebo or medication, significantly more subjects on either orlistat or sibutramine maintained a 5% to 10% weight loss than those on placebo (8–11). Recently, the FDA approved Alli for long-term use. Half the dose of the prescribed orlistat, Alli is first over-the-counter (OTC) medication approved for weight loss. Any future weight-loss medications will also have to adhere to this "gold standard" of proving both safety and efficacy for 2 years or more.

SIGNALING TO REDUCE APPETITE

The nervous system is divided into two major parts: the central nervous system, which consists of the brain and spinal cord, and the peripheral nervous system, which are the nerves throughout the rest of the body and peripheral to the brain and spinal cord. The peripheral nervous system includes the autonomic (automatic reflex) nervous system (ANS), which controls the visceral functions of the body such as arterial pressure, body temperature, gastrointestinal motility, and appetite. The ANS is further subdivided into the sympathetic and parasympathetic systems. Therefore, signals that affect appetite can affect other areas of the body as well, which is why certain weight-loss medications may, for example, affect blood pressure or cause constipation.

Signals (proteins, cytokines, etc) are either afferent (carry information toward the brain from sensory organs, muscles, the circulatory system, and all the organs of the body to the controlling centers in the medulla, pons, and hypothalamus) or efferent (carry information from the brain to the peripheral areas). This constant communication to and from the brain can be interrupted or enhanced by medication.

More than 30% of the American adult population is obese (12). Therefore, it is no surprise that pharmaceutical companies are racing to formulate new weight-loss medications with better efficacy and safety. There are a myriad of peptides and proteins that are being investigated as possible weight loss medications. In brief, there are three important concepts that may help in understanding the potential role of medications for weight loss: (*a*) different peptides work for varying lengths of time; (*b*) one signal may affect many different parts of the brain; and (*c*) one signal can start a cascade of events (13). Using type 2 diabetes as the paradigm, leptin and insulin reflect the basal needs of storage; peptides such as peptide YY_{3-36} (PYY) might be considered for appetite similarly to the way NPH insulin is used for diabetes, working for approximately 12 hours; and a number of short-acting peptides such as cholecystokinin and its competitor ghrelin (the only orexigenic hormone in the gut) or neuropeptide Y (NPY) (an orexigenic peptide in the central nervous system [CNS]) would be the premeal, short-term insulin. When the orexigenic peptides are increased, appetite is stimulated. After a meal, these peptides are decreased. Medication for weight loss would inhibit the orexigenic peptides, or enhance the anorexic peptides (Box 8.1 and Table 8.2). Gastric bypass procedures seem to reduce levels of ghrelin, which may be why patients do not typically complain of hunger after surgery (14). (Refer to Chapter 9 for more information on surgery.)

Box 8.1

Selected Secreted Proteins That Affect Eating Behavior

Fat Cell
- Leptin
- Adiponectin
- Interleukin-6 (IL-6)
- Tumor necrosis factor-α (TNF-α)
- Adipsin
- Plasminogen activator inhibitor-1 (PAI-1)
- Peroxisome proliferator activated ribosomes (PPAR)

Hypothalamus
- Neuropeptide Y (NPY)
- Agouti related protein (AGRP)

- Orexin A and B
- Corticotropin-releasing hormone (CRH)
- Pro-opiomelanocortin (POMC)
- α-melanocyte-stimulating hormone(α-MSH)

Gut
- Cholecystokinin (CCK)
- Glucagon-like peptide-1 (GLP-1)
- Peptide YY
- Ghrelin
- Amylin

Table 8.2

Examples of Cytokines, Hormones, and Enzymes That Must Be Blocked or Enhanced to Reduce Feeding Behavior or Increase Thermogenesis

Block	Enhance
NPY	PYY
PPAR γ	CCK
TNF α	Adiponectin
Ghrelin	MC4
CB-1 receptor	POMC
Resistin	Norepinephrine
AGRP	Serotonin
NPY	Obestatin
Endocannibinoids	MSH
IL-6	GLP-1

Abbreviations: NPY, neuropeptide Y; PYY, peptide YY; PPAR, peroxisome proliferator-activated receptor; CCK, cholecystokinin; TNF, tumor necrosis factor; MC4, melanocortin 4 receptor; CB-1, cannabinoid receptor type 1; POMC, pro-opiomelanocortin; AGRP, agouti related protein; MSH, melanocyte-stimulating hormone; IL-6, interleukin-6; GLP-1, glucagon-like peptide-1.

Leptin is produced primarily by adipose tissue and it targets multiple places in the brain such as the arcuate, dorsomedial, ventromedial, lateral, and paraventricular nuclei of the hypothalamus, as well as the caudal stem and the limbic system. Leptin then directs its signals either to the orexigenic peptides or the anorectic peptides (Table 8.2) (15). The net effect is to inhibit or enhance appetite; stimulate or reduce thermogenesis, enhance either fatty acid oxidation or fat storage, increase or decrease glucose, and modify weight as appropriate.

CASE STUDY: PART 2—JANE TRIES SIBUTRAMINE

Jane decides to try sibutramine (Meridia), and her physician prescribes the standard 10-mg dose for 1 month. In that time, Jane loses only 4 pounds. She had thought that her hunger would disappear and that food would become uninteresting and therefore easier to limit. Although she admits that she thought about food less, she also acknowledges that on bad days she could "eat through" her indifference, and so she is not sure whether Meridia is worth her effort. She now believes she should either stop or try the higher dosage.

The facts of Jane's conundrum are as follows: (*a*) she is obese; (*b*) she is relatively healthy now but exhibiting significant risk for diseases associated with obesity; (*c*) she has tried other avenues for weight loss; and (*d*) she continues to see an RD for behavioral support. Losing 4 pounds in 1 month is considered a success with medication and is an indication that the medication is working (16). Although Jane would like to do better, she has now lost a total of 6 pounds—a considerable accomplishment when she realizes that previously she had been unable to lose any weight. Jane understands that taking a higher dose might increase the adverse effects, but she currently does not admit any effects other than dry mouth and some constipation.

Jane's plan:

- Return to her primary care physician for a blood pressure check and to discuss an increase in the dosage.
- Meanwhile, try taking Meridia closer to the time when she tends to overeat. Meridia has a peak action of 3 to 7 hours, depending on food intake. Therefore, if Jane is most likely to overeat in the evenings, it might be more effective if she takes the medication at lunch.
- Increase fiber and water intake to reduce constipation.
- Be more consistent with physical activity.

SIBUTRAMINE PROFILE

Current FDA-approved medications that affect appetite work by increasing the availability of the monoamine neurotransmitters norepinephrine, serotonin, and, to a lesser degree, dopamine in the central nervous system. There is normal physiologic release of neurotransmitters from a host neuron to receptors on another neuron. Usually the host neuron then immediately takes back the original neurotransmitter for storage until future use. Medications such as sibutramine inhibit the host neuron from taking the neurotransmitter so quickly, leaving it in the system for longer. Selective serotonin-reup-take inhibitors (SSRIs) such as fluoxetine (Prozac) and venlafaxine (Effexor) work this way, and they affect these same monoamines. But SSRIs and weight-loss medications that affect monoamine neurotransmitters are function-specific. Fluoxetine and venlafax-ine, for example, which are prescribed for depression, affect depression, whereas ap-petite suppressants affect only appetite. The ability of SSRIs to affect depression and sibutramine to affect weight loss is attributable to their selectivity (hence the inclusion of the word "selective" in the term "SSRI"). This selectivity distinguishes SSRIs from other and older medications that affect monoamine neurotransmitters, such as tricyclic antidepressants (eg, amitriptyline [Elavil] and imipramine [Tofranil]), and monoamine oxidase inhibitors (eg, phenelzine [Nardil] and tranylcypromine [Parnate]) but do not have the advantage of selectivity and therefore may cause many additional side effects. That said, some of the side effects of medications that affect mono-amines—even selec-tive ones—include arterial blood pressure, body temperature, gastrointestinal motility, and appetite. As clinicians, we must understand the potential adverse effects to ensure that clients are well monitored. For example, if a client has been prescribed an SSRI for 2 years and weight gain has occurred specifically in those 2 years, then it may be effica-cious for the client to try a different SSRI. Likewise, if a client who has just started sibu-tramine has a sudden increase in blood pressure, then trying a different weight loss med-ication may be the appropriate response.

Noradrenergic medications such as sibutramine and phentermine have an increased effect on norepinephrine, compared with their effects on serotonin. Norepinephrine acti-vates the sympathetic nervous system to directly increase heart rate. Therefore, some in-dividuals who take these medications are more susceptible to hypertension, palpitations, insomnia, headache, dry mouth, constipation, or diarrhea (10). This is why these med-ications are contraindicated in individuals with unstable angina or hypertension that is not well-controlled. Medications that have greater effects on serotonin, such as SSRIs, may cause drowsiness, dizziness, reduced libido, and weight gain.

Sibutramine has been FDA-approved since 1997, and its long-term approval status was based on safety and efficacy trials of 2 years or longer (10). It does not stimulate neurotransmitter release and has no incidence of valvular heart disease. Its safety profile is good, but follow-up monitoring is important. The use of sibutramine is associated with small but clinically insignificant increases of less than 1 to 3 mmHg for diastolic blood pressure, as well as an average increase in heart rate of approximately 4 to 5 beats per minute. In a minority of patients, blood pressure and heart rate increase more than this, but the weight loss associated with sibutramine may also attenuate those blood pressure effects. As with any medication that affects noradrenergic receptors, it is important to monitor blood pressure, and it is contraindicated for anyone with unstable hypertension or angina.

Sibutramine is usually prescribed in 10-mg doses but it is also available in 5- and 15-mg doses. It is taken once per day, usually in the morning to avoid insomnia. However, the pharmacokinetics reveal a peak effect of 6 to 7 hours with food; and therefore, al-though the research has never been done, it can by hypothesized that if one timed the peak effect to occur during the time of greatest risk for overeating, one might maximize the effectiveness of the medication. For example, if the client ate more calories in the evening, sibutramine's effectiveness might be greater if the medication were taken at lunch instead of at breakfast, once sleep patterns were restored to normal.

CASE STUDY: PART 3—JANE CONSIDERS PRESCRIPTION ORLISTAT

After 6 months, Jane has lost a total of 15 pounds, which is 7% of her weight and clinically important in helping prevent type 2 diabetes (17). For the last 3 months, she has been on the highest dosage of Meridia: 15 mg. But Jane is not happy with this weight and she is particularly frustrated that her weight loss has plateaued for the last month. Although plateaus are expected and normal, they can be very disheartening for patients who are trying so hard to lose more weight. Jane wants to lose even more weight, and she is sticking to her goal. Even the fact that her serum cholesterol and blood pressure have both decreased does little to appease her. Although Meridia may be helping Jane to maintain her weight loss, this is not enough and Jane asks for information on orlistat, thinking that her lack of success means she needs a new medication. She knows she cannot take both medications at the same time and is willing to stop taking Meridia. She feels that her behavior is good enough to maintain weight but wonders whether hidden fats in her diet could be slowing her progress.

ORLISTAT PROFILE

Unlike other FDA-approved weight-loss medications, orlistat (Xenical) is the first nonsystemic weight-loss medication, acting entirely on the gut, not the brain. Weight loss occurs because of reduced absorption of fat calories. Triglycerides are digested by lipase enzymes into monoglyceride and free fatty acids. These structures attach to bile salt molecules and phospholipids, forming an aggregate called a micelle. The micelles enable the fat to be absorbed into the intestinal epithelium. Orlistat causes a covalent bond to be formed in the lumen of the stomach and the small intestine that inactivates some of the gastric and pancreatic lipases, essentially blocking them from hydrolyzing the triglycerides to free fatty acids and monoglycerides. The undigested fat is then excreted, with approximately 30% of dietary fat eliminated in the stool.

Approved in 1999 for long-term use, orlistat has been evaluated extensively and has a strong safety record (11). Studies have looked at orlistat's effect on fat-soluble vitamins. In one 4-year study without vitamin supplementation, fat-soluble vitamin levels were reduced but remained within normal limits (11). However, orlistat package inserts suggest incorporating a one-a-day vitamin to limit any possible deficiencies. Instructions are to take the multivitamin once per day, either 1 hour before or 2 hours after taking an orlistat pill. It is usually simpler for patients to remember to take a multivitamin before bed so they do not have to worry about timing. Orlistat as prescribed is to be taken three times per day, at meals. Because its mechanism of action is influenced by the amount of fat consumed in the meal, when someone is following a low-fat diet, side effects are few. However, when someone consumes a high-fat meal, side effects can be great and include flatulence, oily stools, severe diarrhea, and stomach cramping. Orlistat is prescribed with advice about following a low-fat diet to reduce side effects. Psyllium with meals may also help attenuate side effects (18).

Orlistat as Xenical is prescribed in 120-mg tablets to be taken three times per day. Orlistat as Alli is over-the-counter, in 60-mg tablets. Alli is at least half the cost of

Xenical and comes with various educational materials to help the dieter with their diet and other behavioral needs (19).

CASE STUDY: PART 4—JANE TRIES OTC ORLISTAT

No matter how the RD feels, Jane is going to do what she wants and, therefore, as long as her choices are not harmful, the RD aims to help Jane as much as possible. But the RD does not see Jane again for 3 months. When Jane does return, her story is quite a saga. She stopped taking Meridia but did not start any other medication and began to regain weight. Desperately ashamed, she went to a new physician and stopped seeing her RD. The new physician prescribed a combination of diethylpropion (Tenuate), furosemide (Lasix), and potassium to help her lose weight. Jane lost some of her regained weight but she was afraid that this mix of medication would have long-term adverse effects. Finally, she decided to try Alli and return to the RD. Jane is very contrite, promising to appreciate a slow weight loss that can be maintained.

After seeing the RD and starting Alli, Jane loses 2½ pounds in the first week, mainly because she was so afraid of the adverse effects that she barely ate anything. By the end of the sixth week, she is testing the medication by eating larger quantities of fat-laden foods to see whether she would experience adverse effects. The RD warns her against this and reminds her that medication can only enhance the behavioral changes Jane makes.

By the end of the third month, Jane has lost another 10 pounds for a total of 20 pounds (10% of her weight). But Jane is now fighting the same issues she faced with Meridia. Weight loss has slowed significantly and her dietary adherence is more difficult. If she could, she would even make a pact with the devil for something magical to help. With encouragement, Jane resigns herself to trying to maintain her weight for a while and relieve herself of some of the pressure. She agrees to continue to see the RD, although less often, and to go to a Weight Watchers group for support that is less expensive than one-on-one counseling. She will also continue taking Alli to help. When she is ready to lose more weight, Jane will start seeing the RD more often to work out a more restrictive plan.

CONCLUSION

Medication is not magic. The hard work of lifestyle change still has to be done. This is something we need to make clear to clients—what are the criteria for success with medication and how does that differ from the client's expectations? (See Chapter 7.) In Jane's case, it was quite clear: she was able to lose enough weight to make a dramatic difference in her health profile, if not in her dress size. Isn't that, at least in part, a success?

References

1. Yanovski SZ. Pharmacotherapy for obesity—promise and uncertainty. *N Engl J Med.* 2005;53:2187–2189.

2. Ryan DH. Use of sibutramine and other noradrenergic and serotonergic drugs in the management of obesity. *Endocrine.* 2000;13:193–199.

3. Clinical Guidelines on the Identification, Evaluation, and treatment of overweight and obesity in adults: the evidence report. National Institutes of Health. *Obes Res.* 1998;6(Suppl 2):51S–210S.

4. Foster GD, Wadden TA, Makris AP, Davidson D, Sanderson RS, Allison DB, Kessler A. Primary care physicians' attitudes about obesity and its treatment. *Obes Res.* 2003;11:1168–1177.

5. Foster GD, Wadden TA, Vogt RA, Brewer G. What is a reasonable weight loss? Patients' expectations and evaluations of obesity treatment outcomes. *J Consult Clin Psychol.* 1997;65:79–85.

6. Fabricatore AN, Wadden TA, Womble LG, Sarwer DB, Berkowitz RI, Foster GD, Brock JR. The role of patients' expectations and goals in the behavioral and pharmacological treatment of obesity. *Int J Obes.* 2007;31:1739–1745.

7. Bray GA. Drug treatment of obesity. *Psychiatr Clin Am.* 2005;28:193–217.

8. James WP, Astrup A, Finer N, Hilsted J, Kopelman P, Rossner S, Saris WH, Van Gaal LF. Effect of sibutramine on weight maintenance after weight loss: a randomized trial. STORM Study Group. Sibutramine Trial of Obesity Reduction and Maintenance. *Lancet.* 2000;356:2119–2125.

9. Gokcel A, Gumurdulu Y, Karakose H, Melek Ertorer E, Tanaci N, Bascil Tutuncu N, Guvener N. Evaluation of the safety and efficacy of sibutramine, orlistat and metformin in the treatment of obesity. *Diabetes Obes Metab.* 2002;4:49–55.

10. Davidson MH, Hauptman J, DiGirolamo M, Foreyt JP, Halsted CH, Heber D, Heimburger DC, Lucas CP, Robbins DC, Chung J, Heymsfield SB. Weight control and risk factor reduction in obese subjects treated for 2 years with orlistat: a randomized controlled trial. *JAMA.* 1999;281:235–242.

11. Bray GA, Ryan DH. Drug treatment of the overweight patient. *Gastroenterology.* 2007;132:2239–2252.

12. Ogden CL, Yanovski SZ, Carroll MD, Flegal KM. The epidemiology of obesity. *Gastroenterology.* 2007;132:2087–2102.

13. Woods SC. Dietary synergies in appetite control: distal gastrointestinal tract. *Obesity.* 2006;14(Suppl 4):171S–178S.

14. Wassan KM, Loojie NA. Emerging pharmacological approaches to the treatment of obesity. *J Pharmacol Pharmaceut Sci.* 2005;8:259–271.

15. Blundell JE. Perspective on the central control of appetite. *Obesity.* 2006;14(suppl): 160S–167S.

16. Wing RR, Hamman RF, Bray GA, Delahanty L, Edelstein SL, Hill JO, Horton ES, Hoskin MA, Kriska A, Lachin J, Mayer-Davis EJ, Pi-Sunyer X, Regensteiner JG, Venditti B, Wylie-Rosett J; Diabetes Prevention Program Research Group. Achieving weight and activity goals among diabetes prevention program lifestyle participants. *Obes Res.* 2004;12:1426–1434.

17. McDuffie JR, Calis KA, Booth SL, Uwaifo GI, Yanovski JA. Effects of orlistat on fat-soluble vitamins in obese adolescents. *Pharmacology.* 2002;22:814–822.

18. Cavaliere H. Floriano I, Medeiros 0, Neto G. Gastrointestinal side effects of orlistat may be prevented by concomitant prescription of natural fibers (psyllium mucilloid). *Int J Obes Relat Metab Disord.* 2001;25:1095–1099.

19. Williams G. Orlistat over the counter. *BMJ.* 2007;335:1163–1164.

CHAPTER 9

SURGERY

PART A: OVERVIEW

STACY A. BRETHAUER, MD, AND PHILIP R. SCHAUER, MD

HISTORY OF BARIATRIC SURGERY

Surgical procedures have been used to treat obesity since the 1950s. The evolution of surgical weight loss has included a myriad of restrictive and malabsorptive procedures. The initial attempts to control obesity with surgery involved the intentional creation of short bowel syndrome and malabsorption. Jejunocolic bypass excluded the entire small bowel except the proximal jejunum and caused severe uncontrollable diarrhea, electrolyte disturbances, and liver dysfunction. This was replaced with jejunoileal bypass (JIB) in which a short segment of small bowel absorptive surface remains in the terminal ileum. JIB gained widespread popularity in the 1960s and 1970s but has since been abandoned due to long-term sequelae of protein-calorie malnutrition, vitamin deficiencies, chronic electrolyte disturbances, chronic renal failure secondary to increased serum oxalate and nephrolithiasis, and irreversible liver failure (1).

Current malabsorptive procedures include the biliopancreatic diversion (BPD) and biliopancreatic diversion with duodenal switch (BPD/DS). These procedures combine a partial gastrectomy with a long intestinal bypass and a 50- to 100-cm common channel to optimize weight loss and durability without incurring many of the long-term risks of JIB.

Another approach to surgical weight loss has been to restrict the size of the stomach. Various types of vertical and horizontal gastroplasties were done during the 1970s, but staple line failures and weight regain due to pouch and stoma dilation were common complications and often required revision. Mason subsequently developed the vertical banded gastroplasty (VBG) in which the narrow outlet between the pouch and distal stomach was reinforced with a nonadjustable ring or mesh (2). The VBG has effective short-term weight loss and was the most common bariatric procedure in the 1980s. However, long-term complications such as weight regain, severe dysphagia, and gastroesophageal reflux occur in 30% to 50% of VBG patients (3–5). Weight regain after VBG is thought to be secondary to disruption of the vertical staple line (common) or changes in eating behavior in which patients consume soft foods and high-calorie liquids to overcome the fixed stenosis at the gastric pouch outlet (6). VBG currently accounts for fewer than 5% of all bariatric procedures (7).

The first gastric banding procedures (without gastroplasty) were done in the early 1980s with nonadjustable bands around the proximal stomach using the open approach. This approach has been modified to a laparoscopically placed adjustable band that avoids the long-term complications of a fixed outlet. The laparoscopic adjustable gastric band (LAGB) has gained popularity worldwide over the last decade due to its excellent safety profile and good weight-loss results.

Sleeve gastrectomy is a restrictive procedure in which the majority of the stomach is removed, leaving a narrow tube or "sleeve" of stomach along the lesser curvature. This vertical gastrectomy has many applications, but is most commonly used as a first stage procedure in high-risk patients or patients with massive hepatomegaly, with conversion to duodenal switch or gastric bypass 1 or 2 years later.

Gastric bypass was first described by Mason and Ito in 1967 (8). After noticing that individuals who underwent gastric resection with a Billroth II reconstruction (loop gastrojejunostomy) for ulcer disease had difficulty maintaining their weight postoperatively, a similar procedure was used with the intention of causing weight loss in obese patients. Many modifications have been made to this original procedure during the last 40 years, resulting in the Roux-en-Y divided gastric bypass used today.

Importantly, the application of laparoscopy to bariatric surgery in the last 15 years has created a greater demand for these procedures and has attracted many surgeons to the field. Currently, Roux-en-Y gastric bypass (RYGB) is the most common bariatric procedure in the United States, and the majority of these are now done laparoscopically.

As minimally invasive techniques continue to evolve, endoscopic bariatric procedures are being developed. Although the role of these endoluminal procedures has yet to be defined, the low-risk nature of this approach will be attractive to many morbidly obese individuals who are reluctant to undergo the currently available procedures.

CURRENT STATUS OF BARIATRIC SURGERY

There have been many changes in the field of bariatric surgery in the last decade. Data demonstrating the relatively low risk associated with modern bariatric procedures, the development of Centers of Excellence programs by leading surgical societies, and the emergence of a new generation of laparoscopic surgeons interested in treating morbidly obese patients have all been important changes. Between 1998 and 2002, there was a 450% increase in the number of bariatric operations done in the United States, a 144% increase in the surgeon membership of the American Society for Metabolic and Bariatric Surgery (ASBS), and a 146% increase in the number of bariatric centers (9). According to the American Society for Metabolic and Bariatric Surgery, an estimated 140,000 bariatric procedures were done in the United States in 2004. This represented a nine-fold increase since 1994. In the next several years, the annual number of bariatric procedures will likely exceed 200,000.

Despite the growing popularity and acceptance of bariatric surgery for the treatment of severe obesity, however, only 1% of patients in the United States who are eligible for bariatric surgery receive this therapy (7). Many socioeconomic factors are responsible for this disparity (10); also, patients and referring physicians continue to be reluctant to accept the potential risks of bariatric surgery despite the well-documented benefits.

CHOOSING A CANDIDATE FOR BARIATRIC SURGERY

The 1991 National Institutes of Health (NIH) consensus conference for the surgical treatment morbid obesity still provides the criteria to accept patients for bariatric surgery (11). These criteria defined morbid obesity as a body mass index (BMI) of 35 or more with severe obesity-related comorbidity, or a BMI of 40 or more with or without comorbidity. Whereas these are the basic eligibility criteria for entrance into a bariatric surgery program and reimbursement by payers, further assessment is required to determine whether an individual is truly a good candidate for surgery (see, for example, criteria in Box 9.1). Preoperative nutrition and psychological evaluations are critical to identify eating behaviors or uncontrolled psychological or substance abuse disorders that may compromise the success of the surgery.

The 1991 NIH guidelines recommended age limits between 18 and 60 years (11). At that time, there was insufficient evidence to make recommendations about surgery for patients at the extremes of age. Although advanced age has been shown to be a predictor of increased mortality after bariatric surgery (12,13), there is some evidence (case series) that bariatric surgery is safe and effective in carefully selected adolescents and elderly patients (14–16).

Individuals who cannot tolerate general anesthesia due to severe medical compromise are not candidates for surgery. Additionally, patients must be able to comply with the extensive preoperative evaluation and the postoperative lifestyle and diet changes, vitamin supplementation, and follow-up program.

The choice regarding which procedure to use is primarily patient-driven. Malabsorptive procedures are done at only a few specialized centers, and individuals interested in BPD or DS seek out those surgeons specifically. Sleeve gastrectomy is used as a primary procedure or selectively in high-risk patients or when intraoperative anatomy (severe hepatomegaly or intestinal adhesions) prohibits safe completion of RYGB or DS. The choice between RYGB and LAGB is based on a discussion with the patient of the risks and benefits of each procedure. Unless there is a clear contraindication to one of these, the ultimate choice lies with the well-informed patient.

Box 9.1
Characteristics of Candidates for Bariatric Surgery

- Body mass index (BMI) > 40, or BMI > 35 with severe obesity-related comorbidities
- Acceptable operative risk
- Documented failure of nonsurgical weight-loss programs
- Psychologically stable with realistic expectations
- Well-informed and motivated
- Supportive spouse/family/social environment
- Absence of uncontrolled psychotic or depressive disorder
- Absence of active alcohol or substance abuse

SURGICAL OPTIONS

Roux-en-Y Gastric Bypass

RYGB combines gastric restriction with a bypass of the proximal small bowel. The technique of RYGB involves creation of a small 15- to 30-mL gastric pouch and a 75- to 150-cm Roux (alimentary) limb (Figure 9.1). The gastrojejunostomy size is typically 1.5 cm or smaller. The mechanism of action of RYGB is primarily restrictive (small pouch and anastomosis) with a limited, and probably transient, degree of malabsorption. Excluding (bypassing) the distal stomach, duodenum, and proximal jejunum from the flow of nutrients seems to have effects on hunger and glucose metabolism, and these mechanisms continue to be investigated. Gastric bypass is the most common bariatric procedure done in the United States (75%) and the majority of these procedures are now done laparoscopically. The advantages of the laparoscopic approach are faster recovery time, less postoperative analgesia requirements, and fewer pulmonary and wound complications compared with open surgery (17,18). The 20% incidence of incisional hernia after open RYGB has been nearly eliminated with the laparoscopic approach.

The early major postoperative risks associated with RYGB include anastomotic leaks, venous thromboembolism, and bleeding. Later complications can include anastomotic strictures, bowel obstruction, ulcers at the gastrojejunostomy (marginal

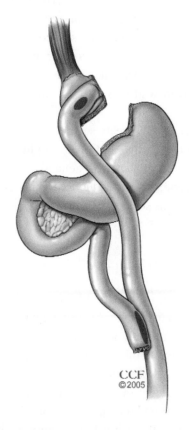

FIGURE 9.1   Roux-en-Y gastric bypass. Reprinted with permission of The Cleveland Clinic Center for Medical Art & Photography © 2007. All Rights Reserved.

TABLE 9.1

Risks of Laparoscopic Bariatric Procedures

Complication	Procedure (References)			
	Laparoscopic Gastric Bypass (17,19–30)	**Laparoscopic Adjustable Gastric Banding (26,31–40)**	**Laparoscopic Sleeve Gastrectomy (41–45)**	**Laparoscopic BPD, BPD/DS (46–50)**
Bleeding	0.4%–4%	0.1%	0%–6.4%	5%–10%
Bowel leak	0%–4.4%	0.5%–0.8%	0%–2.5%	2.5%–3%
Wound infection	0%–8.7%	0.1%–8.8%	NR	2.5%–19%
Deep venous thrombosis	0%–1.3%	0.01%–0.15%	NR	0.5%–2.5%
Pulmonary embolism	0%–1.1%	0.1%	0%–1.6%	0.9%

Abbreviations: BPD, biliopancreatic diversion; DS, duodenal switch; NR, not reported.

ulcer), and micronutrient deficiencies. The incidences of early postoperative complications are listed in Table 9.1 (17,19–50). Lack of nutrient flow through the distal stomach and duodenum impairs absorption of iron and vitamin B-12; the most common deficiencies after RYGB are in these two nutrients. The incidence of these deficiencies after standard or long-limb bypass (longer bypass with increased malabsorption) ranges from 6% to 52% for iron and 3% to 37% for vitamin B-12 (51). Different supplementation regimens and variable patient adherence to long-term supplementation account for the wide ranges in reported deficiencies. Bariatric surgeons agree, however, that these patients require lifelong supplementation and/or monitoring to avoid deficiencies and anemia. Calcium and vitamin D absorption are also decreased after RYGB, and supplements of these nutrients are recommended after surgery to minimize long-term problems with bone loss.

Gastric bypass effectively treats severe obesity and obesity-related comorbidities. This procedure is more invasive and poses slightly higher postoperative risk than the purely restrictive procedures, but it is generally considered a more powerful tool for rapid weight loss and comorbidity reduction. This operation has a favorable risk-benefit profile for most individuals seeking bariatric surgery.

Laparoscopic Adjustable Gastric Banding

Prior to their introduction in the United States, adjustable banding procedures were in use since the early 1990s in Europe, Australia, and South America with good to excellent results. LAGB devices currently available include the Lap Band (Allergan Inc, Irvine, CA) and the Realize Band (Ethicon Endosurgery, Cincinnati, OH). The Food and Drug Administration approved the Lap Band for use in the United States in 2001 and approved the Realize Band in October 2007. LAGB uses a silicone band with an inflatable inner collar, which is placed around the upper portion of the stomach to create a small gastric pouch. The fundus of the stomach is then sewn over the top of the band to prevent band slippage or prolapse of the stomach upward through the band (Figure 9.2). The band is connected to a port that is placed in the subcutaneous tissue of the abdominal wall. Post-

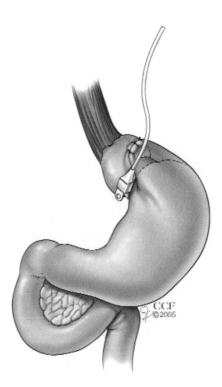

FIGURE 9.2 Laparoscopic adjustable gastric band. Reprinted with permission of The Cleveland Clinic Center for Medical Art & Photography © 2007. All Rights Reserved.

operatively, the inner diameter of the band, and therefore the amount of restriction, can be adjusted by injecting saline through the port.

The adjustable nature of the LAGB is a major advantage that distinguishes it from the vertical banded gastroplasty and nonadjustable bands. Band adjustments are made according to the rate of weight loss and symptoms of dysphagia or regurgitation by injecting or removing saline from a subcutaneous port. Severe complications and mortality rates are lower for LAGB (Table 9.1) than for other bariatric operations. This excellent safety profile makes it an appealing option for many patients and surgeons, and this procedure is growing in popularity. Although early major postoperative complications are rare after LAGB, the long-term reoperation rate for this procedure is 10% to 15% (31).

Reoperations are most commonly needed for gastric prolapse (band slip), tubing or port malfunctions, or band erosion into the gastric lumen. As experience with this procedure increases, the incidence of these complications decreases.

Unlike gastric bypass, a procedure that alters gut hormone physiology, the effects of the LAGB on comorbidities seems to be related solely to weight loss. Weight loss with the LAGB is more gradual than with RYGB. Most patients reach their nadir weight 2 to 3 years after the procedure, and the effectiveness of this procedure is closely related to patient adherence and regular follow-up visits for adjustments (52).

Most bariatric surgeons recommend that LAGB patients take a daily multivitamin and multimineral supplement postoperatively. Because the gastrointestinal tract remains

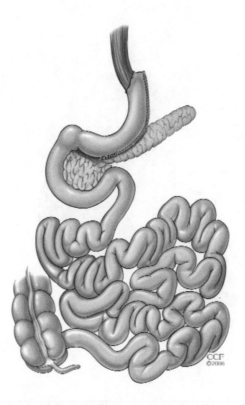

FIGURE 9.3   Sleeve gastrectomy. Reprinted with permission of The Cleveland Clinic Center for Medical Art & Photography © 2007. All Rights Reserved.

in normal continuity, the incidence of vitamin and other micronutrient deficiencies is low.

Sleeve Gastrectomy

Sleeve gastrectomy is a relatively new bariatric surgery procedure. This procedure originated as the gastric restrictive portion of the duodenal switch procedure, in which 75% of the stomach is resected, leaving a narrow gastric tube along the lesser curvature (Figure 9.3).

Currently, sleeve gastrectomy is most commonly done laparoscopically and has several applications. It is still used as the restrictive component of the duodenal switch procedure, but it is also used as a first-stage procedure for high-risk bariatric patients. Patients with multiple severe comorbidities or extremely high BMI (BMI > 60) may not tolerate a longer operation such as BPD/DS or RYGB or a complication such as an anastomotic leak. These patients' risk can be effectively managed by doing a shorter, less risky procedure such as the laparoscopic sleeve gastrectomy with conversion to RYGB or BPD/DS 1 or 2 years later when their comorbidities and functional status have substantially improved (41,42). The early postoperative risks associated with laparoscopic sleeve gastrectomy (LSG) are listed in Table 9.1. Given the high-risk patient population included in most of these series, these complication rates compare favorably with other bariatric procedures.

The most important unanswered question regarding LSG is durability. The current literature describes a heterogeneous patient population, and many are converted to another procedure as part of a planned second stage operation. Therefore, the durability of laparoscopic sleeve gastrectomy beyond 5 years is unknown. Sleeve gastrectomy is being used as a primary procedure in patients with lower BMIs (BMI 35–50) by some surgeons, but long-term results are needed before laparoscopic sleeve gastrectomy is widely accepted as a primary operation. The short-term data currently available for LSG do not allow for a detailed analysis of nutritional complications.

Biliopancreatic Diversion

Biliopancreatic diversion is a malabsorptive procedure done by fewer than 5% of bariatric surgeons in the United States. This procedure, and a modification called the duodenal switch, is designed to limit intestinal energy absorption to the length of the distal common channel. A partial gastrectomy is completed (sleeve gastrectomy for BPD/DS) and the common channel is created 50 to 100 cm from the ileocecal valve by creating a long Roux limb and a very long biliopancreatic limb (Figures 9.4 and 9.5). This short common channel is where all nutrient absorption takes place.

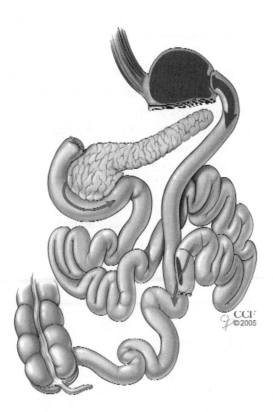

FIGURE 9.4 Biliopancreatic diversion. Reprinted with permission of The Cleveland Clinic Center for Medical Art & Photography © 2007. All Rights Reserved.

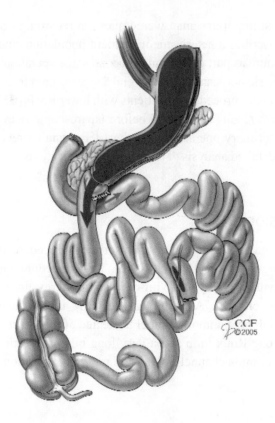

FIGURE 9.5   Biliopancreatic diversion with duodenal switch. Reprinted with permission of The Cleveland Clinic Center for Medical Art & Photography © 2007. All Rights Reserved.

After these malabsorptive procedures, patients experience four to eight loose bowel movements per day. Long-term follow-up with surveillance of nutritional status is imperative after malabsorptive operations. These procedures result in excellent long-term weight loss and comorbidity resolution. Like the RYGB, these procedures bypass the foregut and alter gut hormone physiology and glucose metabolism. Case series of BPD and BPD/DS typically include higher risk patients with higher BMIs than LAGB and RYGB series. This, in part, may explain the higher complication rates reported with malabsorptive procedures (Table 9.1). Although these procedures may offer the most durable weight loss of any bariatric procedure done today, higher complication rates, nutritional deficiencies, and a higher mortality rate have limited their widespread use.

OUTCOMES

Weight Loss and Comorbidity Reduction

Weight loss in the bariatric surgery literature is most commonly reported as percentage of excess weight loss: (% EWL):

$$\% \text{ EWL} = \frac{\text{Preoperative weight} - \text{Current weight} \times 100}{\text{Excess weight}}$$

Excess weight is calculated using the ideal body weight for medium frame from the Metropolitan Life Tables. Weight loss after laparoscopic RYGB ranges from 68% to 80% EWL 1 to 5 years after surgery in large case series (17,19–25,53). Durable weight loss has been demonstrated after RYGB with 67% EWL 10 years after surgery (54).

Most LAGB series report lower weight loss, ranging from 44% to 68% EWL (31,32,33,55,56), and durability has been demonstrated out to 6 years with 57% EWL (31). A randomized controlled trial evaluating the use of the Lap-Band in mild to moderate obesity (BMI 30–35) has demonstrated significantly greater weight loss and comorbidity resolution in the surgical group compared with an aggressive medical weight-loss program. After 2 years, % EWL was 87% in the surgical group and 21% in the nonsurgical group. Metabolic syndrome resolved in 93% of surgical patients and 47% of nonsurgical patients (57).

The large sleeve gastrectomy series report % EWL ranging from 46% to 83% 1 to 2 years after surgery (41-43,45,58,59). In a randomized trial by Himpens et al comparing LAGB to LSG, median % EWL at 3 years was 48% and 66%, respectively (43).

Biliopancreatic diversion and BPD with duodenal switch (BPD/DS) provide excellent long-term weight loss. Hess and Hess have demonstrated 75% EWL in 167 patients 10 years after duodenal switch (92% follow-up) (60). Scopinaro et al (61) reported overall % EWL of 74% at 8 years and 77% at 18 years after open BPD with nearly 100% follow-up and showed no difference in long-term % EWL between morbidly obese (BMI 35–49) and superobese (BMI ≥ 50) patients.

A large prospective matched cohort study (Swedish Obese Subjects Study [SOS]) demonstrated the durability of weight loss and comorbidity reduction 10 years after bariatric surgery (62). The majority of procedures in the SOS study were restrictive operations with relatively few gastric bypass patients (5%) included in the 10-year analysis. At 10 years, the matched control group had a 1.6% weight gain and the surgical group had lost 16.1% of their total weight.

A meta-analysis of 22,094 patients in 136 studies found that for all bariatric procedures, the mean excess weight loss was 61.2% (63). Weight loss and comorbidity resolution data for different procedures reviewed in the meta-analysis are shown in Table 9.2 (63).

TABLE 9.2

Weight Loss and Reduction in Comorbidities after Bariatric Surgery (Summary of Meta-analysis)

	Gastric Banding	Gastric Bypass	BPD or DS	All Procedures
Mean % EWL	47%	62%	70%	61%
Mortality rate	0.1%	0.5%	1.1%	NR
Resolution of diabetes mellitus	48%	84%	99%	77%
Resolution of hyperlipidemia	59%	97%	99%	79%
Resolution of hypertension	43%	68%	83%	62%
Resolution of sleep apnea	95%	80%	92%	86%

Abbreviations: BPD, biliopancreatic diversion; DS, duodenal switch; EWL, excess weight loss; NR, not reported.
Source: Adapted with permission from Buchwald H, Avidor Y, Braunwald E, Jensen MD, Pories W, Fahrbach K, Schoelles K. Bariatric surgery: a systematic review and meta-analysis. *JAMA*. 2004;292:1724–1737. Copyright © 2004, American Medical Association. All rights reserved.

Mortality

The operative mortality for restrictive procedures (banding, VBG), gastric bypass, and BPD in Buchwald et al's meta-analysis was 0.1%, 0.5%, and 1.1%, respectively (63). A review of the international LAGB literature reveals a mortality rate of 0.05% (32). Mortality rates after RYGB vary with the risk of the patient population being studied. Large population-based studies have demonstrated 30-day mortality rates after RYGB as low as 0.3% (64). Mortality after RYGB or BPD is primarily due to pulmonary embolism and anastomotic leak. Early postoperative complications, particularly septic complications, are less common after restrictive procedures such as LAGB.

Life Expectancy

The mortality rate of an individual with a BMI of 40 or more is double that of a normal-weight individual (65). It is estimated that a man in his 20s with a BMI more than 45 will have a 22% reduction (13 years) in life expectancy (66). Most obesity-related deaths are due to complications related to diabetes and cardiovascular disease.

Three large studies have recently demonstrated long-term improvement in survival after bariatric surgery. Adams et al (67) compared 7-year survival rates for nearly 8,000 patients who underwent gastric bypass vs 8,000 severely obese control subjects who were matched for age, sex, and BMI. Gastric bypass patients had an all-cause mortality reduction of 40%. Cause-specific mortality rates decreased in the gastric bypass group by 56% for coronary artery disease, 92% for diabetes, and 60% for cancer. Deaths due to accidents and suicides were 58% higher in the surgical group, however. The SOS study compared 10-year mortality rates for 2,000 bariatric surgery patients (band, gastroplasty, RYGB) and 2,000 matched obese control subjects and found a 29% relative reduction in mortality for the surgical group and sustained weight loss in the surgical group (68). Busetto et al reported a relative risk reduction of 60% 5 years after LAGB compared with a BMI-matched cohort (69). This series of 821 LAGB patients had 40% EWL 5 years after surgery. This data provide a convincing argument that weight loss after common bariatric operations as mentioned earlier is durable and results in improved life-expectancy.

CONCLUSION

Bariatric surgery currently provides the only effective, durable therapy for severe obesity. The benefits of bariatric surgery in terms of weight loss, comorbidity reduction, and improved survival are now well demonstrated. The benefits of the currently available bariatric procedures outweigh the risks for most patients.

The decision to proceed with surgery must be made after careful medical, psychological, and nutrition assessments. When done by experienced surgeons in centers dedicated to the care of obese patients, bariatric surgery is safe, with low perioperative morbidity and mortality rates. Despite the rapid growth of bariatric surgery in the last decade, only a small percentage of patients eligible for bariatric surgery are currently receiving this therapy due to limited or no coverage by most private insurance carriers.

Lower risk options including endoscopic endoluminal bariatric procedures are currently under development.

References

1. DeWind LT, Payne JH. Intestinal bypass surgery for morbid obesity. Long-term results. *JAMA*. 1976;236:2298–2301.

2. Mason EE. Vertical banded gastroplasty for obesity. *Arch Surg*. 1982;117:701–706.

3. Kim CH, Sarr MG. Severe reflux esophagitis after vertical banded gastroplasty for treatment of morbid obesity. *Mayo Clin Proc*. 1992;67:33–35.

4. MacLean LD, Rhode BM, Forse RA. Late results of vertical banded gastroplasty for morbid and super obesity. *Surgery*. 1990;107:20–27.

5. Ramsey-Stewart G. Vertical banded gastroplasty for morbid obesity: weight loss at short and long-term follow-up. *Aust N Z J Surg*. 1995;65:4–7.

6. Brolin RL, Robertson LB, Kenler HA, Cody RP. Weight loss and dietary intake after vertical banded gastroplasty and Roux-en-Y gastric bypass. *Ann Surg*. 1994;220:782–790.

7. Buchwald H, Williams SE. Bariatric surgery worldwide 2003. *Obes Surg*. 2004;14:1157–1164.

8. Mason EE, Ito C. Gastric bypass in obesity. *Surg Clin North Am*. 1967;47:1345–1351.

9. Nguyen NT, Root J, Zainabadi K, Sabio A, Chalifoux S, Stevens CM, Mavandadi S, Longoria M, Wilson SE. Accelerated growth of bariatric surgery with the introduction of minimally invasive surgery. *Arch Surg*. 2005;140:1198–1202; discussion 1203.

10. Livingston EH, Ko CY. Socioeconomic characteristics of the population eligible for obesity surgery. *Surgery*. 2004;135:288–296.

11. National Institutes of Health conference. Gastrointestinal surgery for severe obesity. Consensus Development Conference Panel. *Ann Intern Med*. 1991;115:956–961.

12. Flum DR, Salem L, Elrod JA, Dellinger EP, Cheadle A, Chan L. Early mortality among Medicare beneficiaries undergoing bariatric surgical procedures. *JAMA*. 2005;294:1903–1908.

13. Livingston EH, Huerta S, Arthur D, Lee S, De Shields S, Heber D. Male gender is a predictor of morbidity and age a predictor of mortality for patients undergoing gastric bypass surgery. *Ann Surg*. 2002;236:576–582.

14. Inge TH, Garcia V, Daniels S, et al. A multidisciplinary approach to the adolescent bariatric surgical patient. *J Pediatr Surg*. 2004;39:442–447; discussion 446–447.

15. St Peter SD, Craft RO, Tiede JL, Swain JM. Impact of advanced age on weight loss and health benefits after laparoscopic gastric bypass. *Arch Surg*. 2005;140:165–168.

16. Stanford A, Glascock JM, Eid GM, et al. Laparoscopic Roux-en-Y gastric bypass in morbidly obese adolescents. *J Pediatr Surg*. 2003;38:430–433.

17. Nguyen NT, Goldman C, Rosenquist CJ, Arango A, Cole CJ, Lee SJ, Wolfe BM. Laparoscopic versus open gastric bypass: a randomized study of outcomes, quality of life, and costs. *Ann Surg*. 2001;234:279–289; discussion 289–291.

18. Nguyen NT, Lee SL, Goldman C, Fleming N, Arango A, McFall R, Wolfe BM. Comparison of pulmonary function and postoperative pain after laparoscopic versus open gastric bypass: a randomized trial. *J Am Coll Surg*. 2001;192:469–476; discussion 476–477.

19. DeMaria EJ, Sugerman HJ, Kellum JM, Meador JG, Wolfe LG. Results of 281 consecutive total laparoscopic Roux-en-Y gastric bypasses to treat morbid obesity. *Ann Surg*. 2002;235:640–645; discussion 645–647.

20. Higa KD, Boone KB, Ho T. Complications of the laparoscopic Roux-en-Y gastric bypass: 1,040 patients—what have we learned? *Obes Surg*. 2000;10: 509–513.

21. Higa KD, Boone KB, Ho T, Davies OG. Laparoscopic Roux-en-Y gastric bypass for morbid obesity: technique and preliminary results of our first 400 patients. *Arch Surg*. 2000;135:1029–1033; discussion 1033–1034.

22. Lujan JA, Frutos MD, Hernandez Q, Liron R, Cuenca JR, Valero G, Parrilla P. Laparoscopic versus open gastric bypass in the treatment of morbid obesity: a randomized prospective study. *Ann Surg*. 2004;239:433–437.

23. Nguyen NT, Ho HS, Palmer LS, Wolfe BM. A comparison study of laparoscopic versus open gastric bypass for morbid obesity. *J Am Coll Surg*. 2000;191:149–155; discussion 155–157.

24. Schauer PR, Ikramuddin S, Gourash W, Ramanathan R, Luketich J. Outcomes after laparoscopic Roux-en-Y gastric bypass for morbid obesity. *Ann Surg*. 2000;232: 515–529.

25. Wittgrove AC, Clark GW. Laparoscopic gastric bypass, Roux-en-Y- 500 patients: technique and results, with 3–60 month follow-up. *Obes Surg*. 2000;10:233–239.

26. Biertho L, Steffen R, Ricklin T, Horber FF, Pomp A, Inabnet WB, Herron D, Gagner M. Laparoscopic gastric bypass versus laparoscopic adjustable gastric banding: a comparative study of 1,200 cases. *J Am Coll Surg*. 2003;197:536–544; discussion 544–545.

27. Fernandez AZ, Demaria EJ, Tichansky DS, Kellum JM, Wolfe LG, Meador J, Sugerman HJ. Multivariate analysis of risk factors for death following gastric bypass for treatment of morbid obesity. *Ann Surg*. 2004; 239:698–702; discussion 702–703.

28. Fernandez AZ Jr, DeMaria EJ, Tichansky DS, Kellum JM, Wolfe LG, Meador J, Sugerman HJ. Experience with over 3,000 open and laparoscopic bariatric procedures: multivariate analysis of factors related to leak and resultant mortality. *Surg Endosc*. 2004;18:193–197.

29. Papasavas PK, Hayetian FD, Caushaj PF, Landreneau RJ, Maurer J, Keenan RJ, Quinlin RF, Gagne DJ. Outcome analysis of laparoscopic Roux-en-Y gastric bypass for morbid obesity. The first 116 cases. *Surg Endosc*. 2002;16:1653–1657.

30. Westling A, Gustavsson S. Laparoscopic vs open Roux-en-Y gastric bypass: a prospective, randomized trial. *Obes Surg*. 2001;11:284–292.

31. O'Brien PE, Dixon JB, Brown W, Schachter LM, Chapman L, Burn AJ, Dixon ME, Scheinkestel C, Halket C, Sutherland LJ, Korin A, Baquie P. The laparoscopic adjustable gastric band (Lap-Band): a prospective study of medium-term effects on weight, health and quality of life. *Obes Surg*. 2002; 2:652–660.

32. Chapman AE, Kiroff G, Game P, Foster B, O'Brien P, Ham J, Maddern GJ. Laparo-scopic adjustable gastric banding in the treatment of obesity: a systematic literature review. *Surgery.* 2004;135:326–351.

33. O'Brien PE, Dixon JB. Lap-band: outcomes and results. *J Laparoendosc Adv Surg Tech A.* 2003;13:265–270.

34. Angrisani L, Alkilani M, Basso N, Belvederesi N, Campanile F, Capizzi FD, D'Atri C, Di Cosmo L, Doldi SB, Favretti F, Forestieri P, Furbetta F, Giacomelli F, Giar-diello C, Iuppa A, Lesti G, Lucchese M, Puglisi F, Scipioni L, Toppino M, Turicchia GU, Veneziani A, Docimo C, Borrelli V, Lorenzo M; Italian Collaborative Study Group for the Lap-Band System. Laparoscopic Italian experience with the Lap-Band. *Obes Surg.* 2001;11:307–310.

35. Belachew M, Belva PH, Desaive C. Long-term results of laparoscopic adjustable gastric banding for the treatment of morbid obesity. *Obes Surg.* 2002;12:564–568.

36. Cadiere GB, Himpens J, Hainaux B, Gaudissart Q, Favretti S, Segato G. Laparo-scopic adjustable gastric banding. *Semin Laparosc Surg.* 2002;9:105–114.

37. Dargent J. Laparoscopic adjustable gastric banding: lessons from the first 500 pa-tients in a single institution. *Obes Surg.* 1999;9:446–452.

38. O'Brien PE, Dixon JB. Weight loss and early and late complications—the interna-tional experience. *Am J Surg.* 2002;184(6B):42S–45S.

39. Ren CJ, Horgan S, Ponce J. US experience with the LAP-BAND system. *Am J Surg.* 2002;184(6B):46S–50S.

40. Rubenstein RB. Laparoscopic adjustable gastric banding at a U.S. center with up to 3-year follow-up. *Obes Surg.* 2002;12:380–384.

41. Cottam D, Qureshi FG, Mattar SG, Sharma S, Holover S, Bonanomi G, Ra-manathan R, Schauer P. Laparoscopic sleeve gastrectomy as an initial weight-loss procedure for high-risk patients with morbid obesity. *Surg Endosc.* 2006;20: 859–863.

42. Silecchia G, Boru C, Pecchia A, Rizzello M, Casella G, Leonetti F, Basso N. Effec-tiveness of laparoscopic sleeve gastrectomy (first stage of biliopancreatic diversion with duodenal switch) on co-morbidities in super-obese high-risk patients. *Obes Surg.* 2006;16:1138–1144.

43. Himpens J, Dapri G, Cadiere GB. A prospective randomized study between laparo-scopic gastric banding and laparoscopic isolated sleeve gastrectomy: results after 1 and 3 years. *Obes Surg.* 2006;16:1450–1456.

44. Baltasar A, Serra C, Perez N, Bou R, Bengochea M, Ferri L. Laparoscopic sleeve gastrectomy: a multi-purpose bariatric operation. *Obes Surg.* 2005;15:1124–1128.

45. Lee CM, Cirangle PT, Jossart GH. Vertical gastrectomy for morbid obesity in 216 patients: report of two-year results. *Surg Endosc.* 2007;21:1810–1816.

46. Rabkin RA, Rabkin JM, Metcalf B, Lazo M, Rossi M, Lehmanbecker LB. Laparo-scopic technique for performing duodenal switch with gastric reduction. *Obes Surg.* 2003;13:263–268.

47. Baltasar A, Bou R, Miro J, Bengochea M, Serra C, Perez N. Laparoscopic biliopan-creatic diversion with duodenal switch: technique and initial experience. *Obes Surg.* 2002;12:245–248.

48. Paiva D, Bernardes L, Suretti L. Laparoscopic biliopancreatic diversion: technique and initial results. *Obes Surg.* 2002;12:358–361.

49. Ren CJ, Patterson E, Gagner M. Early results of laparoscopic biliopancreatic diversion with duodenal switch: a case series of 40 consecutive patients. *Obes Surg.* 2000;10:514–523; discussion 524.

50. Scopinaro N, Marinari GM, Camerini G. Laparoscopic standard biliopancreatic diversion: technique and preliminary results. *Obes Surg.* 2002;12:241–244.

51. Bloomberg RD, Fleishman A, Nalle JE, Nalle JE, Herron DM, Kini S. Nutritional deficiencies following bariatric surgery: what have we learned? *Obes Surg.* 2005;15:145–154.

52. Shen R, Dugay G, Rajaram K, Cabrera I, Siegel N, Ren CJ. Impact of patient follow-up on weight loss after bariatric surgery. *Obes Surg.* 2004;14:514–519.

53. Papasavas PK, Gagne DJ, Kelly J, Caushaj PF. Laparoscopic Roux-En-Y gastric bypass is a safe and effective operation for the treatment of morbid obesity in patients older than 55 years. *Obes Surg.* 2004;14:1056–1061.

54. Christou NV, Sampalis JS, Liberman M, Look D, Auger S, McLean AP, MacLean LD. Surgery decreases long-term mortality, morbidity, and health care use in morbidly obese patients. *Ann Surg.* 2004;240:416–423; discussion 423–424.

55. Ponce J, Paynter S, Fromm R. Laparoscopic adjustable gastric banding: 1,014 consecutive cases. *J Am Coll Surg.* 2005;201:529–535.

56. Watkins BM, Montgomery KF, Ahroni JH. Laparoscopic adjustable gastric banding: early experience in 400 consecutive patients in the USA. *Obes Surg.* 2005;15:82–87.

57. O'Brien PE, Dixon JB, Laurie C, Skinner S, Proietto J, McNeil J, Strauss B, Marks S, Schachter L, Chapman L, Anderson M. Treatment of mild to moderate obesity with laparoscopic adjustable gastric banding or an intensive medical program: a randomized trial. *Ann Intern Med.* 2006;144:625–633.

58. Hamoui N, Anthone GJ, Kaufman HS, Crookes PF. Sleeve gastrectomy in the high-risk patient. *Obes Surg.* 2006;16:1445–1449.

59. Moon Han S, Kim WW, Oh JH. Results of laparoscopic sleeve gastrectomy (LSG) at 1 year in morbidly obese Korean patients. *Obes Surg.* 2005;15:1469–1475.

60. Hess DS, Hess DW, Oakley RS. The biliopancreatic diversion with the duodenal switch: results beyond 10 years. *Obes Surg.* 2005;15:408–416.

61. Scopinaro N, Gianetta E, Adami GF, Friedman D, Traverso E, Marinari GM, Cuneo S, Vitale B, Ballari F, Colombini M, Baschieri G, Bachi V. Biliopancreatic diversion for obesity at eighteen years. *Surgery.* 1996;119:261–268.

62. Sjostrom L, Lindroos AK, Peltonen M, et al. Lifestyle, diabetes, and cardiovascular risk factors 10 years after bariatric surgery. *N Engl J Med.* 2004;351:2683–2693.

63. Buchwald H, Avidor Y, Braunwald E, Jensen MD, Pories W, Fahrbach K, Schoelles K. Bariatric surgery: a systematic review and meta-analysis. *JAMA.* 2004;292:1724–1737.

64. Zingmond DS, McGory ML, Ko CY. Hospitalization before and after gastric bypass surgery. *JAMA.* 2005;294:1918–1924.

65. Flegal KM, Graubard BI, Williamson DF, Gail MH. Excess deaths associated with underweight, overweight, and obesity. *JAMA.* 2005;293:1861–1867.

66. Fontaine KR, Redden DT, Wang C, Westfall AO, Allison DB. Years of life lost due to obesity. *JAMA.* 2003;289:187–193.

67. Adams TD, Gress RE, Smith SC, Halverson RC, Simper SC, Rosamond WD, Lamonte MJ, Stroup AM, Hunt SC. Long-term mortality after gastric bypass surgery. *N Engl J Med.* 2007;357:753–761.

68. Sjostrom L, Narbro K, Sjostrom CD, Karason K, Larsson B, Wedel H, Lystig T, Sullivan M, Bouchard C, Carlsson B, Bengtsson C, Dahlgren S, Gummesson A, Jacobson P, Karlsson J, Lindroos AK, Lönroth H, Näslund I, Olbers T, Stenlöf K, Torgerson J, Agren G, Carlsson LM; Swedish Obese Subjects Study. Effects of bariatric surgery on mortality in Swedish obese subjects. *N Engl J Med.* 2007;357:741–752.

69. Busetto L, Mirabelli D, Petroni ML, Mazza M, Favretti F, Segato G, Chiusolo M, Merletti F, Balzola F, Enzi G. Comparative long-term mortality after laparoscopic adjustable gastric banding versus nonsurgical controls. *Surg Obes Relat Dis.* 2007;3:496–502.

PART B: PRACTICAL APPLICATIONS

SUE CUMMINGS, MS, RD

OVERVIEW

The number of weight-loss surgeries, also referred to as bariatric surgery, in the United States has increased substantially over the past decade (1). Increasing numbers of registered dietitians (RD) are specializing in the care of weight-loss surgery patients. In addition, many nonspecialist RDs and other health care providers in both outpatient and inpatient settings are evaluating and counseling patients before and after surgery. Although there is an increasing body of research in the field of bariatric surgery, most current recommendations for the medical, nutrition, and psychological care of patients are based on case reports; nonrandomized, small sample, retrospective studies; and expert opinion. To date, care has not been standardized across surgical centers. Recently, major organizations have been analyzing the existing data and, where evidence is lacking, working to standardize recommendations based on expert opinion (2,3). All weight-loss surgery procedures have nutritional implications, and this section will provide guidance for the nutrition evaluation and care of the weight-loss surgery patient.

WEIGHT-LOSS SURGERY PROCEDURES AND POTENTIAL NUTRITIONAL IMPLICATIONS

Weight-loss surgery procedures are characterized into three broad categories. These categories are (*a*) purely gastric restrictive procedures, such at the laparoscopic adjustable gastric band (LAGB) and vertical banded gastroplasty (VBG); (*b*) gastric restrictive with some malabsorption of micronutrients, such as the Roux-en-Y gastric bypass (RYGBP); and (*c*) gastric restriction with significant intestinal malabsorption, such as the biliopancreatic diversion (BPD) and the BPD with duodenal switch (BPD/DS). The sleeve gastrectomy (SG) is a newer procedure that causes restriction and has neural and hormonal influences that are not fully understood. Although the 5-year data for SG are promising, long-term data are not available for this procedure.

The most common weight-loss surgery in the United States today is RYGBP. Weight loss after RYGBP is most likely caused by some combination of restriction and changes in neural and hormonal pathways. RYGBP leads to malabsorption of some micronutrients, such as vitamin B-12, vitamin B-1 (thiamin), vitamin D, vitamin K, folate, iron, and calcium, but not macronutrients.

The number of LAGB procedures in the United States is increasing. As described in Part A of this chapter, LAGB is a purely restrictive procedure that limits total energy intake; however, because the foregut is not bypassed, absorption of nutrients is not affected. SG is gaining increasing recognition as a restrictive procedure that may be used in patients who are at high risk for more complicated surgical procedures.

BPD and BPD/DS are less commonly done and because of the extensive reconstruction of the intestinal tract, substantial malabsorption of both micro- and macronutrients occur. Individuals undergoing these procedures need very close short- and long-term nutrition monitoring. This section on practical approaches will focus primarily on RYGBP and LAGB.

Most weight-loss surgery procedures today are done laparoscopically. The laparoscopic procedure has several advantages: fewer wound complications, less postoperative pain, shorter hospital stays, and more rapid postoperative recovery (4,5). The choice of bariatric procedures ultimately depends on individual factors related to a risk-benefit analysis. Consideration should be given to body mass index (BMI), perioperative risk, metabolic parameters, comorbidities, surgeon competence, and other patient preferences (6).

REIMBURSEMENT CRITERIA FOR WEIGHT-LOSS SURGERY

In the past 5 years, changes have been made to the criteria used by Medicare/Medicaid and private health care insurance companies for patients to qualify for insurance coverage for bariatric procedures. After an internal, evidence-based review of the bariatric literature and extensive analysis, the Centers for Medicare & Medicaid Services (CMS) concluded that bariatric surgery could be offered to Medicare beneficiaries with a BMI of 35 or more who have at least one comorbidity and have been unsuccessful at previous weight-loss attempts. CMS also require the surgery be done at a Center of Excellence (7). A Center of Excellence (8) meets the standards of multidisciplinary care set by the American Society for Metabolic and Bariatric Surgery (ASMBS) (9) and the American College of Surgeons (ACS) (10). The Center of Excellence must have a dedicated multidisciplinary bariatric team that includes surgeons, nurses, medical consultants, nutritionists, psychologists, and/or exercise physiologists (see Table 9.3). Private insurers often follow the requirements of CMS.

TABLE 9.3

The Surgical Care Team

Discipline	Evaluation
Medical (registered nurse, physician assistant, internist)	• Identify and evaluate comorbidities • Exclude medically treatable causes of obesity • Assess need to adjust medications • Laboratory evaluation for causes and effects of obesity • Determine need for additional presurgical testing • Reduce risks of surgery and increase safety
Mental health (psychologist, psychiatrist)	• Evaluate impact of weight on functioning • Current psychological symptoms and stressors • Psychiatric history • History or presence of eating disorders including binge eating disorder • Interpersonal consequences of weight loss • Identify obstacles to treatment • Assess stability of mental health disease; medications
Nutrition (registered dietitian)	• Height and weight; calculate body mass index • Nutritional factors related comorbidities; medications, and compliance • Dieting history • Weight history • Food intake; supplements • Work, cultural, and social history affecting weight • Eating behaviors • Meal/snack patterns • Eating style • Physical activity and limitations • Knowledge of surgeries including weight expectations, impact on current eating behaviors and habits (all team members); motivation • Nutrition-related laboratory values
Surgery (physician)	• Surgical evaluation • Assess and recommend type of surgery • Consent

PRESURGICAL CONSIDERATIONS

Nutrition Care Process

Nutrition management for weight-loss surgery may be provided by the RD using the Nutrition Care Process (NCP) (11) and according to guidelines established in the American Dietetic Association (ADA) Adult Weight Management Evidence-Based Practice Guidelines (12). The initial nutrition assessment for individuals with obesity is described in detail in the ADA Adult Weight Management Certificate Course and the ADA Adult Weight Management Toolkit (13,14). Table 9.3 lists the additional components of the nutrition assessment for presurgery patients. By synthesizing and classifying client assessment information, RDs can proceed through the NCP to assign nutrition diagnoses, formulate a nutrition prescription, and identify the desired goals and outcomes of nutrition intervention(s) both before and after weight loss surgery. See Part B of Chapter 1 for more information on NCP and *ADA Pocket Guide to Bariatric Surgery* (15) for guidance on using NCP with this patient population.

Specific criteria will need to be included in the insurance Letter of Medical Necessity for approval of weight-loss surgery and should be documented by the RD. These are height, weight, BMI, severity and duration of obesity, weight history, and the patient's dieting history, which includes a brief statement of self-directed attempts, commercial programs, and medically supervised programs.

Presurgery Micronutrients

An individual with obesity does not necessarily have normal levels of vitamins and trace minerals. To the contrary, poor nutritional intake may lead to nutritional deficiencies, and a person with obesity may have malnutrition. Because bariatric surgery procedures that alter nutrient absorption (such as the RYGB, BPD, and the BPD/DS) can lead to nutritional deficiencies, all patients should be tested preoperatively and deficiencies corrected before surgery (16). Box 9.2 (17–20) lists the vitamins and minerals that should be assessed and the deficiencies to detect and correct before surgery.

Vitamins B-12 and D, folate, iron, and calcium should be screened before bariatric surgery and repleted as needed (16). Special considerations should be given to the following:

• Vitamin D deficiency is common in the US population, and patients with obesity are at higher risk (17). Ybarra et al found vitamin D deficiency preceded bariatric surgery (18).
• Thiamin deficiency is not uncommon, especially in African-American and Hispanic patients with obesity. Patients should be screened and repleted prior to surgery (19).

In a review of nutritional consequences of bariatric surgery, Xanthakos and Inge summarize recent advances and understanding and provide guidelines for nutrition screening

---

Box 9.2
Nutrition-related Laboratory Tests Recommended Before Weight-loss Surgery

- Complete blood count with differential
- Glucose, A1C
- Serum lipids
- Serum iron, ferritin and TIBC
- Serum calcium, alkaline phosphatase
- Serum vitamin B-12 (MMA, homocysteine)
- Folate (in women of childbearing age); consider plasma homocysteine
- Parathyroid hormone, 25-hydroxyvitamin D
- Thiamin
- Baseline dual-energy X-ray absorptiometry to assess bone mineral density/content especially in postmenopausal women

Abbreviations: A1C, glycated hemoglobin; TIBC, total iron-binding capacity; MMA, methylmalonic acid.
Source: Data are from references 17–20.

(20). In addition, recent guidelines for the recommended biochemical surveillance of nutritional status after malapsorptive bariatric surgery have been published (3).

Comorbidities

Comorbidities and medications and dosages should also be noted before surgery because these will need to be closely monitored after weight-loss surgery. Monitoring is especially needed for comorbidities with nutritional implications, such as diabetes and hypertension, because postoperative medications may need early adjustment (3).

Nutrition Prescription

Based on the initial nutrition assessment and diagnosis or diagnoses, the RD will then prescribe/recommend a nutrition intervention. This intervention may be for a short presurgery nutrition intervention to reinforce the importance of a balanced diet; to assist the patient in structuring his or her meal patterns; and/or to set presurgery weight or nutrition goals. Depending on the patient's nutrition diagnoses, the RD may determine that the patient would benefit from a comprehensive nutrition program before having weight-loss surgery. In some cases, the RD and surgical team may determine the patient is ready for surgery; however, the insurance provider may require a short or extended presurgical nutrition and psychology program.

Preoperative Weight Loss

Some evidence indicates that a weight loss of at least 5% of total body weight before weight-loss surgery is associated with decreased operative time, which may potentially decrease surgical risk (21,22). One study involving patients who followed a very-low-calorie diet before weight-loss surgery had a substantial decrease in liver volume, resulting in a reduction in reported surgical difficulty and a reduction in conversion from a laparoscopic procedure to an open procedure during surgery (23). However, study results regarding the benefit of presurgical weight loss and reduction of postoperative complications are contradictory, and this is an area of some controversy. More studies are needed to establish the efficacy and ethical implications of mandatory presurgery weight loss (24,25).

Preoperative Insurance-mandated Nutrition Programs

Despite the lack of evidence, a few private insurance providers require documentation that patients have participated in a presurgical nutrition and weight-loss program before they will authorize weight-loss surgery. The program requirements can range from 3 to 12 months. These requirements can be burdensome to patients both financially and time-wise, and delays before surgery can be an obstacle for patients in the most need of effective obesity treatment. RDs can help patients through this process by (*a*) establishing cost-effective programs, (*b*) motivating patients by emphasizing the physical and psychological benefits of presurgical preparation, and (*c*) using this time to shape patient expectations regarding early postsurgical challenges and the lifestyle changes required for long-term success.

When reimbursement for individual medical nutrition therapy (MNT) sessions is not available, group programs are often less expensive and more resource-efficient. Centers may want to consider establishing weekly nutrition group sessions in which the patient can be enrolled for 1, 3, or 6 months, depending on insurance provider requirements. These sessions can be ongoing with rotating nutrition topics focused on preparing patients for surgery. Topics may include the following:

- Obesity etiology and treatments: how weight loss surgery differs from restrictive dieting
- How to structure healthful meals and snacks
- Healthful nutrition
- Preparing for weight-loss surgery: giving up high-calorie beverages, weaning off of caffeine, limiting concentrated sweet intake, increasing daily intake of calorie-free fluids, increasing activities of daily living, and incorporating a walking program
- Reading food labels
- Mindful eating

The order in which patients participate in these sessions should not matter, so that the groups can be open and patient enrollment need not be delayed. The RD running the program can establish visit templates for documentation; all attendance and weights should be documented in the patient's chart for insurance providers that require this.

Preoperative Surgical Information Session

Data indicate that preoperative teaching by a multidisciplinary team improves patient selection and enables patients to choose the surgical procedure most appropriate for them, thus leading to more successful outcomes (26). RDs are important members of the surgical multidisciplinary team. They are uniquely trained in both physical and behavioral sciences, and this training gives them the skills to lead surgical information sessions and help patients make informed decisions about weight-loss surgery.

The surgical information session should be open to all patients considering weight-loss surgery and should minimally contain the following information:

- Definition of obesity (estimated by BMI)
- Education about BMI (provide BMI chart)
- Education regarding indications for weight-loss surgery (National Heart, Lung, and Blood Institute criteria)
- Additional program criteria (program fees, scheduling commitments, etc)
- Contraindications to surgery
- Description of types of surgery, including their risks and benefits
- Review of expectations for weight loss (for each type of surgery), postoperative diet stages, and lifestyle and behavioral changes required for long-term success

- Financial requirements (patients need to research individual insurance policies)
- Postoperative appointments (making the commitment)
- Getting started (what the patient can do now to prepare for surgery)

A surgeon should be available at every session. It is helpful to ask patients who have undergone weight-loss surgery to attend and share their experiences. These patients should be encouraged to share all aspects of their postsurgical experiences, including complications, challenges, and successes.

Preparing for Weight-loss Surgery

Patients should be encouraged to prepare for surgery by accepting surgery as a "tool" and making a commitment to healthful lifestyle changes, such as choosing a healthful meal plan and being physically active. They should start to make healthful changes before surgery.

Physical Activity

Walking after surgery is essential to decrease the risk of developing life-threatening blood clots. Before surgery, encourage all patients who are able to take mini-walks throughout the day to develop strength and stamina.

Eating and Drinking Behaviors

Encourage patients to work on the following changes:

- Stop drinking carbonated beverages.
- Wean off of caffeine, which has a diuretic effect and should be discouraged during the early months after surgery.
- Practice eating very, very slowly and mindfully.
- Get in the habit of drinking 48 to 64 ounces of no-calorie, noncarbonated, noncaffeinated beverages each day.

Mandatory Presurgery Education Classes

The types of surgery procedure offered to patients typically depend on the surgical expertise available, patient preferences, and a risk-benefit analysis of each procedure. The patient and the surgeon select the procedure to use. Once patients have met with the surgeon and the procedure has been selected, a mandatory presurgery nutrition class should be scheduled. At this class, patients should be given printed materials describing the inpatient and discharge diets, including sample meal plans and shopping lists and a list of adequate supplemental vitamins and minerals. In addition, patients should be scheduled for a nutrition visit 1 to 2 weeks after surgery to assess progress and advance the diet.

PERIOPERATIVE PATIENT CARE AFTER WEIGHT LOSS SURGERY

The diet after weight-loss surgery is based on nutritional needs with a strong emphasis on texture. The diet is provided in a staged approach to maximize tolerance. The amount of food patients can eat, and the type and the pace at which they can drink or eat, will vary widely among patients.

While in the hospital, RYGBP patients may be required to undergo a gastrogaffin swallow test to assess for anastomosis leak. Until they take the test, they will remain on intravenous hydration, taking nothing by mouth. After a successful swallow test, patients are started on clear liquids.

Clear liquids after weight-loss surgery should have no calories, no carbonation, and no sugar. When fully awake, LAGB patients should sip fluids to assess tolerance because edema and tissue within a newly placed band can cause obstruction. Patients should be encouraged to sip slowly; ice chips and a pitcher of water should be kept at the bedside.

The staged approach to diet advancement after surgery varies widely among institutions and can contain between four to six diet stages. The diet stages progress from clear liquids inpatient; to clear and full liquids at home; to soft, moist pureed, diced, and/or ground proteins. Vegetables, fruits, and starches are added over time as tolerated. Tables 9.4 and 9.5 provide examples of diet stages for RYGBP and LAGB. Eating style should be addressed with every patient. Chewing well, eating slowly, and eating mindfully are essential to avoid vomiting, dumping syndrome, and/or foods feeling "stuck." Patients undergoing LAGB may adopt poor eating habits postsurgery because soft foods such as ice cream are easily consumed. Therefore, frequent postoperative nutrition counseling, education, and follow-up are important.

Hydration

Adequate hydration is a top priority in the period following surgery. Patients should be encouraged to consume 48 to 64 ounces or more of total fluids per day. They should be taught early signs and symptoms of dehydration and advised to consume salty fluids such as broth if they experience early signs of dehydration or are unable to meet minimum fluid requirements. Patients with early postoperative nausea may find they better tolerate solid liquids (sugar-free ice pops, gelatin) and should be encouraged to keep these available. Early and persistent vomiting may lead to dehydration and is also associated with thiamin deficiency. If dehydration becomes severe, patients will most likely need intravenous hydration. Thiamin should always be administered with intravenous hydration containing glucose because thiamin deficiency can lead to Wernicke's encephalopathy, a serious nonreversible neurologic disorder.

Diet Progression and Supplementation

Patients who have had an uncomplicated laparoscopic RYGBP are often discharged 2 days after surgery. Patients having the LAGB may be discharged the same day as the

TABLE 9.4

Diet Stages for Roux-en-Y Gastric Bypass (RYGBP) Patients

Diet Stage[a]	Begin	Fluids/Food	Guidelines
Stage 1	Post-op Days 1 and 2	**RYGBP clear liquids:** noncarbonated; no calories; no sugar; no caffeine.	• Post-op Day 1, patients undergo a gastrogaffin swallow test for leak; once tested, they can begin sips of RYGBP clear liquids.
Stage 2	Post-op Day 3 (discharge diet)	**RYGBP clear liquids:** variety of no-sugar liquids or artificially sweetened liquids; encourage patients to have salty fluids at home; solid liquids: sugar-free ice pops. *Plus* **RYGBP full liquids:** < 25 g sugar per serving; protein-rich liquids (≤ 20 g protein per serving of added powders).	• Begin supplementation: chewable multivitamin with minerals twice daily; chewable or liquid calcium citrate with vitamin D; 350 mcg crystalline vitamin B-12. • Patients should consume a minimum of 48–64 oz total fluids per day; 24–32 oz or more RYGBP clear liquids plus 24–32 oz of any combination of full liquids: 1% or nonfat milk mixed with whey or soy protein powder (≤ 20 g protein per serving); Lactaid milk or soy milk mix with soy protein powder; light yogurt, blended; plain yogurt; Greek yogurt.
Stage 3: Week 1	Post-op Days 10–14	Increase RYGBP clear liquids (total liquids 48–64 oz/d) and replace full liquids with soft, moist, diced, ground or pureed protein sources as tolerated: eggs; meats, poultry or soft, moist fish with added gravy, bouillon, or light mayonnaise to moisten; cooked beans; hearty bean soups; cottage cheese; low-fat cheese; yogurt.	• Protein food choices are encouraged for 3–6 small meals per day. Patients may only be able to tolerate a couple of tablespoons at each meal/snack. • Encourage patients to not drink with meals and to wait ~30 minutes after each meal before resuming fluids.
Stage 3: Week 2	4 weeks post-op	Advance diet as tolerated. Add well-cooked, soft vegetables and soft and/or peeled fruit. Always eat protein first.	• Adequate hydration is essential and a priority for all patients during the rapid weight-loss phase. • Encourage patients to wait 30 minutes after meals before consuming liquids.
Stage 3: Week 3	5 weeks post-op	Continue to consume protein with some fruit or vegetable at each meal. Some people tolerate salads 1 month post-op. Starches should be limited to whole-grain crackers with protein, potato and/or dry low-sugar cereals moistened with milk.	• May switch to pill-form supplementation. • Patients should **avoid** rice, bread, and pasta until they are comfortably consuming 60 g protein per day and fruits/vegetables.
Stage 4	As hunger increases and more food is tolerated	Healthy solid-food diet.	• Vitamin and mineral supplementation daily. • Healthy, balanced diet consisting of adequate protein, fruits, vegetables, and whole grains. • Calorie needs based on height, weight, age.

[a]Diet stages are not standardized; diet protocols vary with regard to how long patients stay on each stage and what types of fluids/foods are recommended.

Source: Reprinted with permission by Sue Cummings, MS, RD.

TABLE 9.5

Diet Stages for Laparoscopic Adjustable Gastric Band (LAGB) Patients

Stage	Begin	Fluids/Foods	Guidelines
Stage 1	Post-op Days 1 and 2	LAGB clear liquids: noncarbonated, no calories, no sugar, no caffeine	• Post-op LAGB Day 1, patients may begin sips of water, ice chips, and sugar-free powdered drinks. • Avoid carbonation.
Stage 2	Post-op Days 2 and 3 (discharge diet)	**LAGB clear liquids:** variety of no-sugar liquids or artificially sweetened liquids. *Plus* **LAGB full liquids:** < 25 g sugar per serving, and ≤ 3 g fat per serving; protein-rich liquids	• Begin supplementation: chewable multivitamin with minerals twice daily; chewable or liquid calcium citrate with vitamin D. • Patients should consume a minimum of 48–64 oz total fluids per day; at least 24–32 oz LAGB clear liquids plus 24–32 oz any combination of full liquids: 1% or nonfat milk mixed with whey or soy protein powder (≤ 20 g protein per serving); Lactaid milk or soy milk mix with soy protein powder; light yogurt, blended; plain yogurt.
Stage 3: Week 1	Post-op Days 10–14	Increase LAGB clear liquids (total liquids ≥ 48–64 oz/d) and replace full liquids with soft, moist, diced, ground or pureed protein sources as tolerated: eggs; meats, poultry, or soft, moist fish with added gravy, bouillon, or light mayonnaise to moisten; cooked beans; hearty bean soups; cottage cheese; low-fat cheese, yogurt.	• **Note:** Patients should be reassured that hunger is common and normal after LAGB. • Protein food (moist, ground) choices are encouraged for 3–6 small meals per day, to help with satiety. • Mindful, slow, eating is essential. • Encourage patients to not drink with meals and to wait ~30 minutes after each meal before resuming fluids.
Stage 3: Week 2	4 weeks post-op	Advance diet as tolerated. If protein foods are well tolerated in first week, add well-cooked, soft vegetables and soft and/or peeled fruit.	• Adequate hydration is essential and a priority for all patients during the rapid weight-loss phase. • Patients should have protein at every meal and snack, especially if increased hunger noted prior to initial band filling or adjustment. • Very well-cooked vegetables may also help to increase satiety.
Stage 3: Week 3	5 weeks post-op	Continue to consume protein with some fruit or vegetable at each meal. Some people tolerate salads 1 month post-op.	• If patient is tolerating soft, moist, ground, diced and/or pureed proteins with small amounts of fruits and vegetables, may add crackers (eat with protein). • **Avoid** rice, bread, and pasta.
Stage 4	As hunger increases and more food is tolerated	Healthy solid-food diet	• Vitamin and mineral supplementation daily. • Healthy, balanced diet consisting of adequate protein, fruits, vegetables, and whole grains. • Calorie needs based on height, weight, age.
Post-LAGB fill/adjust-ment	~6 weeks after LAGB, and possibly every 6 weeks there-after until satiety is reached	Full liquids for 2 days after fill. Advance to Stage 3: Week 1 guidelines (earlier in table) as tolerated for 4–5 days, then advance through Stages 3 and 4.	• Follow Stage 2 guidelines for liquids for 48 hours (and/or as advised by surgeon). • **Note:** When diet advances to soft solids, patients should pay special attention to mindful eating and chewing foods until liquid—with more restriction, the risk for food getting stuck above stoma of band increases if food is not properly chewed until liquid.

Source: Table reprinted with permission by Sue Cummings, MS, RD.

Box 9.3
Post Weight-loss Surgery Supplementation: Patient Information

Purchase vitamin and calcium supplements before going into hospital and begin taking them when you return to your home.

Multivitamin with iron:
- For the first month following surgery, patients should take *chewable or liquid* vitamins and minerals.
- Take two children's chewable complete multivitamins with iron *or* two chewable *or* liquid adult multivitamins.

Calcium with vitamin D:
- Iron and calcium should not be taken together. It is best to take vitamins a couple of hours apart from calcium.
- It is also important that to take calcium supplements in divided doses for better absorption.
- How much calcium to take:
  - All men: 1,200 mg per day
  - Premenopausal women: 1,200 mg per day.
  - Postmenopausal women: 1,500 mg per day.
- Calcium supplement should contain vitamin D.
- For the first month after Roux-en-Y gastric bypass, patients should use only liquid or chewable forms of calcium with vitamin D.
- Because calcium supplements are usually large, patients undergoing laparoscopic adjustable gastric band may need to choose liquid or chewable forms to keep the pills from getting stuck.
- Calcium citrate is the best source of supplemental calcium after gastric bypass surgery because it does not require an acidic environment for absorption. The new pouch produces little to no acid.

Vitamin B-12:
- Take 350–500 mcg per day as a pill or sublingually.

procedure or 1 day after. Therefore, most patients advance from diet stage 1 (clear liquids) to diet stage 2 (clear liquids plus full liquids) at home and may remain on diet stage 2 for 2 weeks. Patients should begin their vitamin and mineral supplementation at home. Box 9.3 lists the appropriate recommendations for early postoperative supplementation.

Micronutrient Adequacy After RYGBP

Micronutrient deficiencies, a known complication of the RYGBP procedure, are attributed to early restriction of food intake and the bypassing of the major part of the stomach, all the of duodenum, and a variable amount of the jejunum where micronutrients are cleaved from their food source, prepared for absorption, and absorbed. Data suggest that micronutrient deficiencies after RYGBP, with the exception of folate, increase over time. There are numerous case reports, case series, and retrospective studies on micronutrient deficiencies, but few prospective studies. In addition, although long-term follow-up is essential, many patients are lost to follow-up, even at centers that have established follow-up protocols and make great efforts to contact their postoperative patients (27). To measure the incidence of vitamin deficiency in postoperative patients who, by self-report, were compliant with vitamin supplementation, and to examine the progression of vitamin deficiency over time, Clements et al (27) prospectively collected 2 years of follow-up data and assessed the medical records of patients who had undergone RYGBP surgery. Despite many efforts to bring patients back into their center for follow-up, the investigators were able to achieve only 65% at 1-year follow-up and 39% at the 2-year follow-up.

Vitamin D

Vitamin D is absorbed preferentially in the jejunum and ileum. Bypassing these segments of the intestine during bariatric operations leads to malabsorption of vitamin D. Ybarra et al studied 144 patients with severe obesity, including 64 who had undergone RYGBP (18). At the 36-month follow-up, none of the patients were taking vitamin D supplements, and 43% in the RYGBP group and 27.5% of the control group were vitamin D-deficient. Clements et al, whose patients reported compliance with recommended supplementation of a chewable multivitamin that included 400 IU vitamin D as well as calcium and vitamin B-12, found that the incidence of vitamin D deficiency after 1 and 2 years was 7% and 8%, respectively (ie, no significant difference was observed between the 1- and 2-year follow-up) (27). These researchers attribute the low incidence of deficiencies in their studies to vitamin supplementation; however, they recommend a longer term follow-up study to assess whether the incidence increases with time. It is not known whether the 400 IU of vitamin D typically found in a standard multivitamin is sufficient to prevent deficiencies in the long-term.

Recommendations for vitamin D supplementation are as follows (28):

- Multivitamin with 400 IU vitamin D.
- Standard oral calcium citrate with added vitamin D.
- If a patient's 25-OH vitamin D laboratory value is below normal, replete with 50,000 IU weekly for 6 to 8 weeks, then recheck the level in 3 to 6 months. At that point, if vitamin D level is normal, resume baseline postoperative supplements and recheck in 3 months.

Calcium

In RYGB patients, bypassing the duodenum and proximal jejunum, where calcium is primarily absorbed, may contribute to calcium deficiency. The malabsorption of vitamin D further contributes to calcium malabsorption. Intolerance to calcium-rich foods may also limit the intake of dietary calcium. However, calcium deficiency is not always apparent, because serum calcium is kept stable by the release of calcium from the bone (29). When serum calcium is low, the production of parathyroid hormone (PTH) increases, which causes the release of calcium from the bone. This may potentially cause bone loss and long-term risk of osteoporosis in RYGBP patients. Higher turnover of bone in patients after RYGB may be partly due to increased weight loss. Evidence of postoperative metabolic bone disease comes from observations of increased serum and urine markers of bone turnover, including elevated alkaline phosphatase (ALP) and PTH (30).

Recommendations for calcium supplementation and monitoring after RYGBP include the following (28,29,31):

- Oral daily supplementation of 1,200 mg calcium for men and all premenopausal women, and 1,500 to 2,000 mg for postmenopausal women, taken in divided doses (typically 500–600 mg calcium per dose); calcium supplement should contain vitamin D.
- Calcium supplementation with the citrate salt is recommended in post-RYGBP patients.
- Monitor PTH. If abnormal, assess serum calcium and phosphorus. Monitor at 12 months, 18 months, 24 months, and annually thereafter.
- Consider baseline dual-energy X-ray absorptiometry to assess bone mineral density and repeat every 2 years postoperatively. If abnormally low bone density is found at 1 year or bone density has decreased, measure bone density yearly.

Iron

Iron absorption after gastric bypass surgery is impaired because of the bypassing of the major part of the stomach that produces acid; the bypassing of the primary absorption sites, the duodenum and proximal jejunum; and the decreased intake of dietary sources of iron. Anemia usually observed in the setting of chronic sources of bleeding, such as menstruation or stomal ulceration. Deficiency after gastric bypass is most common in menstruating women. Iron deficiency can be seen soon after surgery or later (after 7 years) (32). Measurement of serum iron and ferritin along with a complete blood cell count with differential is recommended after RYGBP surgery. Serum ferritin is the first test to show abnormal results and should be used to diagnose iron deficiency. Patients may have normal hemoglobin but low ferritin after bariatric surgery (20,33).

Recommendations for iron supplementation include the following (28,33):

- Standard high-potency multivitamin with iron (preferably chewable).
- Two 325-mg ferrous sulfate tablets (65 mg elemental per tablet) in high-risk individuals.
- Repletion dose of 325 mg iron sulfate orally 1 to 3 times daily. If oral repletion is unsuccessful, parenteral infusions may be required.
- Adding vitamin C supplementation to iron supplementation substantially increases ferritin levels more than would occur with iron alone.

Vitamin B-12

A review of studies indicates that vitamin B-12 deficiency is fairly prevalent after bariatric operations (30). To be absorbed, vitamin B-12 must first be cleaved from the food source (meat protein); gastric acid facilitates this process. Once freed, vitamin B-12 is bound to R-protein in the stomach, which is then secreted into the duodenum where R-protein is cleaved from the vitamin and bound to intrinsic factor (IF). The B-12-IF complex is absorbed into the circulation in the distal ileum. After RYGBP, the new pouch produces little of the acid needed to cleave B-12 from dietary protein. In addition, the remnant produces IF, which is secreted into the duodenum where IF and B-12 are bound. Because the duodenum is bypassed, this binding does not occur. Also, some patients cannot tolerate meat protein, the primary source of dietary vitamin B-12. Therefore, there is some consensus that RYGBP patients cannot adequately absorb vitamin B-12 from dietary sources alone. There is some passive absorption of vitamin B-12. Clements et al (27) administered 1,000 mcg of intramuscular B-12 every 3 months or 500 mcg of self-administered intranasal B-12 every week and observed an incidence of B-12 deficiency of 3.6% and 2.3% at the 1- and 2-year follow-ups, respectively, which is much less than reported in other studies. The investigators attribute this low incidence to the routine administration of vitamin B-12 (27).

Recommendations for supplementing and monitoring vitamin B-12 are as follows (28,34):

- Supplement with 500 to 1,000 mcg crystalline vitamin B-12 per day to maintain normal serum levels, or supplement with 1,000 mcg of intramuscular B-12 every 3 months.
- Serum increases in methylmalonic acid and homocysteine are more sensitive markers early in vitamin B-12 deficiency.
- Vitamin B-12 can be administered sublingually or with nasal spray.

Folic Acid

Folic acid deficiency can lead to macrocytic anemia, leucopenia, thrombocytopenia, glossitis, megaloblastic marrow, and, in pregnant women, neural tube defects in the fetus. After RYGBP surgery, folic acid deficiency occurs less frequently than iron or vitamin B-12 deficiency. Folic acid is absorbed in the duodenum and most efficiently in the jejunum. Low levels of folate are attributed to low intake of food sources of this vitamin. Folic acid deficiency is usually preventable with a daily multivitamin. Low levels can be treated with 1 mg of folic acid daily.

Recommendations for folic acid supplementation include the following:

- Daily multivitamin containing 400 mcg folic acid.
- If red blood cell folate level is low, take 1 mg folic acid daily for 3 months.

Macronutrients

Protein

To minimize loss of lean body mass during the rapid weight-loss phase, patients must consume adequate protein. There are no evidence-based guidelines for meeting protein needs after surgery. Calculations used for early, noncomplicated weight-loss patients range from 0.8 to 1.2 g protein per kilogram of ideal body weight per day, or more than 80 to 120 g protein per day for patients with a BPD or BPD/DS, and at least 60 g/d for patients undergoing RYGBP. Because patients experience decreased hunger and early satiety, protein foods are encouraged as the primary foods consumed in the period immediately following surgery. Many patients experience protein intolerances in the first year after RYGBP, and even when these issues are resolved, protein intake after RYGBP often does not meet the daily recommendations. However, hypoalbuminemia is rarely seen after a noncomplicated, standard RYGBP (35).

Carbohydrates

Consumption of fruits and vegetables should be encouraged in the early and late periods after weight-loss surgery; however, patients should avoid simple carbohydrates. RYGBP patients may experience "dumping syndrome" after consuming simple sugars. Dumping syndrome produces symptoms such as flushing, fatigue, weakness, vomiting, and/or diarrhea. These symptoms can usually be prevented if patients avoid simple carbohydrates, eat slowly, and include a protein source at each meal or snack. LAGB patients may develop maladaptive eating behaviors because soft foods, especially ice cream and other soft sweets, will pass through the band unrestricted.

Fats

No data address essential fatty acid deficiency in patients undergoing RYGBP or LAGB, which are procedures that do not cause fat malabsorption. There are also no data regarding optimal supplementation with essential fatty acids in bariatric surgery patients.

Fats are an essential part of any healthful diet. Postoperative patients should consume a low-fat diet with the primary fat sources provided by canola, soybean, linseed oils, which are rich in all essential fatty acids.

LAGB Adjustments

Because there is a slow diffusion from the band leading to a decreased restriction over time, patients undergoing an LAGB procedure will need to have their band "filled." These visits are referred to as *band adjustments*. The first fill usually occurs 4 to 6 weeks after band placement. Patients who have undergone LAGB should be seen in the surgical center every 4 to 6 weeks for monitoring, education, and support, and to assess whether they need a band adjustment. The frequency of visits varies among surgical centers.

When patients reach an optimal stable adjustment level, they no longer need regular fills/adjustments. However, all patients should be seen at least once per year for monitoring of weight, nutritional status, and comorbidity assessment.

Weight-loss Surgery Monitoring and Support

The perioperative management of weight-loss surgery patients is typically provided by a multidisciplinary team, with the surgeon, medical specialist, and RD functioning as the primary postoperative caregivers. Patients may also need regular follow-up with other providers if problems occur. Mental health professionals should be available to patients who struggle postoperatively with psychosocial changes. An RD should see each patient early and often to monitor progress, guide diet advancement, and educate about healthful eating and activity.

Diet progression to a full solid-food diet may take from 9 to 18 months. During this time, patients will go through various stages of food intolerances, changes in food preferences, and changes in hunger and satiety.

When their weight is stabilized, patients may need a full re-education about healthful eating, with emphasis on increased consumption of fresh fruits and vegetables, limiting foods high in saturated fats, choosing lean sources of protein, and choosing whole grains. Patients may return to old habits of skipping meals, not planning and preparing foods, and ignoring hunger and satiety cues. Refresher sessions with an RD are extremely valuable during this time.

Many programs provide ongoing monthly support groups; others offer closed cognitive-behavioral programs to address problems and help patients incorporate healthful lifestyle behaviors. Patients should be informed about the possibility of weight regain and encouraged to work with their bariatric team to evaluate and address lifestyle issues with the first 10- to 20-pound regain, rather than waiting until they feel completely out of control and, often, too embarrassed to return.

CONCLUSION

Bariatric surgery procedures have led to a greater understanding of obesity and the weight-regulatory system. Future therapies for overweight and obesity are emerging from this understanding. Currently, weight-loss surgery is the most effective treatment for patients with extreme obesity; however, there is little doubt that patients with less severe obesity who do not have indications for weight-loss surgery will also benefit from the research. Based on the considerable impact of bariatric procedures on comorbidities such as type 2 diabetes, we will likely see a growth in the area of bariatric surgery. New procedures may be introduced and, perhaps, current procedures may become available to a wider range of patients with higher and lower BMIs. The short- and long-term care of patients undergoing weight-loss surgery is critically important to long-term success. Patients and health care providers need to be educated about the nutritional and metabolic implications of these procedures and the need for long-term support, education, counseling, and monitoring.

References

1. Santry HP, Gillen DL, Lauderdale DS. Trends in bariatric surgical procedures. *JAMA*. 2005;294:1909–1917.

2. Aills L, Blankenship MS, Buffington C, Furtado M, Parrott J. ASMBS allied health nutritional guidelines for the surgical weight loss patient. *Surg Obes Relat Disord*. 2008;4(5 Suppl):S73–S108.

3. Mechanick JI, Kushner RF, Sugerman HJ, Gonzalez-Campoy JM, Collazo-Clavell ML, Guven S, Spitz AF, Apovian CM, Livingston EH, Brolin R, Sarwer DB, Anderson WA, Dixon J. American Association of Clinical Endocrinologists (AACE), the Obesity Society, and American Society of Metabolic and Bariatric Surgery

clinical practice guidelines for the perioperative nutritional, metabolic, and nonsurgical support of the bariatric surgery patient. *Endocr Pract.* 2008; 14(Suppl 1):1–83.

4. Schauer PR, Ikramuddin S. Laparoscopic surgery for morbid obesity. *Surg Clin North Am.* 2001;81:1145–1179.

5. Davila-Cervantes A, Borunda D, Dominguez-Cherit G, Gamino R, Vargas-Vorackova F, Gonzalez-Barranco J, Herrera MF. Open versus laparoscopic vertical banded gastroplasty: a randomized controlled double blind trial. *Obes Surg.* 2002;12:812–818.

6. Sauerland S, Angrisani L, Belachew M, Chevallier JM, Favretti F, Finer N, Fingerhut A, Garcia Caballero M, Guisado Macias JA, Mittermair R, Morino M, Msika S, Rubino F, Tacchino R, Weiner R, Neugebauer EA; European Association for Endoscopic Surgery. Obesity surgery: evidence-based guidelines of the European Association for Endoscopic Surgery. *Surg Endosc.* 2005;19:200–221.

7. Centers for Medicare & Medicaid Services. Summary of Evidence—Bariatric Surgery. http://www.cms.hhs.gov/Transmittals/Downloads/R931CP.pdf. Accessed March 4, 2009.

8. Bariatric Surgery Centers of Excellence. Surgical Review Corporation. http://www.surgicalreview.org/pcoe/tertiary/tertiary_requirements.aspx. Accessed August 29, 2007.

9. American Society for Bariatric Surgery Web site. http://www.asbs.org. Accessed July 5, 2007.

10. ACS Division of Research and Optimal Patient Care. American College of Surgeons Bariatric Surgery Center Network (BSCN) Accreditation Program Manual. American College of Surgeons. http://www.facs.org/cqi/bscn. Accessed March 4, 2009.

11. Biesemeier C. Nutrition care process and standardized nutrition language: framework for nutrition care. *On the Cutting Edge.* 2007;28:8–12.

12. American Dietetic Association Evidence Analysis Library: Adult Weight Management Evidence Based Practice Guideline. http://www.adaevidencelibrary.com. Accessed March 4, 2009.

13. American Dietetic Association Adult Weight Management Certificate Training Course. http://www.eatright.org. Accessed March 4, 2009.

14. American Dietetic Association Evidence Analysis Library. Adult Weight Management Toolkit. http://www.adaevidencelibrary.com. Accessed December 28, 2008.

15. Weight Management Dietetic Practice Group. *ADA Pocket Guide to Bariatric Surgery.* Chicago, IL: American Dietetic Association; 2009.

16. Flancbaum L, Belsley S, Drake V, Colarusso T, Tayler E. Preoperative nutritional status of patients undergoing Roux-en-Y gastric bypass for morbid obesity. *J Gastrointest Surg.* 2006;10:1033–1037.

17. Looker AC, Dawson-Hughes B, Calvo MS, Gunter EW, Sahyoun NR. Serum 25-hydroxyvitamin D status of adolescents and adults in two seasonal subpopulations from NHANES III. *Bone.* 2002;30:771–777.

18. Ybarra J, Sanchez-Hernandez J, Gich I, De Leiva A, Rius X, Rodriguez-Espinosa J, Perez A. Unchanged hypovitaminosis D and secondary hyperparathyroidism in morbid obesity after bariatric surgery. *Obes Surg.* 2005;15:330–335.

19. Madan AK, Whitney SO, Tichansky DS, Ternovits CA. Vitamin and trace mineral levels after laparoscopic gastric bypass. *Obes Surg.* 2006;16:603–606.

20. Xanthakos SA, Inge TH. Nutritional consequences of bariatric surgery. *Curr Opin Clin Nutr Metab Care.* 2006,9:489–496.

21. Alvarado R, Alami RS, Hsu G, Safadi BY, Sanchez BR, Morton JM, Curet MJ. The impact of preoperative weight loss in patients undergoing laparoscopic Roux-en-Y gastric bypass. *Obes Surg.* 2005;15:1282–1286.

22. Alami RS, Morton JM, Schuster R, Lie J, Sanchez BR, Peters A, Curet MJ. Is there a benefit to preoperative weight loss in gastric bypass patients? A prospective randomized trial. *Surg Obes Relat Dis.* 2007;3:141–145.

23. Colles SL, Dixon JB, Marks P, Strauss BJ, O'Brien PE. Preoperative weight loss with a very-low-energy diet: quantitation of changes in liver and abdominal fat by serial imaging. *Am J Clin Nutr.* 2006;84:304–311.

24. Jamal MK, DeMaria EJ, Johnson JM, Carmody BJ, Wolfe LG, Kellum JM, Meador JG. Insurance-mandated preoperative dietary counseling does not improve outcome and increases dropout rates in patients considering gastric bypass surgery for morbid obesity. *Surg Obes Relat Dis.* 2006; 2:122–127.

25. Gibbons LM, Sarwer DB, Crerand CE, Fabricatore AN, Kuehnel RH, Lipschutz PE, Raper SE, Williams NN, Wadden TA. Previous weight loss experiences of bariatric surgery candidates. How much have patients dieted prior to surgery? *Obesity.* 2006;14(Suppl 2):70S–76S.

26. Giusti V, DeLucia A, DiVetta V, Calmes JM, Héraïef E, Gaillard RC, Burckhardt P, Suter M. Impact of preoperative teaching on surgical option of patients qualifying for bariatric surgery. *Obes Surg.* 2004;14:1241–1246.

27. Clements RH, Katasani VG, Palepu R, Leth RR, Leath TD, Roy BP, Vickers SM. Incidence of vitamin deficiency after laparoscopic Roux-en-Y gastric bypass in a university hospital setting. *Am Surg.* 2006;72:1196–1202.

28. Shikora SA, Kim JJ, Tarnoff ME. Nutrition and gastrointestinal complications of bariatric surgery. *Nutr Clin Pract.* 2007;22:29–40.

29. Shah M, Simha V, Garg A. Review: long-term impact of bariatric surgery on body weight, comorbidities, and nutritional status. *J Clin Endocrin Metab.* 2006;91: 4223–4321.

30. Bloomberg D, Fleishman A, Nalle JE, Herron DM, Kini S. Nutritional deficiencies following bariatric surgery: what have we learned? *Obes Surg.* 2005;15:145–154.

31. Riedt CS, Brolin RE, Sherrell RM, Field MP, Shapses SA. True fractional calcium absorption is decreased after Roux-en-Y gastric bypass surgery. *Obesity.* 2006;14: 1940–1948.

32. Skroubis G, Anesidis S, Kehagias I, Mead N, Vagenas K, Kalfarentzos F. Roux-en-Y gastric bypass versus a variant of biliopancreatic diversion in a superobese population: prospective comparison of the efficacy and the incidence of metabolic deficiencies. *Obes Surg.* 2006,16:488–495.

33. Brolin RE, Gorman JH, Gorman RC, Petschenik AJ, Bradley LB, Kenler HA, Cody RP. Prophylactic iron supplementation after Roux-en-Y gastric bypass: a prospective, double-blind, randomized study. *Arch Surg.* 1998;133:740–744.

34. Sumner AE, Chin MM, Abrahm JL, Berry GT, Gracely EJ, Allen RH. Stabler SP. Elevated methylmalonic acid and total homocysteine levels show high prevalence of vitamin B-12 deficiency after gastric surgery. *Ann Intern Med.* 1996,124: 469–476.

35. Bock M. Roux-en-Y gastric bypass: the dietitian's and patient's perspectives. *Nutr Clin Pract.* 2003;18:141–144.

CHAPTER 10

WEIGHT MAINTENANCE

PART A: OVERVIEW

RENA R. WING, PHD

Maintenance of weight loss remains a major problem in the treatment of obesity. On average, participants in behavioral weight-loss programs will lose approximately 9 kg (8%–10% of their weight) during the first 6 months of treatment and maintain approximately two thirds of this initial weight loss (5–6 kg) at 1-year follow-up (1). Despite intensive efforts, weight regain seems to continue over the next several years (2). Maintenance of a 4% weight loss at year 4 follow-up has been reported (3), but other studies suggest that participants are back to baseline weight by 5 years (4).

This chapter discusses two approaches to increasing our understanding of long-term weight-loss maintenance. The first approach is to study people who are successful at maintaining weight loss and learn how they have accomplished this feat. The second is to conduct randomized clinical trials of specific strategies aimed at improving maintenance of weight loss (5).

THE NATIONAL WEIGHT CONTROL REGISTRY

The National Weight Control Registry (NWCR) was started by James Hill, PhD, and Rena Wing, PhD, in 1994 to study individuals who have been successful at long-term maintenance of weight loss (5). To enter the registry, participants must be older than 18 years, have lost at least 13.6 kg (30 lb), and have maintained a 13.6 kg weight loss for at least 1 year. Currently there are more than 6,000 individuals in the registry. These individuals have lost 27 kg on average (reducing from a mean body mass index [BMI] of 36.3 to 24.9) and have maintained their weight loss for an average of nearly 6 years. Key findings from the registry are as follows:

- These successful weight-losers have tried to lose weight many times before—but unsuccessfully. Thus, there is nothing inherently different between unsuccessful and successful weight-losers; ie, unsuccessful weight-losers can become successful weight-losers. The variables that seemed to distinguish this successful effort from prior attempts was a greater level of commitment, a stricter diet, and greater reliance on exercise (6).

- Successful weight-losers used a variety of different approaches for weight loss. Approximately half received help from a program, registered dietitian (RD), or physician, whereas the other half lost weight entirely on their own (6). In contrast to the variety of approaches used for weight loss, there seem to be certain common characteristics of the maintenance approach.

- NWCR members consistently report consuming a low-calorie, low-fat diet (1,400 kcal diet, with 24% to 29% of calories from fat). Although more recent NWCR enrollees report higher fat intakes than earlier enrollees reported, the proportion who report consuming a low-carbohydrate regimen, similar to what would be recommended by the Atkins diet, remains low (7).

- NWCR members report regular eating, with five eating episodes per day. Most (78%) report consuming breakfast on a daily basis (8). They continue to eat out, but limit fast-food meals to fewer than once per week (0.74 times/wk) on average (6).

- Physical activity and diet are used in combination to maintain weight loss. On average, NWCR members report weekly energy expenditure through physical activity of approximately 2,800 kcal. That would be equivalent to walking 28 miles/wk (4 miles/d) or 60 to 90 minutes of activity per day (5). Walking is the most popular form of exercise, but bicycling, weight-lifting, and aerobics were also frequently indicated. NWCR members spend less time viewing television than the general population (9).

- Maintaining weight loss seems to require ongoing vigilance. Most (75%) of NWCR members weigh themselves at least weekly. They also exhibit high levels of dietary restraint, resembling individuals who have recently participated in a weight-loss program (10).

- More than 90% of NWCR members report that their weight loss has improved their quality of life, level of energy, mobility, general mood, and self-confidence (6).

- Weight regain in NWCR members is associated with shorter duration of weight-loss maintenance and with decreases in physical activity, self-weighing, and restraint and with increases in television-viewing, fast-food consumption, dietary fat, and disinhibition (11). Thus, long-term maintenance of healthful behaviors is fundamental to weight-loss maintenance.

RANDOMIZED CLINICAL TRIALS

The NWCR is interesting because it involves a large number of highly successful individuals. However, they are a self-selected population and may not be representative of all successful weight-losers. Methodologically, randomized clinical trials are a stronger way to define the variables associated with long-term weight loss. The next section highlights those variables that, based on randomized trials, seem to improve long-term weight-loss maintenance.

Intensive Ongoing Contact

Maintenance of weight loss is improved by providing regular treatment contact. Perri et al (12) compared 20-week and 40-week behavioral treatment programs and found that lengthening the treatment led to larger weight losses and delayed the onset of weight regain. Similarly, after a 6-month weight-loss program, continued biweekly contact with health care practitioners improved long-term weight-loss outcomes (13).

Exercise

A large number of studies have compared diet only, exercise only, and diet and exercise in combination (14). These studies are quite consistent in showing that the combination yields the best long-term weight losses (15). In fact, the clearest benefit of exercise seems to be for the maintenance of weight loss. Exercising at home (rather than in supervised settings) (16) and providing treadmills to patients for the home use (17) both seem to improve maintenance of exercise and, consequently, weight loss. To date, no differences in maintenance of weight loss have been reported from aerobic exercise, strength training, or the combination of these two approaches (16,18).

Recently, attention has focused on the ideal amount of exercise for maintenance of weight loss. Typically, behavioral treatment programs recommend 1,000 kcal of activity per week. However, based on the NWCR and several other studies, investigators have suggested that higher levels of exercise might be preferable. Jeffery et al (19) compared weight loss in participants randomly assigned to 1,000 or 2,500 kcal of energy expenditure from exercise per week. The higher exercise dose was associated with larger weight losses at 12 and 18 months, but even with this higher dose of exercise, maximum weight losses were achieved at 12 months, followed by weight regain. Those participants who maintained high exercise levels (≥ 2,500 kcal/wk) at 30 months maintained the greatest weight losses, averaging 12 kg (20).

Diet

Most studies of dietary interventions have focused on initial weight loss, rather than maintenance. Very-low-calorie diets (diets of 400 kcal per day of lean meat, fish, and poultry or liquid formula) were found to markedly improve initial weight losses (20 kg weight loss after 12 weeks), but the magnitude of weight regain was more than on more balanced, low-calorie regimens (21). Consequently, at the end of 12 to 24 months, there was typically no difference between the two approaches.

Increasing the structure of the diet may improve long-term results. Participants who were given the actual food they should eat or given structured meal plans and grocery lists achieved larger weight losses than those prescribed the same calorie level who followed a self-selected diet (22,23). Of particular note for the maintenance of weight loss is a 4-year trial involving the meal replacement Slimfast (24). Patients who were randomly assigned to drink two Slimfast per day and eat a healthful dinner lost more weight than patients on a self-selected diet at the same calorie level; moreover, the Slimfast group retained their weight losses better over 4 years of follow-up.

Problem-solving

Although ongoing treatment contact is important, it has remained unclear exactly what should occur at these sessions. Recently, Perri et al (25) compared a group given no maintenance contact with a group given a maintenance program that focused on relapse prevention or focused on problem-solving. Both the relapse-prevention and problem-solving groups met biweekly for a year of follow-up. The latter seemed to produce the best long-term weight loss; the problem-solving group maintained a weight loss of 10.8 kg at 17 months, whereas the relapse prevention group averaged 5.8 kg, and the behavioral program with no maintenance contact maintained a weight loss of 4.1 kg.

Social Support

To improve maintenance of weight loss, it may be important to increase social support for diet and exercise changes. The involvement of friends and family members who will be available after the treatment program has ended should be particularly effective. Wing and Jeffery studied two types of social support (26). The first, natural support, was examined by comparing participants who joined a weight-loss program alone vs those who joined the program along with three friends. Experimentally created social support was induced through the use of intragroup cohesiveness activities and intergroup competitions. Both the natural and experimentally created forms of support affected the outcome. The highest number of study completers and the best maintenance of weight loss occurred in participants who entered the program with their friends and were treated in a program with a high level of experimentally created social support.

Increasing Initial Weight Loss vs Setting Modest Weight-loss Goals

There have been several studies exploring the potential benefits of setting more modest weight-loss goals for clients. Clients often expect to lose more weight during treatment than is reasonable (27) and thus may be disappointed by their outcome (and hence likely to regain). Investigators have therefore tried to help subjects accept more "reasonable" weight-loss goals. Such programs have proven to be quite unsuccessful—setting lower expectations seems to limit any weight loss (28). In contrast, in post hoc analyses, Jeffery, Wing, and Mayer (29) have shown that the more individuals lose initially, the better their long-term results. Thus, aggressive approaches that maximize initial weight loss (such as use of meal replacements and 2,500 kcal weekly exercise goals) seem to be more effective for long-term weight loss. See Chapter 2 for more information on meal replacements and Chapter 6 for a discussion of physical activity and weight management.

Self-regulation

Having identified the key strategies of successful weight-loss maintainers through the NWCR, Wing and colleagues (30) conducted a randomized trial to determine whether teaching these strategies to others who had recently lost weight could improve their weight-loss maintenance. A total of 314 participants who had lost at least 10% of their body weight (mean = 18%) within the past 2 years were recruited and randomly assigned to a newsletter control group, a face-to-face intervention group, or an Internet-based intervention. The content of the intervention was the same for the latter two groups and focused on maintaining high levels of physical activity, daily self-weighing, and using the information from the scale to make appropriate adjustments in diet and physical activity. Both groups had weekly sessions for 4 weeks and then monthly for the remainder of the 18-month program, but these sessions were delivered either face-to-face or via the Internet. In addition, participants who experienced weight regains of more than 2.5 kg were offered additional help via telephone or face-to-face or via the Internet, depending on their intervention condition.

This study found that the intervention delivered face-to-face was most effective at reducing the magnitude of weight regain (weight regains over 18 months of 2.5, 4.7, and 4.9 kg for face-to-face, Internet, and control group, respectively). Both the face-to-face and the Internet programs substantially reduced the proportion of participants who regained more than 2.5 kg during the 18 months. Within the intervention groups, continued practice of self-weighing was an important predictor of weight-loss maintenance. Thus, it seems that participants can be taught to self-regulate their behaviors, and these skills can improve their maintenance of weight loss.

CONCLUSION

In conclusion, the National Weight Control Registry provides evidence that it is possible to lose substantial amounts of weight and maintain the weight loss long-term. The key strategies for weight-loss maintenance seem to be a low-calorie, low-fat diet, high levels of physical activity, and vigilance about one's weight.

Randomized controlled trials on weight-loss maintenance yield similar findings. In such studies, the maximum weight loss typically occurs at 6 to 12 months, followed by regain. However, maintenance of weight loss has been improved by (*a*) maximizing contact with participants (which increases the likelihood of ongoing vigilance), (*b*) including high levels of exercise within the intervention, (*c*) providing structured approaches to dietary intake, (*d*) increasing social support and problem-solving techniques, (*e*) increasing initial weight-loss success, and (*f*) teaching self-regulation skills. Clinical approaches to improving maintenance of weight loss are described in the next part of this chapter.

References

1. Wing RR. Behavioral approaches to the treatment of obesity. In: Bray G, Bouchard C, James P, eds. *Handbook of Obesity.* New York, NY: Marcel Dekker, Inc; 1998: 855–873.

2. Diabetes Prevention Program Research Group. Reduction in the incidence of type 2 diabetes with lifestyle intervention or Metformin. *N Engl J Med.* 2002;346: 393–403.

3. Kramer FM, Jeffery RW, Forster JL, Snell MK. Long-term follow-up of behavioral treatment for obesity: patterns of weight regain among men and women. *Int J Obes.* 1989;13:123–136.

4. Wadden TA, Sternberg JA, Letizia KA, Stunkard AJ, Foster GD. Treatment of obesity by very low calorie diet, behaviour therapy, and their combination: a five-year perspective. *Int J Obes.* 1989;13:39–46.

5. Wing RR, Hill JO. Successful weight loss maintenance. *Ann Rev Nutr.* 2001;21:323–341.

6. Klem ML, Wing RR, McGuire MT, Seagle HM, Hill JO. A descriptive study of individuals successful at long-term maintenance of substantial weight loss. *Am J Clin Nutr.* 1997;66:239–246.

7. Phelan S, Wyatt H, Nassery S, DiBello J, Fava JL, Hill JO, Wing RR. Three-year weight change in successful weight losers who lost weight on a low-carbohydrate diet. *Obesity.* 2007;15:2470–2477.

8. Wyatt HR, Grunwald GK, Mosca CL, Klem M, Wing RR, Hill JO. Long-term weight loss and breakfast in subjects in the National Weight Control Registry. *Obes Res.* 2002;10:78–82.

9. Raynor DA, Phelan S, Hill JO, Wing RR. Television viewing and long-term weight maintenance: results from the National Weight Control Registry. *Obesity.* 2006;14: 1816–1824.

10. Klem ML, Wing RR, McGuire MT, Seagle HM, Hill JO. Psychological symptoms in individuals successful at long-term maintenance of weight loss. *Health Psychol.* 1998;17:336–345.

11. Phelan S, Wyatt HR, Hill JO, Wing RR. Are the eating and exercise habits of successful weight losers changing? *Obesity.* 2006;14:710–716.

12. Perri MG, Nezu AM, Patti ET, McCann KL. Effect of length of treatment on weight loss. *J Consult Clin Psychol.* 1989;57:450–452.

13. Perri MG, McAllister DA, Gange JJ, Jordan RC, McAdoo WG, Nezu AM. Effects of four maintenance programs on the long-term management of obesity. *J Clin Psychol.* 1988;56:529–534.

14. National Heart, Lung, and Blood Institute. Clinical guidelines on the identification, evaluation, and treatment of overweight and obesity in adults—the evidence report. *Obes Res.* 1998;6(Suppl 2):51S–209S.

15. Wing R. Physical activity in the treatment of the adulthood overweight and obesity: current evidence and research issues. *Med Sci Sports Exerc.* 1999;31(11 Suppl): S547–S552.

16. Wadden TA, Vogt RA, Foster GD, Anderson DA. Exercise and maintenance of weight loss: 1-year follow-up of a controlled clinic trial. *J Consult Clin Psychol.* 1998;66:429–433.

17. Jakicic J, Winters C, Lang W, Wing RR. Effects of intermittent exercise and use of home exercise equipment on adherence, weight loss, and fitness in overweight women. *JAMA.* 1999;282:1554–1560.

18. Wadden TA, Vogt RA, Andersen RE, Bartlett SJ, Foster GD, Kuehnel RH, Wilk J, Weinstock R, Buckenmeyer P, Berkowitz RI, Steen SN. Exercise in the treatment of obesity: effects of four interventions on body composition, resting energy expenditure, appetite, and mood. *J Consult Clin Psychol.* 1997;65:269–277.

19. Jeffery RW, Wing RW. The effects of an enhanced exercise program on long-term weight loss. *Obes Res.* 2001;9(suppl):100S.

20. Tate DF, Jeffery RW, Sherwood NE, Wing RR. Long-term weight losses associated with prescription of higher physical activity goals. Are higher levels of physical activity protective against weight regain? *Am J Clin Nutr.* 2007;85:954–959.

21. Harris MI. Epidemiological correlates of NIDDM in Hispanics, Whites, and Blacks in the U.S. population. *Diabetes Care.* 1991;14:639–648.

22. Wing RR, Jeffery RW, Burton LR, Thorson C, Sperber Nissinoff K, Baxter JE. Food provision vs. structured meal plans in the behavioral treatment of obesity. *Int J Obes.* 1996;20:56–62.

23. Jeffery RW, Wing RR, Thorson C, Burton LR, Raether C, Harvey J, Mullen M. Strengthening behavioral interventions for weight loss: a randomized trial of food provision and monetary incentives. *J Consult Clin Psychol.* 1993;61:1038–1045.

24. Flechtner-Mors M, Ditschuneit HH, Johnson TD, Suchard MA, Adler G. Metabolic and weight loss effects of long-term dietary intervention in obese patients: four-year results. *Obes Res.* 2000;8:399–402.

25. Perri MG, McKelvey WF, Renjilian DA, Nezu AM, Shermer RL, Viegener BJ. Relapse prevention training and problem-solving therapy in the long-term management of obesity. *J Consult Clin Psychol.* 2001;69:722–726.

26. Wing RR, Jeffery RW. Benefits of recruiting participants with friends and increasing social support for weight loss maintenance. *J Consult Clin Psychol.* 1999;67:132–138.

27. Foster GD, Wadden TA, Vogt RA, Brewer G. What is a reasonable weight loss? Patients' expectations and evaluations of obesity treatment outcomes. *J Consult Clin Psychol.* 1997;65:79–85.

28. Foster G, Phelan S, Wadden TA, Gill D, Ermold J, Didie E. Promoting more modest weight losses: a pilot study. *Obes Res.* 2004;12:1271–1277

29. Jeffery RW, Wing RR, Mayer RR. Are smaller weight losses or more achievable weight loss goals better in the long term for obese patients? *J Consult Clin Psychol.* 1998;66:641–645.

30. Wing RR, Tate DF, Gorin AA, Raynor HA, Fava JL. A self-regulation program for maintenance of weight loss. *N Engl J Med.* 2006;355:1563–1571.

PART B: PRACTICAL APPLICATIONS

SUZANNE PHELAN, PHD

Weight loss and weight maintenance share many requisite behaviors, including consuming a reduced-calorie diet, increasing physical activity, and practicing behavioral strategies. A critical difference between the two processes, however, is the presence of motivators. During weight loss, clients experience a variety of motivating factors: weekly feedback from the scale; compliments from others about their weight loss; and noticeable improvements in mood, energy, body image, and health. During weight maintenance, however, many of these advantages disappear: compliments decline, the scale does not budge, adherence becomes more challenging, and the improvements in health become less salient. In such a context, it is difficult for clients to maintain their weight loss. This section describes specific strategies to help clients achieve successful weight-loss maintenance, including methods to reverse weight regain and increase motivation during challenging times.

SKILLS THAT PROMOTE WEIGHT MAINTENANCE

Sandra has lost 10% of her initial body weight by eating a low-calorie diet, exercising, and consistent self-monitoring of eating and activity. Although ideally she would like to lose more weight, she is now willing to work at weight maintenance because she "can't imagine" consuming less or exercising more than she already does. It is clear that Sandra is well educated about energy balance, exercise, self-monitoring, and other behavioral strategies. Now what? What can be done to keep Sandra engaged in the treatment process and help her remain successful at weight maintenance?

Patients like Sandra who have lost weight already know the skills required for weight control. The goal now is to facilitate their continued practice of weight-control behaviors and to help them take ownership of these behaviors for life.

Frequent Patient-Provider Contact

As stated in the first part of this chapter, frequent contact between the client and the provider seems critical during the maintenance period (1). Contact every 2 weeks is recommended. However, at a minimum, monthly visits should be maintained, and more frequent contact should be scheduled when clients begin to regain weight.

Ironically, when clients are at greatest risk for weight regain (ie, when the maintenance stage begins), contact with treatment providers tends to decrease. Some treatment programs finish when maintenance starts. More often, however, clients gradually drop out of the treatment process by missing treatment visits or by not returning phone calls. Clients may stop attending treatment for a variety of reasons, including financial limitations, feeling bored with the treatment process, or feeling ready to "do it on their own" now that they have lost weight. However, it is generally safe to assume that clients who start reducing contact are doing poorly.

There are several different ways to maintain contact with clients after weight loss. Although bimonthly visits with a registered dietitian (RD) is the ideal, some clients cannot afford this option. Another strategy is for clients to attend community weight-loss groups on a bimonthly basis, with individual meetings with the RD on a quarterly basis. This method can offset treatment costs for the client while providing both group and individual support. Alternatively, telephone check-ins or e-mail contacts with the RD can be used in conjunction with quarterly face-to-face visits. This provides a fast and practical means of maintaining contact with the client; however, some clients may not have easy access to a computer. Other members of the health care team can also help maintain contact with the client. Staff may provide bimonthly "check-ins" or may be available for weigh-ins at the clinic, while individual visits with the RD are scheduled on a quarterly basis.

Self-regulation

A major difference between weight loss and weight maintenance is the reinforcement a person receives from others. Thus, it is important to teach clients how to self-regulate, using skills shown to be effective in preventing weight regain (2). The critical component of effective self-regulation is self-weighing. In addition to being weighed at each treatment visit, the RD should encourage clients to weigh themselves at home, usually on a daily basis (3,4). The rationale for daily weighing is that it keeps clients attentive to their weight and gives them the information they need to make quick adjustments.

In the context of daily self-weighing, teach clients how to respond to the information provided by the scale. If the scale indicates weight loss or maintenance, clients should learn to provide themselves with some form of positive self-reinforcement, such as treating themselves to an earned reward. If the scale indicates a small weight gain (ie, 3–4 lb) from their maintenance weight, help clients use problem-solving skills (as described later in this chapter) to reverse this gain. *The sooner clients respond to any increases in the scale, the better their chances are of maintaining long-term weight loss.* Immediate efforts to reverse even small gains are critical. Clients with more considerable weight gains (ie, 5 lb or more) should be encouraged to restart active weight-loss efforts, using either their initial approach to weight loss or a standard behavioral approach involving a low-calorie, low-fat diet, meal replacements, and increased physical activity. Weekly counseling, if possible, should be instituted until they return to their maintenance weight. See the Coping with Lapse and Relapse section of this chapter for more information on this topic.

Regular Physical Activity

A client's level of physical activity should also be monitored at each clinical encounter. Clients working at weight maintenance are likely already engaged in some form of physical activity. The goal during maintenance is to increase the duration of exercise. At a minimum, clients should be encouraged to accumulate 30 minutes of moderate-intensity physical activity (equivalent to brisk walking) 5 days per week. Once they are comfortable with this minimum level, they should continue to strive to increase their goal to 300 to 400 minutes per week (1 hour per day, 5 to 7 days per week). There are a variety of strategies that can be used to promote higher levels of activity during maintenance. (Several of the following physical activity topics are discussed in greater detail in Chapter 6.)

Self-monitoring

Most clients who have lost weight in standard treatment programs are familiar with self-monitoring—"too familiar," some will say. Until the physical activity goal is reached, it is helpful for clients to continue recording their minutes of activity each day, counting anything that is equivalent to brisk walking and that lasts 10 minutes or more. Once clients have reached their exercise goal, self-monitoring may be reduced to 1 to 2 weeks per month, providing a way for clients to ensure that a high level of physical activity is maintained.

Pedometers

Purchasing a pedometer and recording the number of steps taken each day is also helpful for tracking increases in lifestyle activity. In general, 10,000 steps per day is an effective goal.

Enjoyable Activities

Encourage clients to choose activities that they enjoy. If they enjoy an activity, they may be more likely to continue doing it.

Variety

Some people find that it is easier for them to stay on track when they stick to the same exercise routine. This style works because clients do not have to think much about their routine once becomes an established part of their daily life. Other people, however, are motivated by variety. They are bored following the same routine, and varying their routine with different exercises helps them stay on track. Clients who say they are bored with their exercise may benefit from adding a new variation of their usual activity (eg, instead of taking their usual aerobics class, they can try spinning) or trying a new activity altogether (eg, taking a lesson in something they have always dreamed about, such as ice skating or rock climbing). Of the successful members of the National Weight Control Registry (NWCR), many reported walking as their primary activity; however, many combined walking with other activities (5). Table 10.1 (5) lists the six most frequently reported activities by NWCR participants.

Reduced-calorie, Low-fat Diet

As noted earlier, the successful members of NWCR clearly ate a low-calorie diet (women 843 to 1,750 kcal/day, and men 1,078 to 2,372 kcal/day) that was also low in fat (24%–29% calories from fat). How many calories should clients who are working at weight maintenance eat? The answer to this question depends on the individual's goal. If the goal is truly to maintain weight, the average number of calories eaten each day is a good reference point for what the body needs to stay at its current weight. Given that most clients underreport their dietary intake, however, their reported calorie intake should be considered only an estimate of their actual intake (6). If the client wants to continue losing weight, it is useful to provide fixed-calorie diets of 1,200 kcal/d for clients weighing less than 200 lb, and 1,500 kcal/d for those weighing more than 200 lb.

TABLE 10.1

Activities Reported by Successful Weight Losers of the National Weight Control Registry

Activity	% Reporting Participation in the Activity
Walking	76.6
Cycling	20.6
Weight lifting	20.3
Aerobics	17.8
Running	10.5
Stair climbing	9.3

Source: Data are from reference 5.

Unfortunately, there are many barriers to maintaining a reduced-calorie, low-fat diet. Clients may crave fast foods, feel bored with their diet, feel deprived, or question whether they can eat fewer calories long-term. Under such pressure, attention to calories and portion sizes may wane. Several strategies, however, can help clients remain attentive to their dietary intake and continue to consume a low-fat, reduced-calorie diet.

Self-monitoring

In addition to self-monitoring of exercise; we also recommend that clients self-monitor their calorie intake until they have reached their weight-maintenance goal. After their goal is reached, we recommend periodic self-monitoring (eg, in response to small weight gains), to ensure that small changes in the diet do not go unnoticed. Consider simplifying the self-monitoring process during maintenance. For example, a client who consumes one of three different breakfasts on a regular basis could identify, in advance, the portion size and calorie content of breakfast 1, breakfast 2, and breakfast 3. To record, the client would simply write the number corresponding to the breakfast selection, rather than list the portions and calorie content of the breakfast's individual items. Creating checklists that itemize different food selections may also help simplify recording during maintenance.

Limiting Dietary Variety

Successful participants in the NWCR limit the number of different types of food they consume each day (7) and also tend to eat the same during the week as on the weekends and during holidays as the rest of the year (8). Eating the same foods may make it easier to stay on track with eating. Thus, clients who are bored with their diet should be reassured that they are doing exactly what it takes to maintain weight control. Nonetheless, if feelings of boredom with the diet are leading to episodes of overeating unhealthful foods, clients may benefit from adding a little variety to the diet. With such clients, the RD may explore which meals or snacks are causing boredom and suggest ways to alter the particular eating situation (eg, change breakfast cereals). RDs may also encourage clients to explore new vegetables and fruits (eg, turnips, okra, parsnips, rutabaga, star fruit, or cactus pears) or to try new low-calorie recipes.

Diet Novelty

Sometimes, a more dramatic change in the dietary regimen is needed to keep clients captivated and therefore mindful of dietary intake. For example, if a client is consuming a standard, self-selected diet, the RD can provide guidelines for a vegetarian diet for 6 months, followed by a Mediterranean-type diet. Alternatively, meal replacements and prepackaged frozen entrees may be incorporated into the diet. For example, a client may consume self-selected foods for breakfast, snacks, and dinner, but consume a meal replacement for lunch. Meal replacements are highly recommended for patients who start to regain weight (as described later). See Chapters 2 and 4 for more information on meal replacements and Mediterranean diets, respectively.

Problem-solving

Problem-solving is another useful tool for weight maintenance (9). Practitioners promoting weight maintenance should remind patients of the basic steps of problem-solving and revisit this skill on an ongoing basis throughout treatment. Problem-solving is helpful in identifying solutions to current, past, or future problems related to eating and exercise. Problem-solving can be broken down into three steps.

1. *Defining the problem.* The more specific the client can be in identifying the problem, the easier it will be to identify solutions. Clients should think carefully about when a particular problem started. Many times an exercise lapse or an episode of overeating is at the end of a long chain of problematic behaviors (see Chapter 7 for information on behavior modification). For example, if a client reports eating a box of cookies, the RD should query about how the box of cookies got into the house in the first place. To define the problem, RDs should help clients identify the source, or beginning, of the problematic behavior chain (see Figure 10.1).

2. *Brainstorming possible solutions.* Once a client has identified the problem, the next step is to think about all possible solutions to the problem. Perhaps exercise has decreased because it is getting dark earlier and the client does not want to walk alone at night. Some possible solutions could include exercising in the morning, finding a walking partner, exercising at a shopping mall, or taking a walk during the lunch hour. Many more options could be generated. At this stage, clients should be encouraged to think about all possible solutions, not just the ones that seem most realistic or feasible.

3. *Implementing one of the solutions.* From the list of possible solutions, pick a solution that the client thinks would work best and then try it. At future sessions, revisit the issue and evaluate whether the solution has worked. If it has not, another strategy from the list should be implemented. This process should be repeated until the client is successful.

Anticipating High-risk Situations

Another important skill for patients working at weight maintenance is to identify and anticipate high-risk situations. These include situational or emotional triggers that increase a patient's risk of overeating and/or inactivity.

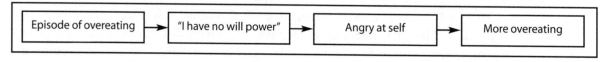

FIGURE 10.1 Example of a behavior chain.

Situational Triggers

Vacations and holidays are, perhaps, the most obvious examples of situational triggers for relapse. Some clients choose to lose a few pounds to create a "buffer" before the impending high-risk period. For example, a client could aim to lose 4 pounds during the month preceding a vacation or holiday. To do this, the client would need a weekly 3,500-calorie deficit (500 kcal/d), to lose 1 pound per week.

Other triggers for overeating may include places (eg, restaurants) or people (eg, relatives). After such high-risk situations are identified, problem-solving may be used to prevent them from leading to weight regain.

Emotional Triggers

It is particularly important for RDs working with clients maintaining their weight to monitor levels of stress and negative affect. Greater depressive symptoms and stress commonly precede weight regain (10,11). Thus, helping clients develop strategies to reduce the potential adverse effects of mood and stress on eating and exercise is critical. Ideally, clients are able to anticipate when stress or dysphoria will occur (eg, during holidays or a particular time of year at work). Problem-solving may be used to identify the specific factors that are likely to trigger regain and the strategies to cope effectively with the upcoming situation. However, the client experiencing an increase in stress or negative mood will often start missing treatment sessions. In these cases, it is important to try to maintain contact with the client (eg, by e-mail or telephone) and use these opportunities to provide support and help with problem-solving. Clients with clinically significant distress should be referred to a mental health professional.

COPING WITH LAPSE AND RELAPSE

Bob arrives at the treatment session with a look of guilt on his face. The scale shows his weight is up a few pounds, and he feels terrible about it. Although Bob continues to weigh himself frequently and to exercise, his eating has been out of control after an incident at work left him feeling angry.

Almost inevitably, patients such as Bob will have times when they eat amounts of food that they do not consider appropriate for long-term weight loss. Before such occasions become more frequent, they need to implement strategies to prevent the lapse from turning into a relapse. This section reviews strategies for coping with lapse (ie, a temporary setback) and relapse (ie, a substantial weight regain). See Table 10.2 for a summary of these strategies, as well as strategies to prevent weight regain.

Responding to a Lapse

Clients who are experiencing a lapse typically have not reverted completely back to their former eating and exercise habits. They have experienced a minor setback that they can be remedy with some immediate intervention. Here are a few strategies that can help clients get back on track.

TABLE 10.2
Strategies for Weight Maintenance, Coping with Lapse, and Coping with Relapse

Weight Status	Strategies
Maintenance	• Frequent patient-provider contact • Frequent weighing • High level of physical activity • Low-calorie, low-fat diet • Problem-solving • Anticipating high-risk situations
Lapse (3–4 lb higher than starting weight)	• Problem-solving • Stop negative thinking • Develop a plan
Relapse (≥ 5 lb above starting weight)	• Simplify the dietary regimen • Meal replacements • Structured meal plans • Self-monitoring • Consider medication

Putting the Lapse in Perspective

First, help clients recognize that they are not alone; everyone experiences lapses. The key is to recognize that a lapse has occurred and take steps quickly to remedy the situation.

Promoting Realistic Thinking

Next, help the client resist the tendency toward negative thoughts and feelings. After a lapse, some clients may say to themselves, "I'm a failure," "I'll never succeed," or "I blew it; why even try?" Such distorted thinking can lead to feelings of discouragement, guilt, and/or anger at being in this position "once again." It is important to identify such thoughts and feelings because they can undermine a client's ability to deal effectively with a lapse. Such thinking should be countered by more realistic thoughts about the situation and the client's success. The person who "blew it" today is the same person who has been successful during many previous weeks. A lapse in behavior is not revealing the real" self. It is simply another occasion of eating behavior from which the person can recover and learn.

To learn from the situation, the client should look closely at it and consider what led to inappropriate eating. Often, lapses coincide with a specific high-risk situation (eg, argument at work, holidays). In such cases, clients can make efforts to alter the high-risk situation (eg, bringing low-calorie foods to a holiday party) or their reactions to it (eg, assertiveness training for interpersonal distress, relaxation techniques). If the situation was temporary, such as a holiday or a wedding, once the client is back in the usual environment, eating and exercise habits may normalize.

Lapses are sometimes the result of a series of subtle behavior changes that are going unnoticed (Table 10.3). Alone, each of these small behaviors may not result in any weight change; together, they may account for a lapse. The key is to recognize the snow-

TABLE 10.3

Subtle Behavior Changes That Contribute to a Lapse

Behavior During Successful Weight Control	Sign of Lapse
Adding nonfat milk to coffee	Adding cream to coffee
Putting jelly on toast	Putting butter on toast
Ordering dressing on the side	Not making healthful requests when ordering at restaurants
Parking farther away at shopping malls	Parking as close as possible to the door
Exercising 30 min/d, 5 d/wk	Exercising 15 min/d, 5 d/wk

ball effect. With time, these small behaviors can accumulate and lead to a loss of control of weight maintenance.

Regaining Control

The third step is for the client to regain control of eating or exercise at the next opportunity. Encourage clients to avoid self-critical statements such as, "Well, I blew it for the day," and waiting until the next day to start controlling their behavior. It is best to make the next meal a controlled one or to make the next opportunity a time to be physically active. This strategy helps keep lapses in perspective—as *temporary* setbacks.

Responding to a Relapse

Despite all best efforts, some clients may end up eating inappropriately on a string of occasions or not exercising for a long period of time, resulting in considerable weight regain. At this point, immediate action is necessary to get back on track. A reduction in calorie intake should be the focus, because it is hard to suddenly increase exercise enough to make a real difference in energy balance. One of the most effective ways to reverse weight regain is to simplify choices and to provide structure. Several options may be considered, alone or in combination, to reduce calorie intake.

Self-monitoring

Clients in relapse should be strongly encouraged to monitor calorie intake (9). Individuals working on maintenance may have taken a "break" from monitoring and found great relief in doing so. Clients may meet an RD's suggestion to start recording again with reluctance. In such cases, emphasize that recording is not a "life sentence" but rather one of many strategies that can help get clients back on track. "Portion distortions" and a general decrease in awareness of intake can occur over time and lead to relapse. Self-monitoring is required to make sure daily calorie totals are in line with goals (12). It is also helpful for clients to record their weight daily.

Meal Replacements

One of the most effective ways to simplify choice and to decrease calorie intake is to start a structured meal plan, using meal replacements (such as shakes) and/or portion-controlled meals. These will help clients meet their calorie-intake goals. Use of meal replacements or any of the prepackaged frozen entrees has many advantages. Such meals save time (clients do not have to spend any time thinking about what to prepare for a meal or preparing it), reduce exposure to foods that might tempt clients to overeat, and avoid problems of underestimating portion sizes. See Chapter 2 for more information on meal replacements.

Structured Meal Plans

Another way to increase structure in the diet is to provide clients with a short-term, low-calorie, low-fat meal plan. Such short-term plans simplify food choices and increase adherence to a daily calorie goal. Clients need to weigh and measure foods to ensure appropriate portion sizes. This short-term structure can give clients a fresh start and break the pattern of relapse.

Self-selected Diet

Another dietary option is to have clients choose foods and calculate their cost with calorie and fat-gram counters. This requires clients to weigh and measure their foods. When using this strategy, clients must be diligent about looking up foods throughout the day so they will know how close they are to reaching their calorie target.

PHARMACOLOGICAL INTERVENTION

Clients who have lost weight via pharmacotherapy will likely benefit from continued use. Those who have difficulty reversing small weight gains using the standard behavioral techniques described earlier may benefit from integrating pharmacotherapy into their program. Currently, sibutramine and orlistat are approved for use in the treatment of obesity in clients with a body mass index (BMI) more than 30 or in those with a BMI more than 27 who also have one or more obesity-related risk factors (eg, hypertension or dyslipidemia) (13,14). Clients for whom these medications are appropriate should follow-up frequently with a physician to monitor the medication and its potential adverse effects (see Chapter 8 for more information on medications for weight loss).

Medication is most effective for maintenance when combined with a comprehensive program of behavior modification that includes frequent client-provider contact (15,16). It is important to communicate to clients that medication is not a "magic bullet." The medication may make it easier to adhere to a low-calorie, low-fat diet, but it also requires substantial effort on the part of the client to eat less, exercise more, and maintain healthful behavior changes.

STRATEGIES TO ENHANCE MOTIVATION

JoAnne's weight has increased for the sixth week in a row, and she is inching closer to her baseline weight. She seems to have lost motivation. What can be done? Clients such as JoAnne who are experiencing a decline in motivation may feel like they have given up some of the positive aspects of eating and leading a sedentary lifestyle and have likely become increasingly aware of the negative aspects of weight maintenance. They often say they are "sick of" the effort it takes to remain physically active and/or bored with trying to select healthful foods. When the negative aspects of maintaining weight loss outweigh the positives, clients may become unmotivated and may begin to regain their weight. The challenge for the RD is to find new ways to help clients stay motivated to maintain their healthful habits. Some suggestions are provided here.

Making a List of Positive Changes

Setting future goals is important. Clients often focus on what they have not yet done or on how much weight they would eventually like to lose rather than on what they have achieved. In such cases, it may be helpful for clients to list the positive changes they have made that have enabled them to lose and maintain their weight loss. Ask clients to recall what eating and exercise was like before they began losing weight. What are they doing differently now? Do they exercise more frequently? Wear different-size clothing? Walk stairs without getting winded? Realizing accomplishments may help boost motivation by increasing awareness of the positive changes.

Renewing Reasons for Maintaining Weight

Clients may also find it helpful to list the reasons why they would like to maintain weight loss. What benefits will occur in terms of their health, looks, or mood if they maintain their habit changes? Some clients may find that looking at a photo of themselves at their lowest weight helps them see the benefits of maintaining their lower weight. Clients may also compare current laboratory test results and/or blood pressure readings with those from before weight loss.

Making the Negative Aspects of Weight-loss Maintenance Less Negative

Why is it particularly difficult for the client to maintain a healthy eating and exercise regimen? What aspects of weight maintenance are the most bothersome? What is getting in the way? Help the client explore ways to make the bothersome things less so. For example, if clients report that they are bored with the foods they are eating, suggest that they buy a new low-fat cookbook or subscribe to a healthful cooking magazine. If they are tired of walking on the treadmill, maybe they could move their workout outdoors, try a new activity, or listen to an audio book while they walk. Suggest at least one change the client could make to reduce the troublesome aspects of weight maintenance.

Setting Goals and Rewards

Setting goals, both large and small, and rewards may be the best means of increasing motivation. Help clients select a long-term challenging goal, such as completing a 5K race or raising money for a charity walk. However, clients should also identify smaller goals that can be achieved sooner. For example, the client could call a friend to set up an exercise date for tomorrow, dispose of the high-calorie foods at home, or pack a healthful salad to bring to work.

Incentives that are tied to goals should be commensurate with the goals achieved. For short-term goals, clients may want to treat themselves to a massage or a manicure, purchase a new book or magazine, or go to a movie. Health-promoting rewards may also be used (Box 10.1). For larger goals, clients could put a sum of money in a box every day that they meet the goal. At the end of the month, the client can buy something with the money.

Finding a Partner

Just having company can sometimes be an effective motivator. Many people find that time passes quickly when exercising with a friend. In addition, clients are likely to stay motivated to continue exercising if they know someone is waiting for them to exercise. Encourage clients to seek out others interested in exercise and weight control by joining weight-loss meetings, biking clubs, aerobic classes, or a gym.

FOR THE CLINICIAN: HANDLING BURNOUT

Practitioners working with clients who are regaining weight may become frustrated or even burned out. Being aware of how frustration could interfere with compassionate care is the first step in coping. Other practitioners are often the best resource for ways to help the client (and yourself) change course. It may be helpful to identify ways to "spice up" the intervention, such as a field trip to investigate the client's cupboards at home, food shopping together, or a change in treatment modalities (eg, from individual to group treatment). Consider introducing other professionals, such as exercise physiolo-

---

Box 10.1

Examples of Health-promoting Rewards for Achieving Goals

- New exercise attire
- A cookbook of healthful recipes
- A quality nonstick skillet
- Audio books or music to listen to while walking
- Registration for a physical activity class (eg, sports or a dance class)
- Registration for class about low-fat, low-calorie cooking
- Tickets for zoos and museums

gists, other RDs, psychologists, or even chefs and wardrobe consultants, to help advise the client. Clients who are regaining weight during a prolonged period of time (eg, 6 months or more), despite the best efforts of the health care team, should consider delaying further weight-control treatment until their circumstances or motivation change to better support continued weight control efforts. Ultimately, instead of feeling frustrated and hopeless, try to accept that the client is having trouble and be sympathetic during these difficult times.

FINAL NOTE

Successful weight maintenance is achievable but requires a consistent effort and diligence at exercising and consuming a low-calorie, low-fat diet. Maintenance may be improved by maximizing client-practitioner contact, including high levels of exercise within treatment, providing structured approaches to dietary intake, and enhancing problem-solving skills. Moreover, revisiting clients' reasons for weight control, setting specific goals and rewards, and increasing social support may help clients stay motivated to maintain their healthful habits long-term.

References

1. Perri MG, Shapiro RM, Ludwig WW, Twentyman CT, McAdoo WG. Maintenance strategies for the treatment of obesity: an evaluation of relapse prevention training and post-treatment contact by telephone and mail. *J Consult Clin Psychol.* 1984;52: 404–413.

2. Wing RR, Tate DF, Gorin A, Raynor HA, Fava JL. A self-regulation program for maintenance of weight loss. *N Engl J Med.* 2006;355:1563–1571.

3. Wing RR, Papandonatos G, Fava JL, Gorin AA, Phelan S, McCaffery J, Tate DF. Maintaining large weight losses: the role of behavioral and psychological factors. *J Consult Clin Psychol.* 2008;76:1015–1021.

4. Butryn ML, Phelan S, Hill JO, Wing RR. Consistent self-monitoring of weight: a key component of successful weight loss maintenance. *Obesity.* 2007;15: 3091–3096.

5. Klem ML, Wing RR, McGuire MT, Seagle HM, Hill JO. A descriptive study of individuals successful at long-term maintenance of substantial weight loss. *Am J Clin Nutr.* 1997;66:239–246.

6. Lichtman SW, Pisarska K, Berman ER, Pestone M, Dowling H, Offenbacher E, Weisel H, Heshka S, Matthews DE, Heymsfield SB. Discrepancy between self-reported and actual caloric intake and exercise in obese subjects. *N Engl J Med.* 1992;327:1893–1898.

7. Raynor H, Wing RR, Phelan S. Amount of food group variety consumed in the diet and long-term weight loss maintenance. *Obes Res.* May; 13:883–890.

8. Gorin AA, Phelan S, Hill JA, Wing RR. Promoting long-term weight control: does dieting consistency matter? *Int J Obes Relat Metab Disord.* 2004;28:278–281.

9. Perri MG, Nezu AM, McKelvey WF, Shermer RL, Renjilian DA, Viegener BJ. Relapse prevention training and problem-solving therapy in the long-term management of obesity. *J Consult Clin Psychol.* 2001;69:722–726.

10. Grilo CM, Shiffman S, Wing RR. Relapse crises and coping among dieters. *J Consult Clin Psychol.* 1989;57:488–495.

11. McGuire MT, Wing RR, Klem ML, Lang W, Hill JO. What predicts weight regain in a group of successful weight losers? *J Consult Clin Psychol.* 1999;67:177–185.

12. Boutelle KN, Kirschenbaum DS. Further support for consistent self-monitoring as a vital component of successful weight control. *Obes Res.* 1998;6:219–224.

13. National Institutes of Health. Clinical guidelines on the identification, evaluation, and treatment of overweight and obesity in adults—the evidence report. *Obes Res.* 1998;6(suppl):51S–209S.

14. National Task Force on the Prevention and Treatment of Obesity. Long-term pharmacotherapy in the management of obesity. *JAMA.* 1996;276:1907–1915.

15. Davidson MH, Hauptman J, DiGirolamo M, Foreyt JP, Halsted CH, Heber D, Heimburger DC, Lucas CP, Robbins DC, Chung J, Heymsfield SB. Weight control and risk factor reduction in obese subjects treated for 2 years with orlistat: a randomized controlled trial. *JAMA.* 1999;281:235–242.

16. James WP, Astrup A, Finer N, Hilsted J, Kopelman P, Rossner S, Saris WH, Van Gaal LF. Effect of sibutramine on weight maintenance after weight loss: a randomised trial. STORM Study Group. Sibutramine Trial of Obesity Reduction and Maintenance. *Lancet.* 2000;356:2119–2125.

Section 2

Special Issues

CHAPTER 11

OBESITY AS A PUBLIC HEALTH ISSUE

THOMAS A. FARLEY, MD, MPH

The field of public health concerns itself with preventing health problems, rather than treating them after they have occurred, and directs its attention not to individual people but to entire populations. Public health was founded in large part in response to epidemics of infectious diseases. Obesity is a health problem for individual people, but it is also a nationwide epidemic, although of a chronic condition. Obesity is therefore a legitimate topic for public health, and public health insights are necessary to solve the problem, not just for society but also for individual people.

THE EPIDEMIC OF OBESITY

Obesity rates in American adults rose fairly slowly through the 1960s and early 1970s but have grown very rapidly in the last 30 years (Figure 11.1) (1,2). By 2005–2006, one-third of Americans were obese, and another third are overweight (2,3). When two-thirds of a population has a condition, that condition can be considered normal, even if it is unhealthy. The increase in body mass index (BMI) during these three decades was not limited to a fraction of the population with greater than average weight; instead, it represented a shift of the entire distribution (Figure 11.2) (3). People who in a previous era, based on their genes and psychological makeup, would have had a healthy weight are now overweight; people who might have been overweight are now obese; and people who might have been obese are more obese. Taken together, these findings suggest that the increase in BMI during the past 30 years does not represent a change in individuals, but rather represents a change in social or environmental factors to which the entire population is exposed. The differences among individuals—such as those arising from genetics or psychological make-up—explain why some people have more adipose tissue than others today, but such interindividual differences have always been present and cannot explain dramatic shift in the population over time. To find the causes of the epidemic, one must start by identifying social or environmental factors that have changed during this time and that influence BMI.

THE MAGNITUDE OF ENERGY IMBALANCE

While the metabolic causes of obesity are complex and are not fully understood, there is no serious disagreement that the problem arises fundamentally from a chronic excess of caloric consumption compared with energy expenditure. A daily energy imbalance does

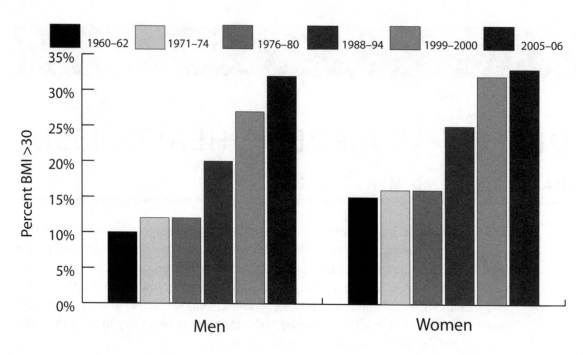

FIGURE 11.1   Trends in obesity prevalence in US adults, 1960–1962 to 2005–2006. Data are from references 1 and 2.

not need to be large to explain substantial weight gain over a year. An individual who drinks one additional 12-ounce can of a soft drink per day (approximately 150 kcal) will gain approximately 15 pounds over 1 year if he or she does not reduce consumption of other food items or increase energy expenditure from physical activity. Taking an elevator instead of climbing two flights of stairs a day can add as much as 6 pounds a year. As weight is gained, energy expenditure increases even if physical activity levels stay the same; therefore, over several years the actual weight gain per year is likely to be somewhat less than this (4), but the observation that small but consistent daily imbalances can account for substantial obesity is still valid. In fact, by one estimate, an imbalance of as little as 100 to 150 kcal per day, or about as much as one cookie, is sufficient to explain the entire obesity epidemic in America (5). An imbalance this small is difficult to identify through surveys of diet or physical activity, which have various inherent inaccuracies. In addition, an imbalance this small could be induced by features in the environment, even if the influence of those features is weak.

WEIGHT LOSS VS PREVENTION OF WEIGHT GAIN

Unfortunately, much of the focus of the response to the obesity epidemic in the United States has been programs to help obese persons lose weight. This idea also has taken hold among the public at large: the majority of Americans consider themselves overweight, and nearly one-third are actively trying to lose weight (including nearly one-quarter of women of normal weight) (6,7). It is a common assumption among those peo-

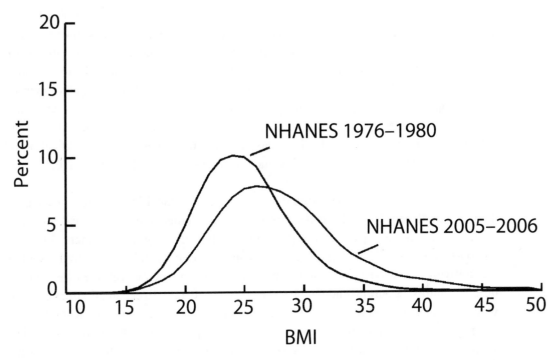

Figure 11.2   Shift in distribution of body mass index in US adults, 1976–1980 to 2005–2006. Reprinted from Ogden CL, Carroll MD, McDowell MA, Flegal KM. Obesity among adults in the United States—no statistically significant change since 2003–2004. *NCHS Data Brief.* 2007;(1):1–6.

ple that the responsibility for obesity and its solution rests with them individually, as evidenced by the multi-billion-dollar industry that sells weight-loss products such as books, programs, and dietary supplements.

However, sustained weight loss is very difficult for people to achieve. While weight-loss programs in controlled research settings are successful over the short term, the overwhelming majority of people in these programs do not maintain their weight loss over the long term (8). Furthermore, outside of research settings, few people have the willpower to adhere to weight-loss programs long enough to lose weight. There are also questions about whether people who lose weight achieve health benefits equivalent to those who do not gain weight in the first place (9). For these reasons, and given the magnitude of the epidemic, <u>public health approaches to obesity should focus on less on weight loss and more on prevention of weight gain.</u>

ENVIRONMENTAL CAUSES, ENVIRONMENTAL SOLUTIONS

There is increasing evidence that features of the social and physical environment influence levels of both physical activity and food consumption (10–12). For example, the availability of televisions and automobiles and the design of cities and towns in ways that make it difficult to walk outdoors are likely to reduce physical activity, and the availability of healthful and nonhealthful food items influence diet (13,14).

Strategies to change health-related behavior can be classified in two broad categories: individual-level approaches and environmental approaches (also known as structural approaches) (15). Individual-level approaches include educational, motivational, or skills-based interventions that attempt to inform, persuade, or provide skills to individuals to modify their behavior within an existing social and physical environment. Environmental approaches attempt to modify the physical or social environment in ways that bring about changes in the behaviors of individuals in response. Examples of environmental approaches to prevent heart disease are building sidewalks (a modification of the physical environment) or banning indoor smoking (a modification of the social environment).

Environmental approaches differ distinctly from individual-level approaches in both their potential benefits and the barriers to their implementation. Individual-level approaches such as individual counseling can be relatively easy to implement for small numbers of people and may have substantial short-term impact, but they are difficult or prohibitively expensive to bring to a population scale, and their effects are often temporary. In contrast, environmental approaches often have a relatively small effect on individual persons but tend to be large in scale, thus having a large potential effect on an entire population. Implementation of environmental approaches often requires political support that may be difficult to organize, but once implemented such interventions are more likely than individual-level approaches to have long-lasting effects. Because the epidemiology of obesity strongly implies that the causes are environmental, it stands to reason that the solutions will need to be environmental as well.

Obesity and its long-term adverse complications, diabetes and cardiovascular disease, can be seen as consequences of unhealthy behaviors (consumption of excess food, inadequate physical activity) in the same way that chronic lung disease, lung cancer, and heart disease are the consequences of the unhealthy behavior of smoking. The history of attempts to reduce smoking rates in the United States provides lessons for attempts to reduce obesity. In the 1960s, smoking prevention programs emphasized individual-level approaches, specifically educating adults in communities and children in schools about the risks of tobacco, with the hope that adult smokers would quit and children would not adopt the habit. At best, these programs had small, temporary effects; more often, they were complete failures (16). On the other hand, smoking rates have fallen by half in the United States during the past 25 years as anti-smoking strategy has shifted from classroom and community education to changes in the physical and social environment, specifically advertising restrictions, counteradvertising, taxes, and restrictions on indoor smoking (17). Today, virtually the entire field of smoking prevention is based on these environmental approaches to behavior change.

A STRUCTURAL MODEL OF HEALTH BEHAVIOR

Different models have been developed for environmental approaches to health promotion through behavior change. One model categorizes environmental factors that influence health-related behavior into four groups (15):

- *Accessibility of products that impact health,* such as the number of liquor stores in a neighborhood, the availability of vending machines selling sweetened beverages in schools, the length of shelf space allotted to salty snacks at grocery stores, and the prices of products

- *Physical structures,* which make it easier or more difficult to engage in a behavior, such as the presence of sidewalks on a street, the availability and visibility of stairways in buildings, and the size of bottles in which soft drinks are sold
- *Social structures,* which are rules established by organizations to regulate the behavior of individuals (eg, indoor smoking bans and mandatory motorcycle helmet laws) and the organizations themselves (eg, recreational sports leagues and walking clubs)
- *Media messages,* which are the words and images delivered to us via a rapidly increasing number of channels (eg, scenes of characters smoking in movies, advertising of food and alcohol, and violence in video games)

This model can be used to identify social and environmental factors that tend to promote obesity and the actions that could be taken to prevent it.

INCREASING ENERGY EXPENDITURE

Infrequent engagement in physical activity and high levels of sedentary behaviors (such as television watching) contribute to low amounts of energy expenditure and weight gain (18,19). Physical activity levels in the United States are far from optimal for health. Activity levels seem to have risen slightly in the past 10 years (20), but more than one in four adults does not participate in exercise at all, and only about one in ten exercise at least 30 minutes five times a week (20,21). Americans spend about 3 hours daily in sedentary activities, particularly watching television and, increasingly, playing video games or using computers (22).

Physical activity can be divided into the following two categories:

- *Exercise*—ie, physically active behavior that people engage in for pleasure or to promote their health, such as jogging, fitness walking, or playing sports games
- *Lifestyle physical activity*—ie, physically active behavior that occurs as a result of activities that have other purposes, such as walking to a store or climbing stairs at a workplace

The distinction between these two categories can sometimes be blurred (eg, some people may walk to a store when they could have driven an automobile because they enjoy the walk), but it is nonetheless often useful in planning. Many people find exercise unpleasant; therefore, the number of people who will exercise regularly or for sufficient time for optimal health is likely to be limited, although those limits can be increased through environmental changes. On the other hand, lifestyle physical activity can theoretically be increased for nearly everyone through changes in the environment.

Promoting Exercise

Exercise can be promoted by changes in physical and social structures and, to a lesser extent, by media messages. Adults are more likely to be physically active if they have access to recreational equipment and facilities and to trails (23), and children are more likely to be physically active if they have a safe playground in their neighborhood (24). Having to drive to a recreational facility is a barrier that is likely to reduce use; therefore, it is probably more effective to have many smaller facilities distributed in residential areas than to have few large sports facilities at greater distances. A reasonable social goal is that everyone lives within a 10-minute walk of a park, playground, trail, or other place to exercise outdoors.

Many people participate in exercise through organizations such as sports leagues and walking clubs, and it has been demonstrated that people are more likely to participate in exercise if they have social support or companions with whom to exercise (23). More public support for recreational and sports organizations may therefore increase the number of individuals who exercise. Instructor-led physical activity programs in workplaces and public parks may also be successful.

Studies have shown that stair use can be promoted when prompts about the benefits of stair-climbing are placed at the point of decision between stairs and escalators (25). When included in community-wide campaigns, media messages have also been successful in promoting physical activity (25). Additional research is needed on ways to use prompts and other media messages to encourage exercise, particularly at the point at which people can choose to be physically active or not.

Increasing Lifestyle Physical Activity

Walking is the most common form of physical activity. A 70-kg adult expends 200 to 300 kcal/hour while walking, compared to about 70 kcal/hour while watching television (26). This suggests that if adults walked an additional 30 minutes per day instead of watching television, weight gain might be cut in half. Unfortunately, our society has engineered walking out of the lives of most of us by building neighborhoods and communities designed for transportation solely by automobiles. In many communities, the separation of residential and commercial areas is too large for people to walk for errands, and the transportation infrastructure (eg, high-traffic streets and lack of sidewalks) often makes walking unpleasant or dangerous. This type of land use and transportation infrastructure is associated with low levels of walking (27), with consequences for obesity. People who live in communities with high degrees of "sprawl" spend more time in their cars and are more likely to be obese (28–31).

This dependence on automobiles for transportation and the environmental barriers to active transportation can be changed, not just in newly-built communities but also in existing communities. Changes in zoning can encourage the development of mixed-use neighborhoods that place retail stores, schools, and workplaces within walking distance. Suburbs could allow higher-density real estate development that can support retail stores with more customers and thereby increase the number of nearby destinations. Policies can be established and funding directed to build sidewalks and bicycle lanes on all streets and create safer intersections for pedestrians and bicyclists. Greater funding for public transit can increase the number of people walking to transit stops, and, over time, transit stops tend to become higher-density hubs with additional destinations to which people can walk. Ending subsidized parking and turning parking spaces into other community uses can discourage driving and, when combined with improvements in pedestrian infrastructure, encourage walking.

Smaller-scale design changes may also promote lifestyle physical activity. Changing building codes and building designs to make stairways accessible and attractive is likely to promote stair use over escalators or elevators.

Use of electronic media, especially television, is particularly important to the development of obesity in both adults and children (32). Children who watch television have a lower metabolic rate than even those who are inactive (33), and both adults and children consume more calories with each additional hour of television watching (32,34). The amount of time children spend watching television is strongly associated with weight gain (19,34,35). With the increasing availability and greater variety of electronic media, from the Internet (where everything from clothes to electronics can be bought while sitting in the comfort of your home) to video games to interactive television, sedentary use of electronic media continues to increase. More research is needed on approaches to reduce this sedentary behavior. Approaches that provide appealing alternative activities may be part of the solution. For example, people may be less sedentary if a greater number of recreational facilities and organized activities are made available.

DECREASING ENERGY INTAKE

Americans eat very differently today than they did 25 years ago. People consume more calories than they did in the 1970s (36,37). According to national survey data, between the late 1970s and the late 1990s, individual daily consumption increased approximately 200 kcal (36,37). Although these data must be interpreted cautiously because the survey methods changed over time, the increase in energy consumption parallels an increase in the caloric content of food distributed through the US food system, as tracked by the US Department of Agriculture (5). This increase seems to have started, after decades of relative stability, in the late 1970s, around the time that the obesity epidemic began to escalate.

Eating patterns have also changed dramatically. Americans are eating a steadily greater proportion of their food away from home—the proportion is currently approaching 50% (37). Somewhat less than one-third of food is consumed in restaurants and most of the rest is purchased from snack counters, other food stores, or vending machines (37). Americans are also increasingly consuming snacks (37). Adults snack approximately two times per day, with an average of about 200 kcal per episode, and total energy consumption rises with each eating occasion (36,38). In fact, data from Nielsen et al suggest that an increase in snacking alone could account for most of the increase in energy consumption from the late 1970s to the late 1990s (37). This is consistent with experimental data suggesting that individuals do not compensate for the energy in food consumed as snacks by eating less at subsequent meals (39).

Nielsen and associates (37) also assessed changes in consumption in individual food items, and among the food items showing the greatest increases were soft drinks, salty snacks like chips, french fries, and pizza. Americans are particularly consuming more soft drinks and other sweetened beverages, and these are especially important to the development of obesity. In cross-sectional and prospective studies, consumption of sweetened beverages contributes to higher levels of energy consumption, weight gain, and diabetes (40–42), and reduction of consumption of sweetened beverages has led to a reduced weight gain in children in two trials (43,44).

The changes in food consumption patterns during the rise of the obesity epidemic are unlikely to have been caused by spontaneous changes in food preferences. They are much more easily explained by changes in the "food environment." Many studies in recent years have demonstrated powerful influences of the environment on the amount of food that people consume. Four factors are likely to be particularly important: food accessibility (including prices), portion sizes, energy density, and advertising.

Accessibility

Food is available at an increasing number of locations, and it is increasingly ready to eat. Fast-food restaurants are rapidly increasing in the United States, both in total number and in the proportion of total restaurants (45). Fast food is relatively inexpensive. For about $5, one can purchase a combination meal with more than 1,300 kcal, or about two-thirds of the energy needs of a teenage girl. Foods sold away from home in general, and fast foods in particular, tend to be more energy dense (46,47). Although studies have not found a relationship between fast-food restaurant availability and obesity at the neighborhood level, states with more fast-food restaurants have higher obesity rates than states with fewer (48–50).

More food is purchased from grocery stores than restaurants. The display of food on shelves in grocery stores has a strong influence on sales. Marketing studies from the 1970s showed that sales of all items are directly related to the length of shelf space allotted to them. One study demonstrated that sales of fruits and vegetables increased by approximately 40% when the shelf space on which they were displayed was doubled (51). Observations at the Tulane University Prevention Research Center (unpublished data) conducted in supermarkets showed that only 9% of the total store shelf space was devoted to fresh fruits and vegetables, whereas 14% was devoted to snack foods (not including beverages) that are very energy dense. The relative prominence of snack foods in grocery stores may be encouraging consumption of energy-dense foods and as a result promoting excess energy consumption.

The accessibility of food in an ever-proliferating number of sources beyond grocery stores and restaurants, such as snack counters, vending machines, bookstores, and near the cash register at other nonfood stores, is also likely to promote increased consumption. One principle is that the amount of food consumed increases as the effort to eat it decreases, even if the differences in effort are tiny. For example, during a workday office workers who had chocolate "kisses" within reach on their desks ate an average of 5.6 more candies (amounting to 136 kcal) per day than workers for whom the candies were on a shelf 2 meters away from their desks (52).

Energy-dense foods are also falling in price relative to other foods. Between 1982 and 1997, the prices of nonalcoholic beverages, sweets, and fats and oils rose about half as much as the prices of fruits and vegetables (53). Intervention trials show that food choices are very much influenced by prices (54). For example, when the prices of healthier items in vending machines were reduced by 10%, sales increased by 9% (55). The lower prices of energy-dense snack foods tend to encourage overconsumption.

Portion Size

Food portion sizes seem to be very important in determining consumption. People served larger portions simply eat more food, regardless of their body weight and regardless of the item, setting, or timing relative to other meals (56–60). For example, when a restaurant served a baked pasta dish that was 50% larger than the normal portion, people ate 43% more, increasing their energy consumption at the meal by 159 kcal (56). Men given 175-g instead of 25-g bags of potato chips tripled the amount of chips they ate, taking in an extra 311 kcal (59). Portion sizes have increased dramatically in recent decades, with the greatest increases occurring at fast-food restaurants (61).

Energy Density

The energy density of foods is a physical structure that strongly influences energy intake. Foods vary more than 10-fold in their calorie density, from fresh vegetables (0.2 to 0.4 kcal/g) to sandwiches (1.3 to 2.8 kcal/g) to potato chips (5.4 kcal/g). People tend to become satiated by food based more on its weight or volume than its energy content. Therefore, it makes intuitive sense that energy-dense foods would likely increase people's energy intake, and, in fact, participants in laboratory studies who are given food of higher density consume more calories, independent of portion sizes (62). Similarly, in national surveys, the energy density of individuals' diets is positively associated with BMI (63).

Advertising

Food companies spend more than $7 billion a year on advertising (64), and the foods advertised tend to be high in sugar and fat (65). Everyone in the United States is exposed to this advertising, so it is very difficult to study its effect on food consumption. Nonetheless, it is hard to imagine that food companies would spend these billions to advertise if they did not believe it increased consumption. While food companies are only interested in increasing sales of their own products, the cumulative effect of this advertising is likely to be an increased consumption of all advertised foods. This effect need not be large to contribute meaningfully to the obesity epidemic.

Environmental Changes to Reduce Energy Consumption

Given these environmental influences on food consumption, what are the actions that could be taken to reduce energy intake? One option is to use taxation to increase the price of foods that seem to be most responsible for causing increased energy consumption. The taxation categories for foods could be selected based on their energy density, availability, or apparent role in increasing weight gain. For example, a tax could be added to food items that are energy-dense, widely available, ready to eat in the form of snacks, and associated in epidemiologic studies with obesity (eg, sweetened beverages and salty snacks like potato chips). This tax would serve several purposes. First, it would

like cigarettes, gambling

reduce purchases by consumers who would be drawn to lower priced (and therefore lower calorie) items. Second, because energy-dense snack foods would be less appealing to consumers, food store managers would have less incentive to use large amounts of shelf space to display these items. Third, the revenue from such a tax could be used for a variety of obesity-prevention actions, such as building playgrounds, subsidizing healthier items such as fruits and vegetables, or media campaigns promoting consumption of fruits and vegetable and counteradvertising against energy-dense snack foods. Taxing cigarettes has proven repeatedly to be an effective way to reduce consumption, even though tobacco is an addictive drug. Therefore, a tax on energy-dense snack food seems very likely to be effective.

Another category of policies that would alter the food environment favorably are regulations on food availability. Currently, many school districts and some states are taking steps to remove sweetened beverages and snack items from vending machines in schools. When such items are in schools, they not only provide a source of excess calories for students during the school day, they also send a powerful message to children that such foods are acceptable to consume at other times. Removing these items can have the opposite, beneficial effect of sending a message that these items should be avoided. Sweetened beverages and energy-dense snack foods can be removed not just from schools but also from workplaces, with the particular justification that employers pay a large percentage of the health care costs stemming from obesity in their employees.

Communities could also reduce the availability of energy-dense, ready-to-eat food in neighborhoods by planning and zoning rules that reduce the number of fast-food restaurants. Since they were first developed, town planning and zoning have been used for health purposes, and they are already the legal mechanisms to regulate the location of commercial outlets like restaurants. Although they have not generally been used for the specific purpose of limiting access to unhealthy foods, they could easily be employed in that way.

Finally, as a society, it is difficult to respond effectively to the proliferation of food advertising, but two strategies may limit the damage. First, advertising of unhealthy food to children could be regulated at the federal level. Second, counteradvertising that points out the health dangers of certain foods can counteract the inappropriately positive images of unhealthy foods shown in advertising. The experience from tobacco control is that counteradvertising can be very effective even if the messages are greatly outnumbered by the industry's advertisements.

CONCLUSION

Obesity is as much of an epidemic as an outbreak of cholera, and it is important to realize the implications of this. Cholera might be highly infectious and immediately more dangerous than obesity, but both epidemics require environmental changes to stop their spread and both originate from an unhealthful environment. Although the metabolic mechanisms that determine food consumption and weight gain are not fully understood, we do understand the environmental causes well enough to act now to remedy them. Public policy is the tool with which we can act to slow or reverse the epidemic.

References

1. Flegal KM, Carroll MD, Kuczmarski RJ, Johnson CL. Overweight and obesity in the United States: prevalence and trends, 1960–1994. *Int J Obes Relat Metab Disord.* 1998;22:39–47.

2. Ogden CL, Carroll MD, Curtin LR, McDowell MA, Tabak CJ, Flegal KM. Prevalence of overweight and obesity in the United States, 1999–2004. *JAMA.* 2006;295:1549–1555.

3. Ogden CL, Carroll MD, McDowell MA, Flegal KM. Obesity among adults in the United States—no statistically significant change since 2003–2004. *NCHS Data Brief.* 2007;(1):1–6.

4. Weinsier RL, Bracco D, Schutz Y. Predicted effects of small decreases in energy expenditure on weight gain in adult women. *Int J Obes Relat Metab Disord.* 1993;17:693–700.

5. Cutler DM, Glaeser EL, Shapiro JM. *Why Have Americans Become More Obese?* Cambridge, MA: National Bureau of Economic Research; 2003. Report no. 9446.

6. Chang VW, Christakis NA. Self-perception of weight appropriateness in the United States. *Am J Prev Med.* 2003;24:332–339.

7. Kruger J, Galuska DA, Serdula MK, Jones DA. Attempting to lose weight: specific practices among U.S. adults. *Am J Prev Med.* 2004;26:402–406.

8. Wing RR, Phelan S. Long-term weight loss maintenance. *Am J Clin Nutr.* 2005;82(Suppl 1):222S–225S.

9. Kassirer JP, Angell M. Losing weight—an ill-fated New Year's resolution. *N Engl J Med.* 1998;338:52–54.

10. Sallis JF, Bauman A, Pratt M. Environmental and policy interventions to promote physical activity. *Am J Prev Med.* 1998;15:379–397.

11. King AC, Jeffery RW, Fridinger F, Dusenbury L, Provence S, Hedlund SA, Spangler K. Environmental and policy approaches to cardiovascular disease prevention through physical activity: issues and opportunities. *Health Educ Q.* 1995;22:499–511.

12. French SA, Story M, Jeffery RW. Environmental influences on eating and physical activity. *Annu Rev Public Health.* 2001;22:309–335.

13. Morland K, Diez Roux AV, Wing S. Supermarkets, other food stores, and obesity: the Atherosclerosis Risk in Communities study. *Am J Prev Med.* 2006;30:333–339.

14. Morland K, Wing S, Diez Roux A. The contextual effect of the local food environment on residents' diets: the Atherosclerosis Risk in Communities study. *Am J Public Health.* 2002;92:1761–1767.

15. Cohen DA, Scribner RA, Farley TA. A structural model of health behavior: a pragmatic approach to explain and influence health behaviors at the population level. *Prev Med.* 2000;30:146–154.

16. Thompson EL. Smoking education programs 1960–1976. *Am J Public Health.* 1978;68:250–257.

17. Levy DT, Chaloupka F, Gitchell J. The effects of tobacco control policies on smoking rates: a tobacco control scorecard. *J Public Health Manag Pract.* 2004;10:338–353.

18. US Department of Health and Human Services. *Physical Activity and Health: A Report of the Surgeon General*. Atlanta, GA: US Department of Health and Human Services; 1996.

19. Berkey CS, Rockett HR, Field AE, Gillman MW, Frazier AL, Camargo CA Jr, Colditz GA. Activity, dietary intake, and weight changes in a longitudinal study of preadolescent and adolescent boys and girls. *Pediatrics*. 2000;105:E56.

20. Centers for Disease Control and Prevention. Prevalence of no leisure-time physical activity—35 states and the District of Columbia, 1988–2002. *MMWR*. 2004;53: 82–86.

21. Steffen LM, Arnett DK, Blackburn H, Shah G, Armstrong C, Luepker RV, Jacobs DR Jr. Population trends in leisure-time physical activity: Minnesota Heart Survey, 1980-2000. *Med Sci Sports Exerc*. 2006;38:1716–1723.

22. Bureau of Labor Statistics. American Time Use Survey, 2006. 2007. http://www.bls.gov/tus. Accessed January 15, 2008.

23. Wendel-Vos W, Droomers M, Kremers S, Brug J, van Lenthe F. Potential environmental determinants of physical activity in adults: a systematic review. *Obes Rev*. 2007;8:425–440.

24. Farley TA, Meriwether RA, Baker ET, Watkins LT, Johnson CJ, Webber LS. Safe play spaces to promote physical activity in inner-city children: results from a pilot study of an environmental intervention. A*m J Public Health*. 2007;97:1625–1631.

25. Kahn EB, Ramsey LT, Brownson RC, Heath GW, Howze EH, Powell KE, Stone EJ, Rajab MW, Corso P. The effectiveness of interventions to increase physical activity. A systematic review. *Am J Prev Med*. 2002;22(4 Suppl):S73–S107.

26. Ainsworth BE, Haskell WL, Leon AS, Jacobs DR, Jr., Montoye HJ, Sallis JF, Paffenbarger RS Jr. Compendium of physical activities: classification of energy costs of human physical activities. *Med Sci Sports Exerc*. 1993;25:71–80.

27. Owen N, Humpel N, Leslie E, Bauman A, Sallis JF. Understanding environmental influences on walking: review and research agenda. *Am J Prev Med*. 2004;27: 67–76.

28. Frank LD, Andresen MA, Schmid TL. Obesity relationships with community design, physical activity, and time spent in cars. *Am J Prev Med*. 2004;27:87–96.

29. Lopez R. Urban sprawl and risk for being overweight or obese. *Am J Public Health*. 2004;94:1574–1579.

30. Ewing R, Schmid T, Killingsworth R, Zlot A, Raudenbush S. Relationship between urban sprawl and physical activity, obesity, and morbidity. *Am J Health Promot*. 2003;18:47–57.

31. Saelens BE, Sallis JF, Black JB, Chen D. Neighborhood-based differences in physical activity: an environment scale evaluation. *Am J Public Health*. 2003;93: 1552–1558.

32. Bowman SA. Television-viewing characteristics of adults: correlations to eating practices and overweight and health status. *Prev Chronic Dis*. 2006;3:A38.

33. Klesges RC, Shelton ML, Klesges LM. Effects of television on metabolic rate: potential implications for childhood obesity. *Pediatrics*. 1993;91:281–286.

34. Crespo CJ, Smit E, Troiano RP, Bartlett SJ, Macera CA, Andersen RE. Television watching, energy intake, and obesity in US children: results from the third National Health and Nutrition Examination Survey, 1988–1994. *Arch Pediatr Adolesc Med*. 2001;155:360–365.

35. Robinson TN. Reducing children's television viewing to prevent obesity: a randomized controlled trial. *JAMA*. 1999;282:1561–1567.

36. Kant AK, Graubard BI. Secular trends in patterns of self-reported food consumption of adult Americans: NHANES 1971–1975 to NHANES 1999–2002. *Am J Clin Nutr*. 2006;84:1215–1223.

37. Nielsen SJ, Siega-Riz AM, Popkin BM. Trends in energy intake in U.S. between 1977 and 1996: similar shifts seen across age groups. *Obes Res*. 2002;10:370–378.

38. Kerver JM, Yang EJ, Obayashi S, Bianchi L, Song WO. Meal and snack patterns are associated with dietary intake of energy and nutrients in US adults. *J Am Diet Assoc*. 2006;106:46–53.

39. Levitsky DA. The non-regulation of food intake in humans: hope for reversing the epidemic of obesity. *Physiol Behav*. 2005;86:623–632.

40. Malik VS, Schulze MB, Hu FB. Intake of sugar-sweetened beverages and weight gain: a systematic review. *Am J Clin Nutr*. 2006;84:274–288.

41. Schulze MB, Manson JE, Ludwig DS, Colditz GA, Stampfer MJ, Willett WC, Hu FB. Sugar-sweetened beverages, weight gain, and incidence of type 2 diabetes in young and middle-aged women. *JAMA*. 2004;292:927–934.

42. Vartanian LR, Schwartz MB, Brownell KD. Effects of soft drink consumption on nutrition and health: a systematic review and meta-analysis. *Am J Public Health*. 2007;97:667–675.

43. Ebbeling CB, Feldman HA, Osganian SK, Chomitz VR, Ellenbogen SJ, Ludwig DS. Effects of decreasing sugar-sweetened beverage consumption on body weight in adolescents: a randomized, controlled pilot study. *Pediatrics*. 2006;117:673–680.

44. James J, Thomas P, Cavan D, Kerr D. Preventing childhood obesity by reducing consumption of carbonated drinks: cluster randomised controlled trial. *BMJ*. 2004;328:1237.

45. Powell LM, Chaloupka FJ, Bao Y. The availability of fast-food and full-service restaurants in the United States: associations with neighborhood characteristics. *Am J Prev Med*. 2007;33(Suppl 4):S240–S245.

46. Bowman SA, Vinyard BT. Fast food consumption of U.S. adults: impact on energy and nutrient intakes and overweight status. *J Am Coll Nutr*. 2004;23:163–168.

47. Guthrie JF, Lin BH, Frazao E. Role of food prepared away from home in the American diet, 1977-78 versus 1994-96: changes and consequences. *J Nutr Educ Behav*. 2002;34:140–150.

48. Jeffery RW, Baxter J, McGuire M, Linde J. Are fast food restaurants an environmental risk factor for obesity? *Int J Behav Nutr Phys Act*. 2006;3:2.

49. Burdette HL, Whitaker RC. Neighborhood playgrounds, fast food restaurants, and crime: relationships to overweight in low-income preschool children. *Prev Med*. 2004;38:57–63.

50. Maddock J. The relationship between obesity and the prevalence of fast food restaurants: state-level analysis. *Am J Health Promot*. 2004;19:137–143.

51. Curhan RC. The effects of merchandising and temporary promotional activities on the sales of fresh fruits and vegetables in supermarkets. *J Marketing Res*. 1974;11:286–294.

52. Painter JE, Wansink B, Hieggelke JB. How visibility and convenience influence candy consumption. *Appetite*. 2002;38:237–238.

53. Putnam J, Gerrior S. Trends in the U.S. Food Supply, 1970–1997. http://www.ers. usda.gov/publications/aib750/aib750g.pdf. Accessed January 16, 2008.

54. French SA. Pricing effects on food choices. *J Nutr*. 2003;133(suppl):841S–843S.

55. French SA, Jeffery RW, Story M, Breitlow KK, Baxter JS, Hannan P, Snyder MP. Pricing and promotion effects on low-fat vending snack purchases: the CHIPS Study. *Am J Public Health*. 2001;91:112–117.

56. Diliberti N, Bordi PL, Conklin MT, Roe LS, Rolls BJ. Increased portion size leads to increased energy intake in a restaurant meal. *Obes Res*. 2004;12:562–568.

57. Levitsky DA, Youn T. The more food young adults are served, the more they overeat. *J Nutr*. 2004;134:2546–2549.

58. Rolls BJ, Morris EL, Roe LS. Portion size of food affects energy intake in normal-weight and overweight men and women. *Am J Clin Nutr*. 2002;76:1207–1213.

59. Rolls BJ, Roe LS, Kral TV, Meengs JS, Wall DE. Increasing the portion size of a packaged snack increases energy intake in men and women. *Appetite*. 2004;42: 63–69.

60. Rolls BJ, Roe LS, Meengs JS. Larger portion sizes lead to a sustained increase in energy intake over 2 days. *J Am Diet Assoc*. 2006;106:543–549.

61. Nielsen SJ, Popkin BM. Patterns and trends in food portion sizes, 1977–1998. *JAMA*. 2003;289:450–453.

62. Ello-Martin JA, Ledikwe JH, Rolls BJ. The influence of food portion size and energy density on energy intake: implications for weight management. *Am J Clin Nutr*. 2005;82(Suppl 1):236S–241S.

63. Kant AK, Graubard BI. Energy density of diets reported by American adults: association with food group intake, nutrient intake, and body weight. *Int J Obes* (Lond). 2005;29:950–956.

64. 2007 Marketer Profiles Yearbook: 100 Leading National Advertisers. 2007. http:// adage.com/images/random/lna2007.pdf. Accessed January 16, 2008.

65. Powell LM, Szczypka G, Chaloupka FJ, Braunschweig CL. Nutritional content of television food advertisements seen by children and adolescents in the United States. *Pediatrics*. 2007;120:576–583.

CHAPTER 12

THE ECONOMICS OF OBESITY

ANNE WOLF, MS, RD, AND PAM MICHAEL, MBA, RD

INTRODUCTION

Government, health care, and business leaders are concerned by the marked increase of overweight and obesity in the United States and the resulting impact on our nation's health, health care costs, and productivity. Most concerning is that excess weight carries major health risks. These conditions are associated with high costs, including both the direct costs of medical care and the indirect costs of lost productivity and disability. A recent report identified the growing prevalence of obesity as one of the primary factors responsible for the growth of private health care spending between 1987 and 2002 (1). In recent years, there have been numerous studies on the cost of obesity. The purpose of this chapter is to review and synthesize the current literature on the cost of obesity and present relevant information regarding the reimbursement for registered dietitian (RD)-provided medical nutrition therapy (MNT) for obesity and lifestyle treatment.

DIRECT MEDICAL COSTS

Direct costs refer to the cost of preventive, diagnosis, and treatment services related to the disease (eg, hospital care, physician services, and medications). According to the most recent direct cost of obesity estimate (1998), overweight- and obesity-related medical spending was approximately $51.5 billion—or $78.5 billion if nursing home costs were included (2). In 2008 dollars, the estimates would be $77.3 billion and $117.8 billion, respectively. Costs associated with overweight represented 3.7% of the national health care expenditures whereas those associated with obesity were an additional 5.3%. Hence, the combined costs of overweight and obesity were 9.1% of that year's total medical expenditure. The inflation-adjusted per capita health care spending increased by $1,110 from 1987 to 2001 (3). Twenty-seven percent of this growth was attributed to obesity—12% to the increase in the number of obese people and the remainder to faster growth in health care expenses among obese people. Evaluating only the private health care sector, spending attributable to obesity increased ten-fold between 1987 and 2002, raising spending to more than $36 billion in this health sector alone in 2002 (1).

Health Care Costs by Overweight and Obesity Class

Health care costs increase as weight increases. Among the overweight and obese, per capita medical spending increases by 14.5% and 37.4%, respectively, compared with people with a healthy body weight (body mass index [BMI] 18.5–24.9) (2). The monotonic increase in medical spending by weight class has also been reported in various populations (3–5). In the Health and Retirement Survey of Americans in their 50s, people with obesity class I (BMI 30–35) had health care costs about 25% above those with a healthy weight; those with class II obesity (BMI 35–40) had costs about 50% greater; and costs were double for those with class III/extreme obesity (BMI ≥ 40) compared with healthy-weight peers. The increased costs seemed to be driven largely by increased use of outpatient services (4). Among a more general age cohort, Arterburn et al report that health care expenditures for individuals with BMI ≥ 40 were 81% greater than for healthy-weight adults and were disproportionate to prevalence (5). Thorpe also reported that in 2002, 25% of people with severe obesity were treated for six or more medical conditions—an increase of 11% since 1987 (3).

Health Care Costs of Obesity by Race, Age, and Gender

Wee et al examined the interaction of weight with race and age in determining health care expenditures (6). Although there was a clear age effect of overweight and obesity on costs for whites, none was apparent for blacks or Hispanics. Among whites, no effect of weight on health care costs was found in the 18- to 35-year age group, but obesity had a significant effect in the age groups older than 35 and overweight had a significant effect in people older than age 55. This pattern presumably reflects the time required for chronic diseases associated with overweight and obesity to make their appearance in the white population.

Among an older population, Andreyeva et al found significant differences by gender within specific BMI categories. However, the differences were not consistent in direction and overall do not provide strong evidence for gender-associated differences in the costs of obesity (4).

Health Care Costs of Obesity Compared With Other Lifestyle Issues

The cost of obesity is greater than that of many other prominent health risks. In a study using data from the Health Care for Communities, a national household telephone survey of adults between 18 and 65 years, Strum found that obesity increased health care costs by $395/year, compared with $230/year for current or former smoking, $150/year for problem drinking, and $255/year for 20 years' aging (7). Obesity raised expenditure on medical services by 36% and on medications by 77%.

Health Care Costs of Overweight and Obesity by Type of Insurance

The costs of obesity vary by type of insurance. In 1998, the percentage of total medical expenditures due to overweight varied between 2.2% for Medicaid participants to 4.6%

for Medicare participants; the costs for obesity ranged from 3.9% for out-of-pocket payers to 6.7% for Medicaid participants (2). For private health insurers, overweight accounted for 3.4% and obesity accounted for 4.7%; together they equaled 8.2% of private health insurer's total health care costs. Overweight and obesity accounted for almost 20% of Medicaid and Medicare's total health care expenditures. Out of all of the types of health insurance—private, out-of-pocket, and government-sponsored—Medicaid and Medicare combined pay the largest percentage (48%) of the cost of obesity (2).

Health Care Costs Within Managed Care

Studies among members of large managed care organizations, including two divisions of Kaiser Permanente (KP), have shown similar obesity-related increases in health care costs. Quesenberry et al found that, compared with nonobese members of KP of Northern California, costs were 25% higher for members with BMI 30 to 34.9 and 44% higher for those with BMI equal to or greater than 35 (8). The authors observed significantly higher annual rates for inpatient days, number and cost of outpatient visits, and laboratory and outpatient pharmacy costs.

In KP of Colorado, Raebel et al similarly reported that obese patients had more hospitalizations ($P < .001$), prescription drug use ($P < .001$), and outpatient visits ($P < .001$) compared with matched nonobese patients. After controlling for age, gender and chronic diseases, individuals with BMI equal to or greater than 27.9 had median costs that were $250 per person/year more than nonobese individuals (9). Independent of the cost of associated disease (eg, diabetes); every 1% increase in BMI was associated with a 2.3% increase in health care costs among KP members.

Initial weight is not the only factor that matters. Elmer et al found that among a group of managed care patients who were initially mildly obese (mean BMI 31.5), those who gained at least 20 pounds over a 3-year period had health care costs $561 greater than those who did not gain weight (10).

COSTS TO US BUSINESS

Indirect costs represent the value of lost output due to cessation or reduction of productivity caused by morbidity and mortality. Morbidity costs are wages lost by people who are unable to work because of illness and disability. Because of escalating health care costs in the United States, employers are making efforts to identify and contain the both direct and indirect costs associated with chronic health conditions. Thompson et al estimated the cost of overweight and obesity to US business in 1994 was $12.7 billion, 80% of which was due to moderate to severe obesity (BMI ≥ 29) (11). The greatest component of this expenditure was health insurance, representing $7.7 billion. Paid sick leave, life insurance, and disability insurance amounted to $2.4 billion, $1.8 billion, and $800 million, respectively. This may be an underestimate, however, because only eight diseases were included in the analysis.

Among 175,000 General Motors' employees in 1996–1997, mean annual charges were 7% higher among the overweight employees and 46% higher among obese employees compared with the healthy-weight group (12). There was a monotonic increase in medical charges with increasing BMI within this worksite population. Results were consistent across gender and age groups, except for men 75 years and older.

Burton et al evaluated the direct and indirect costs of overweight/obesity to First Chicago National Bank (FCNB, now Chase) (13). "High risk" was defined as a BMI equal to or greater than 27.3 for women and equal to or greater than 27.8 for men. A high-risk BMI increased mean health care costs by 52% over a 3-year period—$6,822 compared with $4,496 for employees with weights less than the aforementioned cut-points. The increase was more striking in women ($3,817) than in men ($440), with the greatest difference in employees older than age 45. Employees with a BMI greater than 30 represented 18.7% of this population but had 28.9% of the total health care costs and 26.3% of the total number of health care claims.

Lost Productivity

In addition to the direct medical costs paid by insurers and patients, overweight and obesity affect productivity, with resulting costs being borne by employers and society in general. Within FCNB, overweight and obese employees had twice as many sick days (mean 8.45 days/year) as employees with a lower body weights (mean 3.73 days/year). The employer's excess employee sick-leave cost for each moderately overweight/obese employee was $863 over a 3-year period; this increased to $1,379 among older (> 45 years) overweight employees (13).

Similarly, Narbro et al found that obese Swedish women had rates of sick leave 50% to 90% higher than their normal-weight counterparts (14). Among the obese women, 12% were drawing disability pensions, more than twice the frequency for normal-weight women. Trends for increased disability among the obese population in the United States have also been reported (11).

Tucker and Friedman reported that among 10,825 employed adults, obese individuals were more than twice as likely as lean employees to experience high absenteeism (≥ 7 days per 6 months) and 1.5 times as likely to have moderate absenteeism (3 to 6 absences) (15). Shell Oil Company found similar results (16). Finkelstein recently aggregated all of the direct and indirect costs of overweight and obesity to the employer and reported that the additional costs due to weight ranged from $175 (overweight) to $2,027 (class III obesity) in men and $588 (overweight) to $2,164 (class III obesity) in women (17).

Disability

Obesity also imposes limitations while at work. Data from the 2002 National Health Interview Survey (NHIS) show that 6.9% of obese workers have work limitations, compared with 3.0% of healthy-weight workers (18).

Worksite injuries are also significantly higher among overweight employees. Among Shell Oil employees, low back injuries were 1.42 times higher and nonback musculoskeletal injuries were 1.53 times higher among overweight/obese employees compared with healthy-weight employees (19).

Additionally, acute back pain may be more likely to develop into chronic back pain among the overweight and obese. Fransen et al followed employees who filed a claim for

for a nutrition class to prevent or delay comorbidities that includes topics such as low-fat cooking and restaurant dining tips.

The education and training codes were added to the CPT code system in 2006, and the extent to which payers are accepting and paying for services billed under them is not yet known. CMS has indicated the education and training CPT codes are not covered for Medicare services. Depending on payer policies, non-Medicare payers may allow RDs to use the codes for classes that may be used in conjunction with a weight management program or for prevention of obesity. RDs should check payer policies and/or fee schedules to determine whether the education and training codes may be used for preventive type nutrition services.

Resources and Information for RDs Regarding Reimbursement

Recognizing RDs' interest in codes, coverage, and reimbursement for nutrition services, ADA has developed resources to help advance RDs' business practice skills, improve members' compliance with payer regulations, and provide tools for expanding local coverage for nutrition services. Unless otherwise noted, the following resources are posted in the MNT section of ADA's Web site (http://www.eatright.org/mnt):

- **Evidence-based Nutrition Practice Guidelines/Nutrition Care Process.** ADA provides members with practice tools and resources to provide quality, safe and effective MNT services for a variety of conditions and diseases, including weight management. RDs can use ADA Evidence-Based Nutrition Practice Guidelines to apply cutting-edge, synthetic research to practice. Among other conditions, nutrition practice guidelines are available for adult and pediatric weight management. For additional information, access ADA's Evidence Analysis Library (http://www.ada evidencelibrary.com).
- **Third-party payer brochure.** A brochure RDs can use with local insurance payers to advocate for increased coverage of RD-provided nutrition services.
- **MNT Works Kit.** A marketing tool designed for payers, medical directors, and health care decision makers to increase MNT coverage and consumer access to MNT services provided by RDs.
- *ADA Guide to Private Practice: An Introduction to Starting Your Own Business.* A guide for private practice that also includes information on payment and reimbursement considerations for RD services (51). Available for sale in ADA's publications catalog (http://www.eatright.org/catalog).
- **ADA Reimbursement Community of Interest (COI) .** The reimbursement COI listserv is available to ADA members who desire to learn more about coverage for MNT and exchange best practices to help advance coverage of nutrition services with health plans, employers, and third-party payers.
- **ADA state dietetic association and dietetic practice group (DPG) reimbursement representatives.** These representatives are available to assist with local coverage and coding issues. Representatives are listed in ADA's leadership directory in the Policy Initiatives & Advocacy Committees/Task Forces section (http://www. eatright.org/leaderdirectory).

- **The Weight Management DPG.** This DPG (http://www.wmdpg.org) and others have resources to aid members. Members of the Weight Management DPG can post questions related to reimbursement on the electronic mailing list.
- **Nutrition Entrepreneurs DPG.** Members of this DPG (http://www.nedpg.org) can use its mentoring service, in which a seasoned practitioner provides advice to RDs new to the private practice arena.
- **ADA staff from the Nutrition Services Coverage Team.** Provides another resource for code, coverage, and compliance information. Contact ADA staff at *reimburse@ eatright.org.*

SUMMARY

The costs of overweight and obesity in the United States are well documented. Obesity greatly increases direct medical costs and decreases worker productivity. The cost-effectiveness and return on investment of obesity treatment is in the initial stages of evaluation. Finally, reimbursement for MNT for obesity is occurring but varies by health insurance companies and state regulations. It is up to the registered dietitian to contact the health insurance company to obtain its policy regarding coverage of MNT for obesity. The American Dietetic Association provides many tools and resources to help registered dietitians expand coverage and obtain reimbursement for their services.

References

1. Thorpe KE, Florence CS, Howard DH, Joski P. The rising prevalence of treated disease: effects on private health insurance spending. *Health Affairs.* 2005;25:317–325.
2. Finkelstein EA, Fiebelkorn IC, Wang G. National medical spending attributable to overweight and obesity: how much and who's paying? *Health Affairs.* 2003;23:219–226.
3. Thorpe KE, Florence CS, Howard DH, Joski P. The impact of obesity on rising medical spending. *Health Affairs.* 2004;24:480–486.
4. Andreyeva T, Sturm R, Ringel JS. Moderate and severe obesity have large differences in health care costs. *Obes Res.* 2004;12:1936–1943.
5. Arterburn DE, Maciejewski ML, Tsevat J. Impact of morbid obesity on medical expenditures in adults. *Int J Obes.* 2005;29:334–339.
6. Wee CC, Phillips RS, Legedza ATR, Davis RB, Soukup JR, Colditz GA, Hamel MB. Health care expenditures associated with overweight and obesity among US adults: importance of age and race. *Am J Public Health.* 2005;95:159–165.
7. Strum R. The effects of obesity, smoking, and drinking on medical problems and costs. *Health Affairs.* 2002;21:245–253.
8. Quesenberry CP Jr, Caan B, Jacobson. A. Obesity, health services use, and health care costs among members of a health maintenance organization. *Arch Intern Med.* 1998;158:466–472.
9. Raebel MA, Malone DC, Conner DA, Xu S, Potter JA, Lanty FA. Health services use and health care costs of obese and nonobese individuals. *Arch Intern Med.* 2004:164:2135–2140.

10. Elmer PJ, Brown JB, Nichols GA, Oster G. Effects of weight gain on medical care costs. *Int J Obes Relat Metab Disord*. 2004:28;1365–1373.

11. Thompson D, Edelsberg J, Kinsey KL, Oster G. Estimated economic costs of obesity to U.S. business. *Am J Health Promot*. 1998;13:120–127.

12. Wang F, Schultz AB, Musich S, McDonald T, Hirschland D, Edington DW. The relationship between National Heart, Lung, and Blood Institute weight guidelines and concurrent medical costs in a manufacturing corporation. *Am J Health Promot*. 2003;17:183–189.

13. Burton WN, Chen CY, Schultz AB, Edington DW. The economic costs associated with body mass index in a workplace. *J Occup Environ Med*. 1998;40:786–792.

14. Narbro K, Jonsson E, Larsson B, Waaler H. Wedel H, Sjostrom L. Economic consequences of sick-leave and early retirement in obese Swedish women. *Int J Obes Relat Metab Disord*. 1996;20:895–903.

15. Tucker LA, Friedman GM. Obesity and absenteeism: an epidemiologic study of 10,825 employed adults. *Am J Health Promot*. 1998;12:202–207.

16. Tsai SP, Gilstrap EL, Colangelo TA, Menard AK, Ross CE. Illness absence at an oil refinery and petrochemical plant. *J Occup Environ Med*. 1997;39:455–462.

17. Finkelstein, EA Fiebelkorn IC, Wang G. The costs of obesity among full-time employees. *Am J Health Promot*. 2005;20:45–51.

18. Hertz RP, Unger AN, McDonald M, Lustik MB, Biddulph-Krentar J. The impact of obesity on work limitations and cardiovascular risk factors in the U.S. workforce. *J Occup Environ Med*. 2004;46:1196–1203.

19. Tsai SP, Gilstrap EL, Cowles SR, Waddell LC, Ross CE. Personal and job characteristics of musculoskeletal injuries in an industrial population. *J Occup Med*. 1992;34:606–612.

20. Fransen M, Woodward M, Norton R, Coggan C, Dawe M, Sheridan N. Risk factors associated with the transition from acute to chronic occupational back pain. *Spine*. 2002;27:92–98.

21. Pavlovich WD, Waters H, Weller W, Bass EB. Systematic review of literature on the cost-effectiveness of nutrition services. *J Am Diet Assoc*. 2004;104:226–232.

22. Pritchard DA, Hyndman J, Taba F. Nutritional counseling in general practice: a cost-effective analysis. *J Epidemiol Community Health*. 1999;53:311–316.

23. Brownell KD, Stunkard AJ, McKeon PE. Weight reduction at the work site: a promise partially fulfilled. *Am J Psychiatry*. 1985;142:47–52

24. Myers AW, Graves TJ, Whelan JP, Barclay DR. An evaluation of a television-delivered behavioral weight loss program: are the ratings acceptable? *J Consult Clin Psychol*. 1996;64:172–178.

25. Nichols G, Brown J, Stevens V, Crawford J. Medical care costs reductions resulting from intentional weight loss. *Obesity Res*. 2004;125:67.

26. American Dietetic Association. Evidence Analysis Library. MNT Cost-effectiveness. http://www.adaevidencelibrary.com/topic.cfm?cat=3675. Accessed March 9, 2009.

27. Pritchard DA, Hyndman J, Taba F. Nutritional counseling in general practice: a cost effective analysis. *J Epidemiol Community Health*. 1999;53:311–316.

28. Wolf AM, Conaway MR, Crowther JQ, Hazen KY, Nadler JL, Oneida B, Bovbjerg VE. Translating lifestyle intervention to practice in obese patients with type 2 diabetes: improving control with activity and nutrition (ICAN). *Diabetes Care*. 2004;27:1570–1576.

29. Wolf AM, Siadaty M, Yaeger B, Crowther JQ, Conaway M, Nadler J, Bovberg VE. Effects of lifestyle intervention on health care costs: improving control with activity and nutrition (ICAN). *J Am Diet Assoc*. 2007;107;1365–1373.

30. Wolf AM, Siadity M, Crowther JQ, Nadler JL, Wagner DL, Cavalieri S, Elward K, Bovbjerg VE. Impact of lifestyle intervention on lost productivity and disability: improving control with activity and nutrition (ICAN). *J Occup Environ Med*. 2009;51:139–145.

31. Wolf AM, Crowther JQ, Nadler JL, Bovbjerg VE. The return on investment of a lifestyle intervention: the ICAN program. Accepted for presentation at the American Diabetes Association 69th Scientific Sessions (169-OR), 7 June, 2009, New Orleans, Louisiana.

32. Herman WH, Brandle M, Zhang P, Williamson DF, Matulik MJ, Ratner RE, Lachin JM, Engelgau MM. The Diabetes Prevention Program Research Group. Costs associated with the primary prevention of type 2 diabetes mellitus in the Diabetes Prevention Program. *Diabetes Care*. 2003;26:36–47.

33. Palmer AJ, Roze S, Valentine WJ, Spinas GA, Shaw JE, Zimmet PZ. Intensive lifestyle changes or metformin in patients with impaired glucose tolerance: modeling the long-term health economic implications of the diabetes prevention program in Australia, France, Germany, Switzerland, and the United Kingdom. *Clin Ther*. 2004;26:304–321.

34. Caro JJ, Getsios D, Caro I, Klittich WS, O'Brien JA. Economic evaluation of therapeutic interventions to prevent type 2 diabetes in Canada. *Diabet Med*. 2004;21:1229–1236.

35. Josse RG, McGuire AJ, Saal GB. A review of the economic evidence for acarbose in the prevention of diabetes and cardiovascular events in individuals with impaired glucose tolerance. *Int J Clin Pract*. 2006;60:847–855.

36. Eddy DM, Schlessinger L, Kahn R. Clinical outcomes and cost-effectiveness of strategies for managing people at high risk for diabetes. *Ann Intern Med*. 2005;143:251–264.

37. White JV, Ayoob KT, Benedict MA, Chynoweth MD, Gregoire M, Howard RL, McCool A, Parrott S, Ramsey SH, Thiessen C, Thomsen KN, Bender T, Myers E, Michael P. Registered dietitians' coding practices and patterns of code use. *J Am Diet Assoc*. 2008;108:1242–1428.

38. Fitzner K, Myers EF, Caputo N, Michael P. Are health plans changing their views on nutrition service coverage? *J Am Diet Assoc*. 2003;103:157–161.

39. Baranoski CL, King SL. Insurance companies are reimbursing for MNT. *J Am Diet Assoc*. 2000;100:1530–1535.

40. Medicare Carrier's Manual. http://216.239.39.104/search?q=cache:RVlNKf60tQkJ:www.cms.hhs.gov/manuals/pm_trans/R1793B3.pdf+Medicare+Manual+Incident+to+services&hl=en&ie=UTF-8. Accessed December 8, 2008.

41. Tsai A, Asch DA, Waddent TA. Insurance coverage for obesity treatment. *J Am Diet Assoc*. 2006;106:1651–1655.

42. Kaplan LM, Fallon JA, Mun EC, Harvey AM, Kastrinakis WV, Johnson EQ, Nierman RS, Keroack CR. Coding and reimbursement for weight loss surgery: best practice recommendations. *Obes Res*. 2005;12:290–300.

43. Medicare Coverage Determination Process. http://www.cms.hhs.gov/DeterminationProcess. Accessed December 8, 2008.

44. US Government Accountability Office (GAO) Report to Congressional Requesters: Managing Diabetes—Health Plan Coverage of Services and Supplies. http://www.gao.gov/new.items/d05210.pdf. Accessed December 19, 2007.

45. Stern J, Kazaks A, Downey M. Future and implications of reimbursement for obesity treatment. *J Am Diet Assoc.* 2005;105(suppl):S104–S109.

46. Israel D, McCabe M. Using disease-state management as the key to promoting employer sponsorship of medical nutrition therapy. *J Am Diet Assoc.* 1999;99:583–588.

47. Centers for Medicaid & Medicare Services Glossary. http://www.cms.hhs.gov/apps/glossary/default.asp?Letter=I&Language=English#Content. Accessed December 8, 2008.

48. American Medical Association. *International Classification of Diseases; ICD-9-CM 2009; Physician; Volumes 1 and 2; 9th Revision—Clinical Modification.* Chicago, IL: American Medical Association Press; 2008.

49. American Medical Association. *CPT 2009 Professional Edition.* Chicago, IL: American Medical Association Press; 2008.

50. Centers for Medicaid & Medicare Services. 2009 Alpha-Numeric HCPCS File. http://www.cms.hhs.gov/HCPCSReleaseCodeSets/ANHCPCS/list.asp. Accessed December 5, 2008.

51. Litt AS, Berger Mitchell F. *American Dietetic Association Guide to Private Practice: An Introduction to Starting Your Own Business.* Chicago, IL: American Dietetic Association; 2004.

Client-related Issues

As already noted, although culturally influenced attitudes and practices about food, eating, and weight are important considerations in obesity management, it is misleading to focus only on these variables when evaluating the scope and nature of needed interventions. Many other distinctive characteristics of ethnic minority groups can affect energy intake and expenditure. Socioeconomic variables differ by ethnicity; most ethnic populations have lower incomes, more poverty, and less education than whites (41).

Socioeconomic variables directly affect food intake and physical activity and also modify the expression of cultural influences. For example, differences in body image between black and white women may be more prominent in higher-income brackets than in lower-income ones (23). Other demographic variables that vary among and within ethnic groups and potentially influence obesity management include the following: whether US- or foreign-born, family size and household arrangements (eg, intergenerational or female-headed households), types of occupations, personal assets, health insurance coverage, and interactions with the health care system (41–44).

To understand cultural influences, one must take into account factors related to age and gender (eg, cultural differences between teens and their parents and grandparents), which may be shaped by American culture generally as well as within particular ethnic groups. Age-related differences may be especially prominent in families in which parents are immigrants and children are US-born or immigrate at a young age. In these instances, the children may be heavily exposed throughout development to cultural influences distinct from and perhaps contradictory to those of their ethnic group.

Ethnic minorities should *not* be considered as homogeneous populations. For example, people classified as Hispanics may have origins in Central or South America, Mexico, Puerto Rico, Cuba, or Spain and may have resided in the United States for several generations or recently immigrated. People who came to the United States as migrant workers have vastly different experiences and options than people who immigrated under different economic or employment circumstances. Cultural diversity within an ethnic group may include country or region of origin, language or dialect, generation and age of migration, and socio-political history within the United States, as well as the degree to which ethnic social and cultural traditions have been disrupted. Health care providers should consider whether certain traditions have been reinforced or discouraged, or whether they have been altered through blending with processes in the society at large and with what result. Clinicians should also understand whether a client's ethnic traditions are relatively compatible with, or contradictory to, the dominant US culture and whether the client is part of an immigrant group that is undergoing very rapid social and economic transitions. In addition, some variables associated with minority status do not relate to ethnic traditions as such but may relate to how cultural norms, beliefs, and values of minority populations interact with their socio-political and economic circumstances (26,36,37).

Provider-related Issues

The professionals and institutions that offer obesity management services also introduce cultural influences into the social exchanges in treatment or programmatic settings. A cultural competence framework focuses on what the health care provider brings to the treatment relationship, rather than viewing cultural issues only as potential issues posed by the client. Moreover, because obesity carries a negative stigma in our society, all professionals who work with obese clients have the additional challenge of managing their own culturally influenced attitudes about obesity and obese people (45). The cultural backgrounds and personal experiences of clinicians shape the knowledge, skills, and expectations they bring to treatment interactions. The professional's socioeconomic status, political opinions, values, moral codes, and worldviews are also relevant.

Limited cross-cultural experience or lack of a cosmopolitan attitude may generally circumscribe one's ability to work effectively in multicultural settings. The health care provider's ability to provide services to clients or client groups of a particular ethnic background will be affected if he or she lacks experience with or is biased toward members of that ethnic group. Professional training alone will not eliminate such characteristics in the clinician.

Professional and organizational cultures also have a significant impact on the treatment interaction. Professional cultures define codes of conduct, expectations about both peers and clients, and systems of rewards and sanctions that foster public confidence and trust in the profession (46,47). However, current professional training and standards may not keep pace with recent mandates for cultural competence, and some professional conventions may pose barriers to the motivation and ability of clinicians to provide services in a culturally competent manner. For example, professionals are often trained to keep a certain emotional distance in the treatment encounter; however, in a cross-cultural interaction, expression of emotion may be necessary for establishing trust and rapport (48).

In treatment settings, several forces that tend to be incompatible may be at work. The challenge for clinicians is to find solutions that bridge these forces and create "win-win" scenarios. For example, registered dietitians (RDs) have been trained to use expert knowledge that is based on scientific understanding of specific nutrients and dietary constituents. However, the dominance of the nutrient-based approach may limit the RD's desire or ability to tailor expert knowledge sufficiently to fit with the client's way of thinking about food and eating. Professional styles or jargon may exclude or create discomfort for people outside a profession, including one's clients (49), but these conventions are not easy to change. RDs may feel discouraged or less enthusiastic about working with certain clients if they need to use different language and personal styles to reach these clients effectively.

When contextual issues cannot be addressed through clinical or interpersonal interventions, this can potentially pose considerable challenges. The treatment and adherence models common to clinical treatment settings are much less appropriate for lifestyle change than they are for pharmacologic interventions (50). As discussed previously, most of the factors that determine success of efforts to change the lifestyle behaviors are beyond the control of the clinician, and some are beyond the control of the client, too. From an organizational perspective, quality standards and financial considerations may limit the level of services that institutions offer to some clients and may also lead to concerns about taking on clients who are viewed as potential treatment "failures." This scenario could become self-perpetuating: clients who are not adequately served reinforce concerns about minority populations being hard-to-reach, leading to less effort to reach them.

Achieving Cultural Sensitivity with Individuals and Groups

In practical terms, culturally sensitive clinicians attempt to fit the service or program to the client or client group, rather than expecting that clients will benefit from services that were not designed with their needs in mind. As suggested above, cultural sensitivity requires clinicians who are both willing and able to incorporate the client's perspective. For the individual practitioner, critical domains of cultural competence include (*a*) becoming aware of one's own cultural values; (*b*) obtaining adequate knowledge of client views and perspectives and, particularly, of the social and economic contexts in which they live; and (*c*) developing skills for designing and delivering services in ways that are culturally appropriate (3). Subobjectives within these three domains are described in references 3 and 51. To achieve these objectives, the clinician must engage in various processes of personal reflection and skill-building to increase readiness to engage in cross-cultural interactions (2,48). Above all, you must learn how to value and be comfortable with differences and to find common ground with people from other cultures. It is useful to have a sense of how people from other cultures might view you or people from your cultural background, and to be attuned to potential cross-cultural issues or learning (2,48). Such awareness should include considerations of status and power gradients that influence counseling interactions (eg, clients viewing professionals as authority figures). It is also critical to develop strong cross-cultural communication skills—both verbal and nonverbal (2,3,48).

Cultural competency is also a concern for clinicians who are from the same ethnic group as the client population or another ethnic minority population. Experiences and views vary within ethnic groups, particularly when there are differences in region of residence or country of origin or in social privilege. Also, differences in income levels and social positions between professionals and clients may present challenges for mutual understanding even when the clinician and client are from the same ethnic background.

Techniques used to adapt programmatic approaches for greater cultural sensitivity may be referred to as *cultural tailoring* or *cultural targeting*. Kreuter et al (52) provide a useful differentiation of these two terms. They use *tailoring* to refer to the adaptation of programs or services at the level of the individual, based on data obtained from individual assessments. *Targeting* refers to services designed for a particular group and based on group characteristics—eg, a weight-loss program designed for African Americans or Latinos based on general cultural knowledge about the group as well as information from focus groups (33,34,39,40,53–59). Targeting implicitly assumes within-group homogeneity whereas tailoring takes into account the person-to-person variation within the group. Tailoring and targeting strategies can be combined (eg, a group program includes opportunities for individualized counseling and feedback). Examples of individual tailoring in culturally targeted programs include the use of a multidisciplinary case management approach in primary care weight-loss counseling of African-American women (58) and an Internet-based program with African-American girls (59) in which individualized information could be captured electronically and used to generate personal feedback.

Approaches to cultural adaptation of group programs—reflected in many studies cited in this chapter—may focus on settings (using convenient and familiar community-based locations), providers (employing providers from the same ethnic group as the clients or employing peer counselors or lay health workers), program content (using bilingual program materials, foods, music, activities, illustrations, and risk-information specific to the particular group), or combinations of these approaches (60–62). Church- or faith-based programs that combine a setting-based approach with culturally relevant content (eg, including a spiritual component in the intervention) are a commonly used strategy for reaching African Americans (39,40). Most targeted programs address issues at the level of surface structure, as defined by Resnicow et al (1). Some attempt to reach "deep structure" (1) by incorporating core values or ethnic heritage through the integral involvement of constituents and by using cultural concepts in framing the program content and process. The previously cited programs with native Hawaiians (33) and American Indians (34) are examples.

IMPLICATIONS FOR RESEARCH AND PRACTICE

Culturally targeted and tailored programs may increase the appeal, salience, and sustainability of programs to clients for whom the program is designed (1,52). However, research to date has not clearly demonstrated the benefits of cultural adaptations for improving weight loss (60–62). Some culturally adapted programs have reported very modest weight losses, and only a few studies have compared programs with and without cultural adaptations (39,40,63). Research is greatly needed to indicate which types of approaches will not only achieve maximum client participation and satisfaction but also facilitate success in weight loss or weight maintenance.

Research is also needed to improve the success of ethnic minority participants in programs that are *not* targeted toward a particular ethnic group. Targeted programs are not always appropriate or possible, and they may not be desired by clients from ethnic minority populations. Clinical trials that included African Americans have reported smaller weight losses in African Americans compared with whites (64–67). Strategies to improve the cultural sensitivity of multi-ethnic studies might be able to close this gap.

Currently, the provision of services that are sensitive to the cultural perspectives and day-to-day social and economic contexts of ethnic minority populations can be justified on ethical and theoretical grounds; furthermore, current guidelines call for cultural competence in the delivery of health services generally (68). Key points to remember can be summarized as follows:

- Cultural differences are usually also associated with differences in social and economic circumstances. Cultural sensitivity, therefore, requires attention to a broader set of factors beyond culturally influenced attitudes and values. Needs assessment to directly elicit issues and perspectives of the client or client group is essential and should be an ongoing process from the initial client encounter onward.
- Although members of ethnic minority populations may differ on average from the white population, there is tremendous heterogeneity among and within these populations. One should be on guard against the tendency to stereotype. In addition, general knowledge about ethnic groups cannot substitute for individualized attention, which is also needed to achieve success in weight management.
- Professionals may require special training or retraining to become comfortable and skilled in providing culturally sensitive services. Culturally sensitive approaches require a certain level of cultural competence; they reframe the role of the professional

to be less authoritative and more supportive; and they involve more understanding of and possibly interaction within the social and economic contexts in which the client or client group operates on a day-to-day basis.

These three themes provide the practical underpinnings for achieving cultural sensitivity in obesity management.

References

1. Resnicow K, Baranowski T, Ahluwalia JS, Braithwaite RL. Cultural sensitivity in public health. Defined and demystified. *Ethn Dis*. 1999;9:10–12.

2. Kumanyika SK, Morssink CB. Working effectively in cross-cultural and multicultural settings. In: J Owen AL, Splett PL, Owen GM, eds. *Nutrition in the Community: The Art and Science of Delivering Services*. 4th ed. New York, NY: McGraw Hill; 1998:542–567.

3. Harris-Davis E, Haughton B. Model for multicultural nutrition counseling competencies. *J Am Diet Assoc*. 2000;100:1178–1185.

4. Grieco EM, Cassidy RC. Overview of Race and Hispanic Origin: 2000. US Census Bureau. Census 2000 Brief. C2KBR/01–1. http://www.census.gov/prod/2001pubs/cenbr01-1.pdf. Accessed January 29, 2006.

5. Last J. *A Dictionary of Epidemiology*. 4th ed. New York, NY: Oxford University Press; 2001.

6. Ogden CL, Carroll MD, Curtin LR, McDowell MA, Tabak CJ, Flegal KM. Prevalence of overweight and obesity in the United States, 1999–2004. *JAMA*. 2006;295:1549–1555.

7. Adams PF, Schoenborn CA. Health behaviors of adults: United States, 2002–04. National Center for Health Statistics. *Vital Health Stat*. 2006;10(230):1–140.

8. Wang Y, Beydoun MA. The obesity epidemic in the United States—gender, age, socioeconomic, racial/ethnic, and geographic characteristics: a systematic review and meta-regression analysis. *Epidemiol Rev*. 2007;29:6–28.

9. Kumanyika S. Ethnicity and obesity development in children. *Ann NY Acad Sci*. 1993;699:81–92.

10. Kumanyika S. Obesity in minority populations: an epidemiologic assessment. *Obes Res*. 1994;2:166–182.

11. WHO Expert Consultation. Appropriate body-mass index for Asian populations and its implications for policy and intervention strategies. *Lancet*. 2004;363:157–163.

12. Smith SC, Clark LT, Cooper RS, Daniels SR, Kumanyika SK, Ofili E, Quinones MA, Sanchez EJ, Saunders E, Tiukinhoy SD. Discovering the full spectrum of cardiovascular disease: Minority Health Summit 2003 Report of the Obesity, Metabolic Syndrome, and Hypertension Writing Group. *Circulation*. 2005;15:111:e134–e139.

13. Thomas PR, ed. *Weighing the Options Criteria for Evaluating Weight-Management Programs*. Washington, DC: National Academy Press; 1995.

14. Bandura A. Social cognitive theory. An agentic perspective. *Annu Rev Psychol*. 2001;52:1–26.

15. Stokols D. Translating social ecologic theory into guidelines for community health. *Am J Health Promotion*. 1996;10:282–298.

CHAPTER 14

PREJUDICE AND DISCRIMINATION

REBECCA M. PUHL, PHD

WEIGHT BIAS IN HEALTH CARE SETTINGS

Obese individuals are vulnerable to bias, stigma, and discrimination in many domains of daily life (1). Negative attitudes or unfair treatment that an individual experiences as a result of being overweight or obese, commonly referred to as *weight bias,* exist in employment settings, educational institutions, the mass media, and even close interpersonal relationships with family members and friends (2,3).

Weight bias is also common in health care settings, where overweight and obese clients are prone to stigma, stereotypes, and prejudice from a range of health care providers including physicians, medical students, registered dietitians (RDs), nurses, and psychologists; even health professionals who specialize in obesity can be prone to bias (3,4–8). Common stereotypes reported by health care providers include perceptions that obese clients are lazy, noncompliant, undisciplined, unsuccessful, unintelligent, and dishonest (2).

Weight bias can take multiple forms, including inappropriate verbal comments (eg, derogatory remarks, negative stereotypes, insults, or jokes) or nonverbal behaviors (eg, inappropriate gestures, facial expressions) by clinicians. It can also include inadequate medical equipment to accommodate obese clients (eg, lack of appropriately sized patient gowns, blood pressure cuffs, or scales) and denial of medical procedures or diagnostic assessments for obese clients without reasonable justification.

Beliefs about the causes of obesity may play an important role in the formation and expression of weight bias. A number of studies demonstrate that perceptions of personal responsibility for obesity may negatively affect behavioral and societal responses to obese persons (9–12). Specifically, the greater the individual responsibility assigned to obesity, the worse the affective reaction is to an obese person, and the lower the stated intentions are to help that person (13,14). Obese individuals are also more likely to be blamed, negatively stereotyped, and perceived as undisciplined and self-indulgent when there is no external cause (eg, a thyroid condition) to account for their weight, but they receive less blame and more favorable attitudes when their obesity can be attributed to a physical cause outside of their personal control (11,12). Experimental research shows that providing individuals with information that emphasizes personal responsibility for obesity worsens negative stereotypes and stigma toward obese persons, whereas information that highlights the complex etiology of obesity, including biological and genetic contributors to weight, improves negative attitudes and reduces weight-based stereotypes (15). Among health care professionals, studies show that clinicians assume obesity can be prevented by self-control, that a client's inability to lose weight is due to treatment noncompliance, and that obesity is caused by emotional problems (16,17). These beliefs are suggestive of attributions of personal responsibility for obesity, which may reinforce biased attitudes.

RDs are not immune to negative attitudes about obese individuals. In a recent study that interviewed more than 2,000 overweight and obese women about the sources of weight bias in their lives, 37% reported being stigmatized by an RD (3). This is of particularly concern because RDs are now working with overweight and obese populations more than ever before. Although research in this area is still in its infancy, several studies have examined weight bias among individuals in the field of dietetics. One study examined attitudes among RDs (n = 234) and dietetics students (n = 64). Both samples reported negative attitudes toward obesity, and those who rated themselves as a "healthful weight" or "underweight" expressed more negative attitudes toward obesity than those who rated themselves as "overweight" (18).

Another study surveyed 439 RDs about their attitudes toward overweight clients and found that RDs believed that overweight clients could not set realistic goals for weight loss and that their excess weight was due to emotional problems (19). Interestingly, RDs who perceived themselves as overweight endorsed negative attitudes, such as blaming themselves for their weight. This parallels other research showing that some overweight individuals may internalize negative stereotypes toward themselves and in turn express anti-fat attitudes (20).

Harvey and associates examined anti-fat attitudes and weight management practices among 187 British dietitians (21). Overall, the participants reported generally positive attitudes toward overweight and obese people, but they endorsed worse attitudes toward obese compared to overweight people and reported that obese individuals were more responsible that those who are overweight for their excess weight. The belief that obesity is caused by a "lack of willpower" was associated with a range of management practices reported by the dietitians.

Most recently, in a study comparing attitudes toward obesity among dietetics and nondietetics students (n = 76), both groups expressed equally negative attitudes toward obese people, including beliefs that obese people have poor self-control (71%), are insecure (73%), are lazy (51%), lack willpower (51%), and are self-indulgent (42%). The authors concluded that a dietetics education may neither promote nor reduce weight bias among students (22).

These few studies reflect mixed findings, and more work is needed to determine the nature of weight bias among RDs and how it affects their treatment practices. However, the existing findings raise concerns, and it seems warranted to include RDs in stigma-reduction interventions to increase sensitivity toward overweight and obese clients, especially because the number of obese clients in treatment with RDs is increasing.

CONSEQUENCES OF WEIGHT BIAS FOR OBESE CLIENTS

Weight bias has a range of negative consequences for the emotional and physical health of obese individuals.

27. Thompson JK, Coovert MD, Richards KJ, Johnson S, Cattarin J. Development of body image, eating disturbance, and general psychological functioning in female adolescents: covariance structure modeling and longitudinal investigations. *Int J Eat Disord*. 1995;18:221–236.

28. Eisenberg ME, Neumark-Sztainer D, Story M. Associations of weight-based teasing and emotional well-being among adolescents. *Arch Pediatr Adolesc Med*. 2003;157:733–738.

29. Ackard DM, Neumark-Sztainer D, Story M, Perry C. Overeating among adolescents: prevalence and associations with weight-related characteristics and psychological health. *Pediatrics*. 2003;111:67–74.

30. Eaton DK, Lowry R, Brener ND, Galuska DA, Crosby AE. Associations of body mass index and perceived weight with suicide ideation and suicide attempts among US high school students. *Arch Pediatr Adolesc Med*. 200;159:513–519.

31. Falkner NH, Neumark-Sztainer D, Story M, Jeffery RW, Beuhring T, Resnick MD. Social, educational, and psychological correlates of weight status in adolescents. *Obes Res*. 2001;9:32–42.

32. Carpenter KM, Hasin DS, Allison DB, Faith MS. Relationships between obesity and DSM-IV major depressive disorder, suicide ideation, and suicide attempts: results from a general population study. *Am J Public Health*. 2000;90:251–257.

33. Neumark-Sztainer D, Falkner N, Story M, Perry C, Hannan PJ, Mulert S. Weight-teasing among adolescents: correlations with weight status and disordered eating behaviors. *Int J Obes*. 2002;26:123–131.

34. Haines J, Neumark-Sztainer D, Eisenberg ME, Hannan PJ. Weight teasing and disordered eating behaviors in adolescents: longitudinal findings from Project EAT (Eating Among Teens). *Pediatrics*. 2006;117:209–215.

35. Garner DM, Olmstead MP, Bohr Y, Garfinkel PE. The Eating Attitudes Test: psychometric features and clinical correlates. *Psychol Med*. 1982;12:871–878.

36. Fairburn CG, Doll HA, Welch SL, Hay PJ, Davies BA, O'Connor ME. Risk factors for binge eating disorder: a community-based, case-control study. *Arch Gen Psychiatry*. 1998;55:425–432.

37. Fairburn CG, Welch SL, Doll HA, Davies BA, O'Connor ME. Risk factors for bulimia nervosa: a community-based, case-control study. *Arch Gen Psychiatry*. 1997;54:509–517.

38. Jackson TD, Grilo CM, Masheb RM. Teasing history, onset of obesity, current eating disorder psychopathology, body dissatisfaction, and psychological functioning in binge eating disorder. *Obes Res*. 2002;8:451–458.

39. Striegel-Moore RH, Dohm F-A, Pike KM, Wilfley DE, Fairburn CG. Abuse, bullying, and discrimination as risk factors for binge eating disorder. *Am J Psychiatry*. 2002;159:1902–1907.

40. Storch EA, Milsom VA, DeBraganza N, Lewin AB, Geffken GR, Silverstein JH. Peer victimization, psychosocial adjustment, and physical activity in overweight and at-risk-for-overweight youth. *J Pediatric Psychol*. 2007;32:80–89. Epub April 6, 2006.

41. Faith MS, Leone MA, Ayers TS, Moonseong H, Pietrobelli A. Weight criticism during physical activity, coping skills, and reported physical activity in children. *Pediatrics*. 2007;110:e23.

42. Vartanian LR., Shaprow JG. Effects of weight stigma on motivation to exercise and exercise behavior: a preliminary investigation among college-aged females. *J Health Psychol.* 2008;13:131–138.

43. Amy NK, Aalbord A, Lyons P, Keranen L. Barriers to routine gynecological cancer screening for white and African-American obese women. *Int J Obes Relat Metab Disord.* 2006;30;147–155.

44. Puhl R. Preventing Weight Bias: Helping Without Harming in Clinical Practice. Module 1: Increasing Self-Awareness of Weight Bias. http://www.yaleruddcenter. org/what/bias/toolkit. Accessed November 20, 2008.

45. Wadden TA, Didie E. What's in a name? Patients' preferred terms for describing obesity. *Obes Res.* 2003;11:1140–1146.

46. Puhl R. Preventing Weight Bias: Helping Without Harming in Clinical Practice. Module 4: Office Environment Strategies to Reduce Weight Bias. http://www. yaleruddcenter.org/what/bias/toolkit. Accessed November 20, 2008.

47. Ahmed SM, Lemkau JP, Birt SL. Toward sensitive treatment of obese patients. *Fam Pract Manage.* 2002;9:25–28.

48. Kushner RF. Roadmaps for Clinical Practice: Case Studies in Disease Prevention and Health Promotion—Assessment and Management of Adult Obesity: A Primer for Physicians. Booklet 9: Setting up the Office Environment. Chicago, IL: American Medical Association; 2003.

49. WIN: Weight-control Information Network. Medical Care for Obese Patients; NIDDK Weight Control Information Center. http://win.niddk.nih.gov/publications/ medical.htm. Accessed December 5, 2007.

50. Barr SI, Yarker KV, Levy-Milne R, Chapman GE. Canadian dietitians' views and practices regarding obesity and weight management. *J HumNutr Diet.* 2004;17: 503–512.

CHAPTER 15

SCHOOL-BASED PREVENTION OF CHILDHOOD OVERWEIGHT AND OBESITY

GARY D. FOSTER, PHD, EILEEN G. FORD, MS, RD, LEIGH ROSEN, MUEP,

SARA SOLOMON, MPH, RD, AND AMY VIRUS, RD

INTRODUCTION

Childhood obesity rates are increasing worldwide and have tripled over the past few decades. Recent National Health and Nutrition Surveys (NHANES) data (1) estimated that 17.1% of children aged 2 to 19 years were obese and 16.5% of children aged 2 to 19 were overweight. For the same age group, Mexican-American and non-Hispanic black children had higher rates of obesity, at 19% and 20% respectively (1). Among a recent sample of 6,358 predominantly African-American and Latino 8th graders in school settings, nearly half (49.3%) were at or above the 85th percentile for body mass index (BMI) for their age and sex, with 19.7% overweight and 29.6% obese (2). Effective prevention strategies are needed because of the serious health and social consequences of overweight and obesity in youths as well as the increased likelihood that obese children, especially obese older children, will become obese adults (3–5).

The Institute of Medicine (IOM) report defines overweight in children as a BMI equal to or greater than the 85th percentile for age and gender, and obesity as a BMI equal to or greater than the 95th percentile (6) whereas the Centers for Disease Control and Prevention (CDC) uses the terms "at risk of overweight" and "overweight" for these same BMI categories (7). In this chapter, we will use the IOM definitions of overweight and obesity (6).

RATIONALE FOR SCHOOLS AS SETTINGS FOR OBESITY PREVENTION

The school environment presents significant opportunities for obesity prevention. Over 90% of US children are enrolled in schools and spend a substantial amount of their time there (8). No other institution has as much contact with children (9). US children attend school for 13 years, (kindergarten through 12th grade) for at least 180 days spanning 10 months per year. Children who participate in the School Breakfast Program (SBP) and National School Lunch Program (NSLP) receive up to two-thirds of their daily calorie requirements from these meals (10). A study of Texas middle schools assessed the potential impact of school food policies that reduced sweetened beverages and high-fat, salty, and sweet food portions offered at snack bars (11). Policy changes could reduce a student's daily energy intake by 47 kcal, a modest decrease but one with the potential to affect long-term energy balance. Schools also provide a broad platform for obesity prevention, including classroom learning opportunities (eg, health and science classes), physical education programs, and health services such as nursing and a growing number of health and dental clinics (9).

Given the adverse effects of childhood obesity on academic performance and attendance, administrators may be open to school-based strategies (12–16). Using self-reported heights and weights to calculate BMI in 5,810 Icelandic 14- and 15-year-old students, Sigfusdottir et al (14) concluded that children with a higher BMI, poorer diet, and lower levels of self-reported physical activity did not perform as well academically (based on self-reported grades). Further, these variables explained up to 24% of the variance in academic performance when controlled for gender, parent education, family structure, and absenteeism. In addition, Geier et al (15) examined relative weight and student absenteeism from a cross-sectional sample of 1,069 4th to 6th grade students in Philadelphia. After adjusting for age, race/ethnicity, and gender, obese children were absent significantly more often than normal-weight students.

REVIEW OF INTERVENTION STUDIES

Schools are a viable and logical target for obesity prevention. It is less clear whether these programs have reliable effects on BMI (17). Several systematic reviews in the literature (17–21) have found either modest or no intervention effects on BMI-based outcomes. Some reviews have suggested that combined physical activity and nutrition interventions work better than isolated interventions, but the number of studies are small (17,18). Durant has suggested that the field consider novel approaches and the use of smaller efficacy studies before proceeding with large-scale implementation (22).

The following section describes the designs and findings of school-based research to prevent obesity. The purpose is not an exhaustive literature review, but rather a description of the most current and representative school-based trials showing various approaches, target populations, and findings. Overall, these data demonstrate that, although it is feasible to conduct interventions related to food service or physical activity in schools, few interventions, to date, have been effective in changing targeted weight outcomes such as BMI.

The Child and Adolescent Trial for Cardiovascular Health (CATCH) study (1991–1994) assessed a multi-component, 3-year coordinated school health promotion program in 96 randomized schools (56 intervention, 40 control) in four states and included more than 5,100 students. CATCH was designed to decrease fat and sodium in children's diets, increase physical activity, and prevent tobacco use. The food service intervention was designed to provide foods lower in total fat and saturated fat. The physical education (PE) intervention aimed to increase moderate to vigorous physical activity (MVPA) to at least 40% of class time. Although CATCH has been widely implemented and disseminated among thousands of schools nationwide (http://www.catchinfo.org), it did not affect weight outcomes in the original study (23,24).

Additional school-based obesity prevention programs have positively influenced various nutrition and activity outcomes but not BMI or other measures of adiposity (25–28). Three of the best-known trials include APPLES, Pathways, and New Moves. APPLES was a randomized, controlled study in five intervention and five comparison schools in Leeds, England. Participants were children 7 to 11 years of age (314 intervention, 322 control). The intervention tested whether school action plans delivered by trained teachers influenced dietary and physical activity behaviors and affected BMI. After 1 year, students in the intervention schools modestly increased vegetable consumption, but there were no significant differences in BMI compared with the control schools (25,26).

Pathways was a 3-year randomized, controlled trial in 41 schools and 1,704 Native American children (879 intervention, 825 control). Intervention students received a four-component intervention: classroom curriculum to promote healthful eating and physical activity behaviors; low-fat school menu changes; a 30-minute comprehensive physical education program delivered three times a week; and family take-home materials and events. After 3 years, there were no differences in body weight or body fatness between children in intervention and control schools, despite marked differences in self-reported measures of energy and fat intake (27).

Finally, New Moves was a 16-week school-based feasibility intervention among six schools (three intervention, three control) and 201 high school girls (89 intervention, 112 control). The intervention consisted of a girls-only alternative physical education program, delivered four times a week with bimonthly nutrition and social support sessions. While New Moves received strong satisfaction ratings by schools, participants, parents, and teachers, there were no differences in BMI between intervention and control schools (28).

One of the few studies to find positive effects on weight outcomes, James et al (29) conducted a cluster-design, randomized controlled trial in 15 intervention and 14 control classes from six elementary schools (each school had three to six classes, randomly assigned to intervention or control). The authors acknowledged possible contamination because classes and not schools were the unit of randomization. Participants were 7 to 11 years of age. The study compared the prevalence of children above the 91st percentile according to the 1990 British percentile growth charts. The intervention discouraged children from drinking carbonated beverages, using four 1-hour health education classes, taste tests, music competitions, and art presentations to reiterate the main theme. After 1 year, the number of children above the 91st percentile increased 7.5% in the control classes, and decreased 0.2% in the intervention classes (29). These effects, however, did not persist 2 years after the intervention ended (30).

El Paso CATCH (31) was an adapted version of the national CATCH program (23). The El Paso CATCH program directed materials toward a predominantly (93%) Hispanic population in four intervention and four control schools in El Paso, Texas. Participants were observed for 2 years, from 3rd to 5th grade. Unlike the national CATCH program, intervention schools demonstrated a lower incidence of children above the 85th percentile for BMI for age and sex compared with the control schools (31). The authors speculated that the success of El Paso CATCH could be due to the fact that intervention schools were allowed to implement each component of the intervention in a way that suited the school environment and included ethnic variations on curricula, and particular school- and district-based variations (31).

Another randomized trial (32) evaluated the effects of a school nutrition policy initiative among 1,349 4th through 6th graders in 10 elementary schools (five intervention, five no-treatment control) in Philadelphia. The intervention consisted of a school self-assessment, staff training, nutrition education, nutrition policy, and social marketing. After 2 years, the incidence rates of overweight (ie, crossing the 85th percentile threshold for BMI for age and sex) were 7.5% in the intervention group and 14.9% in the control schools. There was also a significant difference between intervention and control schools in the prevalence of overweight at 2 years (14.6% and 20.0%, respectively). The intervention was even more effective for African American students. (Details of this intervention are available at http://www.thefoodtrust.org.)

Shape Up Somerville (33) was a multifaceted, community-based, nonrandomized, control trial comparing 1,178 1st to 3rd graders in three low-income communities for 3 years. Somerville, MA, was the intervention community, and two sociodemographically matched cities served as no-treatment control communities. The intervention increased healthful eating and physical opportunities within the school, home, and community. Changes included increases in fruits, vegetables, and whole grains in school food service; 30-minute weekly health lessons; development of a school "wellness" policy; bi-monthly parent newsletters; parent nutrition forums; and community advisory councils, fitness fairs, and resource guides. After 1 year, there was a significantly greater decrease in BMI z-score in the intervention community compared with the control communities.

Kain et al (34) examined changes in BMI z-scores and obesity prevalence from a 2-year nutrition and physical activity intervention in five Chilean primary schools (three intervention, two control) with 1st to 8th grade students (1,700 intervention, 671 control). Intervention components included 4 to 10 hours of nutrition education, two parent education lessons, 90 minutes of weekly physical education, active recess, and a behavioral physical activity program. After 1 year, BMI z-scores decreased significantly from baseline to follow-up in the intervention schools and remained unchanged in the control schools for boys but not girls (34). After 2 years, despite the fact that some intervention components were discontinued or modified during the second year, intervention schools had greater reductions for both boys and girls in obesity prevalence and BMI z-scores compared with the control schools (35).

The WAY (Wellness, Academics & You) program (36) was a 1-year intervention in 1,013 4th to 5th grade students in 69 classes and 16 schools from four states (intervention and comparison classes were randomly selected at each school). The WAY program was designed to improve academic performance by engaging students in behavioral-based health promotion activities that lasted 20 minutes to 1 hour and were delivered throughout the school year by trained teachers in seven modules. Modules 1 and 2 enabled students to examine their own health behaviors, and modules 3 and 4 focused specifically on physical activity and nutrition. Subsequent modules enhanced understanding and encouraged students to bring home the information and skills learned in class. After each module, intervention classes followed a 10-minute aerobic exercise routine each day during class time. After 1 year, prevalence of overweight was significantly lower for students in the intervention classes compared with the controls.

Some researchers have promoted curriculum and interventions to decrease children's "screen time" (ie, time spent watching TV, playing video games, and using computers) in an attempt to affect weight outcomes. Gortmaker et al (37) examined weight outcomes of a 2-year randomized, controlled health behavior intervention known as Planet Health. The study consisted of 10 middle schools randomly assigned to either intervention (n = 5) or control (n = 5). Planet Health sessions were included within existing curricula in four major subject areas and focused on decreasing television viewing, decreasing consumption of high-fat foods, increasing fruit and vegetable intake, and increasing moderate to vigorous physical activity. After 2 years, both obesity prevalence and obesity remission (ie, being obese at baseline but not at follow-up) were significantly lower in girls, but not boys, in the intervention schools vs the controls.

Robinson et al (38) conducted a randomized controlled trial in 192 4th grade students in two elementary schools (one intervention, one control). Intervention students received an 18-lesson, 6-month classroom curriculum to reduce television, videotape, and video game use for 1 school year. Relative BMI and skinfold thickness decreased significantly more in children in the intervention school compared with the control.

Finally, Goran and Reynolds (39) developed and tested IMPACT, a novel computer-based, multimedia program in schools for promoting physical activity in children. The program combined eight interactive media lessons (45 minutes per lesson) and five classroom lessons (45 minutes per lesson), along with four family-based assignments, for a total of 12 hours of contact delivered over 8 weeks. Girls in the intervention schools had significantly lower BMI z-scores than the control schools, but there was no intervention effect for boys.

INSIGHTS FOR PLANNING, IMPLEMENTATION, AND EVALUATION

Context of School Environment

School environments are complex, and obesity prevention initiatives should be part of coordinated, comprehensive, and integrated efforts that address key elements in these environments. Many different conceptual frameworks have been used to guide school-based obesity prevention research studies. Based on a systematic review of this literature, Summerbell et al (21) suggest that environmental approaches may change the environment but must be tied into individual behavior change for sustainable and purposeful results.

Story identified and described an integrated comprehensive model for school-based obesity prevention (9). The components included (*a*) health education through curriculum and instruction; (*b*) school health services for weight screening; (*c*) school counseling and psychological services for weight counseling and weight management; (*d*) school food service with lunches and breakfasts eligible for federal reimbursement; (*e*) the total school nutrition environment, including all food available in various locations such as stores, fund-raising, vending machines, school parties, and rewards;

(*f*) physical education; (*g*) school worksite health promotion for the adult population of the schools; and (*h*) community programs reaching outside of the school.

Challenges Within the School Environment

There are many opportunities in schools to influence the determinants of obesity, but there are also many challenges. Financial constraints exist for many schools, particularly those that serve low-income communities with a limited tax base and depend on limited state support. Under the No Child Left Behind regulations, schools must improve test scores and demonstrate adequate yearly progress (AYP) to qualify for federal funding of basic programs (40). Although it is important to increase the proficiency of US children in academic areas, No Child Left Behind requirements can compete with efforts to influence health in a school setting.

There is growing support for obesity prevention programs in schools, but these same initiatives have potential costs. They may present a burden to administrators with respect to the time needed for planning and supervision in their school; a burden to teachers for training and implementation time; a burden to students if the interventions take time away from academic studies; and a burden to families who may find it economically or emotionally stressful to provide healthier food and safer physical activities. Efforts to understand and appreciate the school environments and cultures can help limit the extent to which programs are burdensome (41).

Engaging School Stakeholders

School-based obesity prevention programs need to exert a fundamental shift in the school culture. School culture is set by stakeholders (students, families, teachers, administration, and staff), the location, external political influences and mandates, and the local school board's mission. To establish prevention interventions in a school, it is important to identify the stakeholders involved and understand their interrelated roles. School stakeholders can be divided into four categories: (*a*) external influences (eg, political leaders, health promotion groups); (*b*) structural/administrative levels (eg, school board, superintendant/chief executive officer, and specific departments such as school food services); (*c*) internal school layers (eg, principals and deans, teachers, school health councils); and (*d*) the local school community (eg, parents, recreation centers, after-school communities). The intervention or program cannot appear to sweep into the school without regard for the existing programs and demands of these stakeholders. Careful relationship-building with all of these groups is paramount to success. The CDC's School Health Index (SHI), explained later in this chapter, is a recommended starting point. Developing lasting partnerships is an active and ongoing process.

External Influences

External influences on schools include local, state, and federal politicians, mandates, and initiatives. The No Child Left Behind Act is a current example. For full federal funding, schools must implement academic initiatives, which may be incompatible—or perceived as incompatible—with physical education and health education needs.

Structural/Administrative Levels

All school districts have their own structure, and the administrative organizational structure varies from one district to the next. To better understand and work with the school district, it is useful to develop partnerships with key identified decision makers. Ideally, these key decision makers include the school district superintendent or chief executive officer and the chief academic officer, but access to these individuals may be limited. Therefore, program introduction needs to take place in the middle levels of the district administration—eg, director of student services, director of special services (those who oversee nurses and health educators), director of food service, and director of physical education—as well as with individual school principals. These individuals can help navigate the district structure and keep the program politically afloat. To keep obesity prevention programs and interventions on the administrative agenda, it is useful to identify school board directors who have voiced concern about student health issues.

Internal School Layers

Once a program or intervention has district-wide approval or acceptance, it is important to work within the internal school layers. Meetings and information sessions, as well as formal advisory boards, can assist in keeping all stakeholders informed and serve as a feedback mechanism. If the school already has a school health council, plans should be made to work with that group.

Although the principal is necessary and responsible for all school activities, the support of the teachers and staff is also essential. It is imperative to recognize the principal's role and importance while continuing to communicate with other relevant staff individually. McDonnell et al (42) found a major gap between principals' and foodservice directors' perceptions of the existence and/or enforcement of nutrition policies. For example, more principals than school foodservice directors reported the existence of enforced policies—a difference that illustrates the need for effective communication and dialogue with multiple parties.

Despite the recent proliferation of information about the increased prevalence of childhood obesity, Nollen et al (43) found that school administrators still did not always perceive it to be a concern for their school. The authors reported the following themes from interviews with school principals: (*a*) obesity was a problem, but not at their school; (*b*) schools have been unfairly targeted more than the community or homes for obesity causation and interventions; (*c*) interventions need to start before high school; (*d*) student health competes with other demands, but academic achievement remains the priority; and (*e*) legislation should be informed by educators and incorporate the school's perspective. Themes from interviews with key school foodservice personnel included (*a*) obesity is not a problem at their school; (*b*) school food service is not a cause of obesity; (*c*) food offerings prepare students for the real world by providing choice, and the options are dictated by the need for high participation rates; (*d*) a la carte options keep lunch participation high and prices low but should be used as a supplement, not re-placement, for meals; and (*e*) vending provides additional revenue to the school; it is not part of food service and is appropriate as long as it does not interfere with the lunch program.

When programs focus on dietary change, all foodservice employees need to be in-cluded in planning and implementing any proposed changes. The foodservice director makes the decisions, but the foodservice employees interact with the students on a daily basis and can exhibit influence.

Focus groups or informal meetings with students can increase the likelihood of stu-dent acceptance of the program. Enabling students to have a voice in some decisions will facilitate program ownership for this critical audience. For example, students could be involved in the selection of music or incentives for school-wide events, or they could be allowed to name the program or its local component. To effectively use student input, program staff should conduct preliminary research and present the students with top choices for names or incentives. Students cannot be expected to undertake the initial stages of these processes.

Local School Community

If the total school environment is to change, the intervention program will need to in-clude efforts at home, in the community, and/or by parent volunteers. School stores and parties are usually organized and staffed by parents. Therefore, including these groups from the beginning will enhance engagement and decrease competitive messages. After-school programs, either at the school or local recreation centers, need to be coordinated as well.

Total School Food Environments

The total school food environment has changed over recent years. Figure 15.1 describes the multiple components of the total school food environment.

Federally Regulated Meals

The US Department of Agriculture (USDA) provides federally defined standards based on the Dietary Guidelines for Americans for the breakfast and lunch programs (44). The standards dictate that meals are to be planned in one of the approved menu planning ap-proaches that limit calories from fat to less than 30% of total calories and calories from saturated fat to less than 10%. Lunches must provide one-third of the Recommended Di-etary Allowances (RDAs) for protein, calcium, iron, vitamin A, vitamin C, and calories (10). Breakfast must contain one-fourth of the RDAs for the same key nutrients (45). Local schools and school districts choose which specific food to serve and how to pre-pare them. Seventy percent of school systems use the food-based and enhanced food-based menu planning approach, which requires school meals to offer set numbers of servings from specific food groups, with minimum portion sizes that vary by age (46).

Box 15.1

Institute of Medicine Recommendations for Schools

USDA, state, and local authorities, and schools should:
- Develop and implement nutrition standards for all competitive foods and beverages sold or served in schools.
- Ensure that all school meals meet the Dietary Guidelines for Americans.
- Develop, implement, and evaluate pilot programs to extend school meal funding in schools with a large percentage of children at risk of obesity.

State and local educational authorities and schools should:
- Ensure that all children and youth participate in a minimum of 30 minutes of moderate to vigorous physical activity during the school day.
- Expand opportunities for physical activity through physical education classes; intramural and interscholastic sports programs and other physical activity clubs, programs, and lesson; after-school use of facilities, use of schools as community centers; and walking- and biking-to-school programs.
- Enhance health curricula to devote adequate attention to nutrition, physical activity, reducing sedentary behaviors, and energy balance, and to include a behavioral skills focus.
- Develop, implement, and enforce school policies to create schools that are advertising-free to the greatest extent possible.
- Involve school health services in obesity prevention efforts.
- Conduct annual assessments of each student's weight, height, and gender- and age-specific BMI percentile and make this information available to parents.
- Perform periodic assessments of each school's policies and practices related to nutrition, physical activity, and obesity prevention.

Federal and state departments of education and health professional organizations should:
- Develop, implement, and evaluate pilot programs to explore innovative approaches to both staffing and teaching about wellness, healthful choices, nutrition, physical activity, and reducing sedentary behaviors. Innovative approaches to recruiting and training appropriate teachers are also needed.

Source: Adapted from reference 6.

Many interventions have been attempted in school settings. With some notable exceptions, most interventions have not affected students' BMI. The reasons for this are unclear, but they may include insufficient time and/or resources allotted to the intervention, or programs that were too broad, focused more on individual behavior than on policy change, or were not sufficiently comprehensive. While top-down, protocol-driven efforts are useful for proof-of-concept in laboratory settings or efficacy studies, schools may also be well served by policy-driven approaches that have their roots in the local school culture. The importance of continued evaluation cannot be overstated. Ultimately, if BMI or similar adiposity outcomes remain largely unaffected by a new generation of studies, it may be time to conclude that school-based interventions are necessary but not sufficient to prevent overweight and obesity among children.

References

1. Ogden CL, Carroll MD, Curtin LR, McDowell MA, Tabak CJ, Flegal KM. Prevalence of overweight and obesity in the United States, 1999-2004. *JAMA*. 2006;295: 1549–1555.

2. The HEALTHY Study Group; Kaufman, FR., Hirst K, Linder B, Baranowski T, Cooper DM, Foster GD, Goldberg L, Harrell J, Marcus MD, Trevino R. Risk Factors for type 2 diabetes in 6th grade muliti-racial cohort: The HEALTHY Study. *Diabetes Care.* 2009;32:953–955.

3. Guo SS, Chumlea WC. Tracking of body mass index in children in relation to overweight in adulthood. *Am J Clin Nutr.* 1999;70(suppl):145S–148S.

4. Daniels SR, Arnett DK, Eckel RH, Gidding SS, Hayman LL, Kumanyika S, Robinson TN, Scott BJ, St. Jeor S, Williams CL. Overweight in children and adolescents: pathophysiology, consequences, prevention and treatment. *Circulation.* 2005;111: 1999–2012.

5. Wang Y, Beydoun MA. The obesity epidemic in the United States—gender, age, socioeconomic, racial/ethnic, and geographic characteristics: a systematic review and meta-regression analysis. *Epidemiol Rev.* 2007;29:6–28.

6. Institute of Medicine. *Preventing Childhood Obesity: Health in the Balance.* Washington, DC: National Academies Press; 2005.

7. Kuczmarski RJ, Ogden CL, Guo SS, Grummer-Strawn L, Flegal KM, Mei Z, et al. CDC growth charts for the United States: methods and development. *Vital Health Stat 11.* 2002;246:1–190.

8. Baranowski T, Cullen KW, Nicklas T, Thompson D, Baranowski J. School based obesity prevention: a blueprint for taming the epidemic. *Am J Health Behav.* 2002;26:486–493.

9. Story M. School-based approaches for preventing and treating obesity. *Int J Obes Relat Metab Disord.* 1999;23(Suppl 2):S43–S51.

10. Nutrition standards and menu planning approaches for lunches and requirements for afterschool snacks. *Fed Register.* 7 CFR 210.10.

11. Cullen KW, Thompson DI. Texas school food policy change related to middle school a la carte/snack bar foods: potential savings in kilocalories. *J Am Diet Assoc.* 2005;105:1952–1954.

12. Fu M, Cheng L, Tu S, Pan W. Association between unhealthful eating patterns and unfavorable overall school performance in children. *J Am Diet Assoc.* 2007;107: 1935–1943.

13. Taras H. Physical activity and student performance at school. *J Sch Health.* 2005;75:214–218.

14. Sigfusdottir ID, Kristjansson AL, Allegrante JP. Health behaviour and academic achievement in Icelandic school children. *Health Educ Res.* 2007;22:70–80.

15. Gier AB, Foster GD, Womble LG, McLaughlin J, Borradaile KE, Nachmani J, Shermann S, Kumanyika S, Shults J. The relationship between relative weight and school attendance among elementary schoolchildren *Obesity.* 2007;15:2157–2161.

16. Sallis JF, McKenzie TL, Kolody B, Lewis M, Marshall S, Rosengard P. Effects of health-related physical education on academic achievement: Project SPARK. *Res Q Exerc Sport.* 1999;70:127–134.

17. Katz DL, O'Connell M, Njike VY, Yeh MC, Nawaz H. Strategies for the prevention and control of obesity in the school setting: systematic review and meta-analysis. *Int J Obes (Lond).* 2008;32:1780–1789.

18. Doak CM, Visscher TLS, Renders CM, Seidell JC. The prevention of overweight and obesity in children and adolescents: a review of interventions and programmes. *Obes Rev.* 2006;7:111–136.

19. Budd GM, Volpe SL. School-based obesity prevention: research, challenges and recommendations. *J Sch Health.* 2006;76:485–495.

20. Harris KC, Kuramota LK, Schulzer M, Retallacj JE. Effect of school-based physical activity interventions on body mass index in children: a meta-analysis. *CMAJ.* 2009;180:719–726.

21. Summerbell CD, Waters E, Edmunds LD, Kelly S, Brown T, Campbell KJ. Interventions for preventing obesity in children. *Cochrane Database Syst Rev.* 2005;3: CD001871.

22. Durant N, Baskin ML, Thomas O, Allison DB. School-based obesity treatment and prevention programs: all in all, just another brick in the wall? *Int J Obes (Lond).* 2008;32:1747–1751.

23. Luepker RV, Perry CL, McKinlay SM. Outcomes of a field trial to improve children's dietary patterns and physical activity: the Child and Adolescent Trial for Cardiovascular Health (CATCH). *JAMA.* 1996;75:768–776.

24. Nader PR, Stone EJ, Lytle LA. Three-year maintenance of improved diet and physical activity. *Arch Pediatr Adolesc Med.* 1999;153:695–704.

25. Sahota P, Rudolf MC, Dixey R, Hill AJ, Barth JH, Cade J. Evaluation of implementation and effect of primary school-based intervention to reduce risk factors for obesity. *BMJ.* 2001;323:1027–1029.

26. Sahota P, Rudolf MC, Dixey R, Hill AJ, Barth JH, Cade J. Randomised controlled trial of primary school based intervention to reduce risk factors for obesity. *BMJ.* 2001;323:1029.

27. Caballero B, Clay T, Davis SM, Ethelbah B, Rock BH, Lohman T, Norman J, Story M, Stone EJ, Stephenson L, Stevens J, Pathways Study Research Group. Pathways: a school-based, randomized controlled trial for the prevention of obesity in American Indian schoolchildren. *Am J Clin Nutr.* 2003;78:1030–1038.

28. Neumark-Sztainer D, Story M, Hannan PJ, Rex J. New Moves: a school-based obesity prevention program for adolescent girls. *Prev Med.* 2003;37:41–51.

29. James J, Thomas P, Cavan D, Kerr D. Preventing childhood obesity by reducing consumption of carbonated drinks: cluster randomized controlled trial. *BMJ.* 2004;328:1236.

30. James J, Thomas P, Kerr D. Preventing childhood obesity: two year follow-up results from the Christchurch Obesity Prevention Programme in Schools (CHOPPS). *BMJ.* 2008;335:762–765.

31. Coleman KJ, Tiller CL, Sanchez J, Heath EM, Sy O, Milliken G, Dzewaltowski DA. Prevention of epidemic increase in child risk of overweight in low-income schools. *Arch Pediatr Adolesc Med.* 2005;159:217–224.

32. Foster GD, Sherman S, Borradaile KE, Grundy, K, Vander Veur SS, Nachmani J, Karpyn A, Kumanyika S, Shults J. A policy-based school intervention to prevent overweight and obesity. *Pediatrics.* 2008;121:794–802.

33. Economos CD, Hyatt RR, Goldberg JP, Must A, Naumova EN, Collins JJ, Nelson ME. A community intervention reduces BMI *z*-score in children: Shape UP Somerville first year results. *Obesity.* 2007;15:1325–1336.

34. Kain J, Uauy Albala R, Vio F, Cerda R, Leyton B. School-based obesity prevention in Chilean primary school children: methodology and evaluation of a controlled study. *Int J Obes Relat Metab Disord.* 2004;28:483–493.

35. Kain J, Leyton B, Cerda R, Vio F, Uauy R. Two-year controlled effectiveness trial of

a school-based intervention to prevent obesity in Chilean children. *Public Health Nutr.* 2008; 23:1–11.

36. Spiegel SA, Foulk D. Reducing overweight through a multidisciplinary school-based intervention. *Obesity.* 2006;14:88–96.

37. Gortmaker SL, Peterson K, Wiecha J, Sobol AM, Dixit S, Fox MK, Laird N. Reducing obesity via a school-based interdisciplinary intervention among youth: Planet Health. *Arch Pediatr Adolesc Med.* 1999;153:409–418.

38. Robinson TN. Reducing children's television viewing to prevent obesity: a randomized controlled trial. *JAMA.* 1999;282:1561–1567.

39. Goran MJ, Reynolds K. Interactive multimedia for promoting physical activity (IMPACT) in children. *Obes Res.* 2005;13:762–771.

40. No Child Left Behind Act 2001. (USC) Public Law 107-110.115 STAT. 1425 (2002).

41. Franks A, Kelder SH, Dino GA, Horn KA, Gortmaker SL, Wiecha JL, Simoes EJ. School-based programs: lessons learned from CATCH, Planet Health, and Not-On-Tobacco. *Prev Chron Dis.* 2007;4:A33.

42. McDonnell E, Probart C, Weirich E, Hartman T, Bailey-Davis L. School competitive food policies: perceptions of Pennsylvania public high school foodservice directors and principals. *J Am Diet Assoc.* 2006;106:271–276.

43. Nollen NL, Befort CA, Snow P, Daley CM, Ellerbeck EF, Ashluwalia JS. The school food service environment and adolescent obesity: qualitative insights from high school principals and food service personnel. *Int J Behav Nutr Phys Act.* 2007;4:18–29.

44. US Department of Health and Human Services and US Department of Agriculture. Dietary *Guidelines for Americans.* 6th ed. Washington DC: Government Printing Office; 2005.

45. School Breakfast Program: Nutrition Standards and menu planning approaches for breakfast. *Fed Register.* 7 CFR 220.08.

46. Gordon A, Crepinsek MK, Nogales R, Condon E. *School Nutrition Dietary Assessment Study—III: Volume 1: School Food Service, School Food Environment, and Meals Offered and Served.* Princeton, NJ: Mathematica Policy Research; 2007.

47. *The Road to SMI Success: A Guide for School Foodservice Directors.* Alexandria, VA: US Department of Agriculture, Food and Nutrition Service; 2007.

48. Ralston K, Newman C, Clauson A, Guthrie J, Buzby J. *The National School Lunch Program: Backgrounds, Trends, and Issues.* Washington, DC: US Department of Agriculture Economic Research Service; 2008. Economic Research Report no. 61.

49. National School Lunch Program: Subpart—Requirements for school food authority participation: competitive food services. *Fed Register.* 7 CFR 210.11.

50. Centers for Disease Control and Prevention. Competitive foods and beverages available for purchase in secondary schools—selected sites, United States, 2004. *MMWR.* 2005;54:917–921.

51. Alliance for a Healthier Generation. Memorandum of Understanding. May 3, 2006. http://www.healthiergeneration.org. Accessed February 26, 2009.

52. American Beverage Association. School Beverage Guidelines Progress Report, 2008–2008. http://www.schoolbeverages.com/index.aspx. Accessed February 26, 2009.

53. Institute of Medicine, Food and Nutrition Board. Review of National School Lunch and School Breakfast Program Meal Patterns and Standards. 2008. http://www8.nationalacademies.org/cp/projectview.aspx?key=48910. Accessed April 7, 2009.

54. Institute of Medicine. Review of National School Lunch and School Breakfast Program Meal Patterns and Nutrient Standards. http://www.iom.edu/CMS/3788/54064.aspx. Accessed February 26, 2009.

55. National Center for Chronic Disease Prevention and Health Promotion. *Physical Activity and Health: A Report of the Surgeon General*. Atlanta, GA: US Department of Health and Human Services; 1996.

56. American Academy of Pediatrics. Physical fitness and activity in schools. *Pediatrics*. 2000;105:1156–1157.

57. US Department of Health and Human Services; US Department of Education. *Promoting Better Health for Young People Through Physical Activity and Sports: A Report to the President from the Secretary of Health and Human Services and the Secretary of Education*. Atlanta, GA: US Department of Health and Human Services; 2000.

58. Centers for Disease Control and Prevention. Guidelines for school and community programs to promote lifelong physical activity among young people. *MMWR*. 1997;46:1–36.

59. Burgeson CR, Wechsler H, Brener ND, Young JC, Spain CG. Physical education and activity: results from the School Health Policies and Programs Study 2000. *J Sch Health*. 2001;71:279–293.

60. Story M, Kaphinst KM, French S. The role of schools in obesity prevention. *Future Child*. 2006;16:109–142.

61. Jago R, Baranowski T. Non-curricular approaches for increasing physical activity in youth: a review. *Prev Med*. 2004;39:157–163.

62. US Department of Agriculture. Child Nutrition and WIC Reauthorization Act of 2004 Section 204 of Public Law 108–265; 2004. http://www.fns.usda.gov/TN/Healthy/108-265.pdf. Accessed February 26, 2009.

63. Donze Black J. Local wellness policies and the Dietary Guidelines: what does it mean to you? *J Am Diet Assoc*. 2005;105:891–894.

64. Kumanyika S, Jeffrey RW, Morabia A, Ritenbaugh C, Antipatis VJ. Obesity prevention: the case for action. *Int J Obes Relat Metab Disord*. 2002;26:425–436.

65. Gittelsohn J, Kumar KM. Preventing childhood obesity and diabetes: is it time to move out of the school? *Pediatr Diabetes*. 2007;8(Suppl 9):S55–S69.

66. Robinson TN, Sirard JR. Preventing childhood obesity: a solution-oriented research paradigm. *Am J Prev Med*. 2005;28(Suppl 2):S94–S201.

CHAPTER 16

PREGNANCY AND MENOPAUSE

JENNIFER C. LOVEJOY, PHD

INTRODUCTION

The significance of obesity as a global health problem is widely recognized. It is less well recognized, however, that the prevalence of obesity in most populations around the world tends to be higher in women than in men, and that obesity confers somewhat differential health risks in women.

According to the 2003–2004 National Health and Nutrition Examination Survey (NHANES), the prevalence of obesity in the United States is slightly higher in women (33%) than in men (31%) (1). The prevalence of extreme obesity (body mass index [BMI] > 40), however, is more than twice as high in US women compared with men (6.9% vs 2.8%). Obesity and overweight are particularly common among minority women in the United States: among African-American, Mexican-American, and some Native American women, the prevalence of BMI greater than 25 exceeds 75% (1,2). It should also be noted that, at any BMI, women have a greater percentage of body fat that do men, indicating that a woman's risk of being "overfat" (as opposed to overweight) is higher, even at when BMI is within the normal range.

Regional fat distribution is a strong predictor of health risks associated with obesity. The National Institutes of Health (NIH) clinical guidelines for obesity recommend the use of sex-specific waist circumference cutoffs to identify individuals at risk for disease (3). According to the guidelines, a waist circumference of more than 88 cm (35 inches) in a woman places her at increased health risk. Distribution of body fat is partially controlled by hormones in both men and women. As reviewed below, decreased estrogen in women (eg, at menopause) and/or increased androgens are associated with greater abdominal body fat distribution (4,5), whereas use of postmenopausal estrogen therapy reduces abdominal fat gain (6).

In addition to the well-known health effects of obesity, including diabetes, heart disease, osteoarthritis, and gallbladder disease, that are risks for all individuals, women face other unique risks. Women who are overweight have a greater risk for postmenopausal breast cancer, endometrial cancer, and premenopausal ovarian cancer compared with women who are lean, and treatment outcomes for these cancers are worse in obese women (7,8). Obesity is associated with polycystic ovarian syndrome (PCOS) and PCOS-related infertility. Significantly reduced fecundity has also been observed in overweight and obese women with apparently normal menstrual cycles (9). Furthermore, obesity during pregnancy (discussed in detail later in this chapter) substantially increases the risk for poor maternal and fetal outcomes.

Thus, obesity is truly a women's health issue, both from the perspective of sex differences in prevalence and in terms of sex-specific obesity-related health risks. The remainder of this chapter will address the high-risk times for weight gain that are due in part to sex hormone fluctuations in women's life cycles: pregnancy and menopause.

PREGNANCY AND OBESITY

Pregnancy and Obesity Risk

The concept of "maternal obesity," or obesity resulting from childbearing, was first introduced in the 1940s (10). Since then, a number of studies (11–13) have found an association between increasing parity and increased body weight (see references 14 and 15 for more information).

After adjusting for the effects of aging per se, the typical amount of weight retained after pregnancy is relatively small, ranging from 0.5 to 2.4 kg depending on the population studied (11,13,16). However, roughly 15% to 25% of women gain substantial amounts of excess body weight as a result of pregnancy, and this effect may increase with sequential pregnancies (11,16). For example, in a study of 540 women in upstate New York with a range of pre-pregnancy body weights, the subjects were on average 1.51 ± 5.95 kg heavier 1 year postpartum compared with early pregnancy, but approximately 25% of the women experienced what the investigators considered a major weight gain (> 4.55 kg) as a result of pregnancy (16). Among 128 obese women attending a weight-loss clinic, rates of excess weight gain due to pregnancy were even higher, with 73% reporting weight retention of more than 10 kg 1 year postpartum (17). Given these findings, it is not surprising that excess pregnancy weight gain and/or failure to lose pregnancy weight postpartum have been associated with long-term (10 to 15 years after delivery) obesity for mothers (18,19).

A large number of studies have confirmed that the absolute amount of weight gained during pregnancy is the primary predictor of the amount of weight retained postpartum. In 1990 the Institute of Medicine (IOM) issued guidelines on weight gain during pregnancy that vary depending on a woman's pre-pregnancy BMI. These IOM weight gain guidelines for pregnant women are as follows (20):

- Underweight: 28–40 pounds
- Normal weight: 25–35 pounds
- Overweight: 15–25 pounds
- Obese: at least 15 pounds

Since the IOM guidelines were issued, studies have shown that women who gain more than the recommended amounts during pregnancy are at significant risk for excess weight retention and postpartum obesity. For example, in a longitudinal study of nearly 500 women after pregnancy, those who gained within the IOM targets during pregnancy weighed 6.7 kg more at 15-year follow-up compared to their pre-pregnancy weight, whereas those who gained more than the IOM recommendations weighed 10.0 kg more (19). Among low-income women, those who gained more than the IOM recommendations during pregnancy retained nearly 4 kg more 1 year postpartum than women who gained within the recommended range, and the former group were five times more likely to experience major weight gain of 4.55 kg or more after pregnancy (16).

Women who are overweight or obese before pregnancy seem to be at higher risk of excess weight gain during pregnancy and may therefore require closer monitoring and nutrition counseling (21,22). Other factors that are associated with excess pregnancy weight retention are less well understood, although some studies suggest that diet and exercise habits, quitting smoking during pregnancy, older or younger maternal age, and low socioeconomic status are significant influences on excess weight retention after delivery (17,22). Box 16.1 summarizes factors that have been associated with excess weight retention following pregnancy.

Racial and Ethnic Variations in Risk Levels

As is the case with obesity prevalence in general, minority women are at greater risk for excessive weight retention due to pregnancy compared with white women (12,23–25). African-American women tend to gain more during pregnancy than do white women, and they also retain more weight following pregnancy—in the National Maternal and Infant Health Survey of approximately 1,600 women, the median weight retention was 7.2 vs 1.6 pounds, respectively, for African-American and white women who gain the recommended amount of weight in pregnancy (23). In a study of first-time African-American mothers, the women at 2 months postpartum weighed on average 18 pounds more than their pre-pregnancy body weights, and by 6 months postpartum they had not

---

Box 16.1
Factors Associated with Excess Body Weight Retention After Pregnancy

- Excess weight gain during pregnancy
- High pre-pregnancy body mass index
- Early (1st trimester) weight gain
- Ethnicity (African American, Hispanic, Native American)
- Unemployment
- Limited pregnancy/postpartum exercise
- Maternal age (< 20 or > 35 years)
- Early menarche (< 12 years)
- Breastfeeding duration
- High snacking frequency
- Low educational level
- Higher parity
- Shorter interval between pregnancies
- Quitting smoking
- Dietary patterns[a]

---

[a]Evidence is suggestive, but not conclusive, for multiple dietary patterns.

lost any additional weight (24). Similarly, in a population-based study of nearly 9,000 Hispanic women in southern California, Siega-Riz and associates found that 37% of normal-weight Hispanic women vs 75% of obese Hispanic women had pregnancy weight gains in excess of the recommended IOM range (25).

Importantly, compared with white women, African-American women not only have higher rates of excess postpartum weight retention in general, they also seem to be particularly at risk for postpartum obesity if they gain in excess of the IOM recommendations (23). Among women in the National Maternal and Infant Health Survey who gained more than the IOM recommendations, 45% of white women retained less than 4 pounds 10 to 18 months postpartum, compared with 25% of African-American women. Also, the median retained weight was 4.9 pounds for white women vs 12.7 pounds for African-American women (23). It is not clear how much the overall elevation in obesity prevalence in minority female populations is due to excess pregnancy-related weight gain.

Relationship of Risk to Energy Intake and Energy Needs

Given the importance of excess pregnancy weight gain as a risk for postpartum obesity, it is essential to understand factors that may influence weight gain during pregnancy. Obviously, one important factor is how many calories are consumed relative to energy needs. Data from Goldberg and colleagues (26) suggest that some women are more efficient than others at storing energy during pregnancy. This study used the doubly labeled water method to measure 24-hour energy expenditure in 12 free-living healthy white women (BMI 23 ± 3.3) before conception and every 6 weeks throughout pregnancy. The results showed considerable interindividual variability in the metabolic response to pregnancy. In some women (ie, "energy-profligate" participants), energy expenditure immediately increased in the first trimester and continued to increase steadily throughout pregnancy. In other women, energy expenditure did not increase until the third trimester, and the metabolic rate in some "energy-sparing" participants actually decreased from the first to second trimesters (26). Clearly, if "energy-sparing" women follow the commonly recommended dietary advice to increase daily energy intake by 300 kcal throughout pregnancy, they will be at risk for gaining weight, particularly early in pregnancy. More recently, Butte et al (27) also reported that the increase in metabolic rate with pregnancy varies tremendously among individuals, with some women actually decreasing energy expenditure relative to pre-pregnancy values. In general, the increases in metabolic rate in pregnancy were higher in women with high BMI, who gained the most weight and fat-free mass during gestation. This study also confirmed that any increases in energy requirements for women with normal BMI in the first trimester are negligible (~80 kcal/d), whereas the requirements for women with high BMIs increase to a slightly greater extent (27). Thus, it is important to customize dietary recommendations for energy intake in pregnancy based on each individual woman's weight-gain targets.

Relationship of Risk to Timing of Weight Gain

Timing of weight gain is another important factor that may influence excess weight gain in pregnancy. In a study of 371 white women, Muscati et al (28) measured maternal weight gain before 20 weeks, from 21 to 30 weeks, and from 31 weeks to term, as well as postpartum weight retention. On average, 86% of the weight gained in the first 20 weeks of pregnancy was retained by the mothers at least 6 weeks postpartum, regardless of whether the women retained excess postpartum weight or not. The women who retained the most weight 6 weeks postpartum had gained on average 6.2 kg during the first 20 weeks of pregnancy, compared with 3.3 kg gained by women who did not retain excess weight. Importantly, maternal weight gain in the first 20 weeks contributed the least to the birth weight of the infant, whereas maternal weight gain in weeks 21 to 30 had the greatest impact on infant weight. While it is obviously important to maintain good nutrition throughout pregnancy, these data suggest that restricting weight gain early in pregnancy, when there is not likely to be a deleterious effect on infant growth, may help prevent maternal obesity. Additional research is needed to determine the role of excess weight gain early in pregnancy on postpartum obesity.

Relationship of Risk to Appetite and Eating Behaviors

Although the data directly relating dietary patterns to excess weight gain during pregnancy are limited, some data suggest that appetite and eating behaviors may play a role in postpartum weight retention. In a retrospective case-control study examining dietary and behavioral factors in healthy women who had normal BMI prior to pregnancy, those women who retained excess weight after pregnancy had higher scores on both the Disinhibition and Hunger scales of the Three-Factor Eating Questionnaire, compared with those who returned to their lean, pre-pregnant weight (29). These results suggest that women who develop postpartum obesity may have had greater difficulty controlling food intake. Theoretically, hormonal changes during pregnancy could result in changes in the neuroendocrine regulation of eating behavior such that women who may have successfully controlled intake pre-pregnancy are no longer able to do so.

Breastfeeding and Postpartum Weight

It may seem logical to assume that breastfeeding would help women lose excess body weight following pregnancy, but research has not clearly demonstrated an association between lactation and postpartum weight retention (see reference 30 for review). In addition to observational studies that found no effect of breastfeeding on postpartum weight loss, one randomized controlled study of calcium supplementation during lactation found that nonlactating women lost body fat at a faster rate from 2 weeks to 6 months postpartum than lactating women (31). Calcium supplementation had no effect on postpartum weight loss in either lactating or nonlactating women in this study.

Some of the discrepancies in the literature may be due to the populations studied. A large Brazilian study found an effect of lactation on postpartum weight loss in women who had less than 30% body fat, but not in women who had a higher percentage of body fat (32). In contrast, other observational studies and those that assessed long-term (> 6 months) exclusive breastfeeding suggest that lactation helps to reduce maternal body fat, although the effect is generally small (33–35). Epidemiologic data from the Stockholm Pregnancy and Women's Nutrition (SPAWN) study, including a 15-year longitudinal follow-up of body weight after pregnancy, indicate that women who become overweight following pregnancy have lower lactation scores, which suggests that breast-feeding may help prevent maternal obesity (35). Unfortunately, research has consistently shown that obese women are less likely than lean women to breastfeed, or they breast-feed for shorter durations (36,37); thus, obese women are less likely to reap the potential benefits of lactation on postpartum weight loss.

Because milk production has a definable energy cost, the most likely explanation for why lactating women do not lose weight is that they exceed their energy requirements. In a study by Lovelady et al (38), overweight lactating women restricted energy intake by 500 kcal/d by limiting intake of fat, sweetened drinks, desserts, and snack foods, and this restriction had little impact on maternal micronutrient status or breastfeeding effective-ness. Thus, it is reasonable to advise women not only to consider breastfeeding for at least 6 months for the multiple benefits it confers, but also to consider restricting fat and simple sugar intake postpartum to facilitate postpartum weight loss.

Obesity During Pregnancy and Maternal and Fetal Risks

Unfortunately, excess weight gain and obesity during pregnancy not only pose long-term risks for women, they also significantly increase the likelihood of pregnancy complica-tions and poor fetal outcomes. In an Italian retrospective cohort study, Druil et al found that women who were obese at the time of conception had a higher incidence of cae-sarean section (odds ratio [OR] = 2.17) and preterm deliveries (OR = 4.86) (39). Meta-analyses have confirmed that obesity in pregnancy confers increased risk for miscar-riage, stillbirth, and caesarean section (40–42).

It is well documented that the incidence of gestational diabetes mellitus (GDM) is higher in women who are obese. Risk of GDM also seems to increase as the rates of ma-ternal weight gain prior to conception and between successive pregnancies increase. For example, women who gain between 2.3 and 10.0 kg/year in the 5 years prior to preg-nancy as well as those who increase BMI by three or more units between pregnancies have a significantly increased risk for GDM (43,44). Women with high interpregnancy weight gain also have significantly increased risk for pre-eclampsia, stillbirth, and large-for-gestational age infants (44).

In addition to increased risk for complications during pregnancy and delivery, ma-ternal obesity may have possible intergenerational consequences. Most studies in this area use animal models, and these studies have clearly shown that "fetal programming" occurs in relation to maternal nutritional variables, including obesity. A number of stud-ies in rats, for example, suggest that maternal obesity increases risk for obesity in the offspring, particularly when the offspring are fed a high-fat diet (see, for example, refer-ence 45). In humans, large-for-gestational-age infants (which occur more often in preg-nancies complicated by obesity) have a higher risk for both childhood and adult obesity (see reference 46 for review).

Although it is not clear whether fetal programming is involved, another risk of ma-ternal obesity may be attention deficit hyperactivity disorder (ADHD) in offspring. In a recent study, women who were overweight or obese prior to pregnancy had a signifi-cantly greater likelihood of having children later diagnosed with ADHD, and women who were both obese prior to pregnancy and had excess pregnancy weight gain had more than twice the risk of having a child with ADHD compared with lean women (47). This finding has led some to speculate that there may be a relationship between the increasing prevalence of ADHD and the obesity epidemic.

Nutrition Interventions to Manage Obesity in Pregnancy

Given the significant risks to women and infants of obesity during pregnancy, it is important to consider nutrition interventions to ameliorate the adverse impact of gaining too much pregnancy weight. Weight loss during pregnancy is not recommended. However, it is certainly advisable, when possible, to recommend that women attain a healthy body weight prior to conception.

Once a woman becomes pregnant, efforts should be directed toward limiting pregnancy weight gain to the recommended levels. Several studies have suggested that nutrition interventions during pregnancy can be effective in this regard. For example, a behavioral intervention program for pregnant women that included education about pregnancy weight gain, healthful foods, and exercise resulted in a significant decrease in the number of normal-weight women who gained more than the IOM recommended ranges (from 58% to 33%) (48). However, this effect was not seen in obese women, which suggests that a more intensive intervention may be required for these women. In a Swedish study, an intervention for obese pregnant women that involved weekly educational sessions and water aerobics resulted in lower weight gains during pregnancy and a significantly smaller percentage of women gaining more than 7 kg compared with obese pregnant women in a control group (49).

In summary, risks of excess weight retention following pregnancy are closely tied to excess weight gain during the pregnancy. Close spacing between pregnancies and failure to return to baseline weight before the next pregnancy compound the problem and probably explain the association between parity and obesity observed in epidemiological studies. Nutrition interventions to limit pregnancy weight gain to healthy ranges and to facilitate postpartum weight loss can be effective in preventing pregnancy-induced obesity.

MENOPAUSE AND OBESITY

Menopause and Weight Gain

It has been understood for nearly a century that ovariectomy increases food consumption and causes significant weight gain in female rodents (50). This effect has subsequently been identified in a wide variety of species, including nonhuman primates. This effect of ovariectomy on body weight and eating behavior is controlled by estradiol, and replacement of physiological levels of estrogen reduces excess weight and restores normal eating patterns (see reference 51).

Although there have been fewer studies in women, most studies suggest that the impact of decreased estrogens in women is similar to that observed in nonhuman females. Wing et al (52) studied 485 women who were initially premenopausal and followed them for 3 years, at which time 61 were defined as postmenopausal (without a menstrual period for 12 months), 94 were perimenopausal (having missed 3 to 11 menstrual periods in the year before follow-up), and 279 were still premenopausal. The mean weight gain in the group was 2.25 kg, and 20% of the population had gained 4.5 kg or more. Similarly, Pasquali et al (53) reported that BMI was significantly higher among perimenopausal and postmenopausal women compared with premenopausal women in an Italian population study, and Toth et al (54) found that body weight was 6% higher and percentage of body fat was 17% higher in age-matched postmenopausal vs premenopausal women. The Study of Women's Health Across the Nation (SWAN), a US survey of approximately 13,000 women of varying ethnicities, found that BMI was significantly higher in women who had surgical menopause than in premenopausal women, but the study did not find a significant difference in weight related to natural menopause independent of aging (55).

Recently, in a longitudinal study of middle-aged women going through the menopause transition, Lovejoy et al showed that both total 24-hour energy expenditure and sleeping energy expenditure declined to a greater extent in women who became menopausal than age-matched women who remained premenopausal at a 4-year follow-up visit (56). Sleeping energy expenditure was reduced approximately 100 kcal/d in women who became postmenopausal (a drop of 6.6%) compared to a decrease of approximately 50 kcal/d (3.3%) in women who remained premenopausal. One possible explanation for the observed postmenopausal decline in energy expenditure is the loss of the typical luteal phase increase in energy expenditure (~100 kcal/d) that occurs in women with normal menstrual cycles (57). Another possible reason for decreasing energy expenditure is loss of lean body mass, which occurs more rapidly at menopause than would be expected due to aging per se (54). Regardless, given the magnitude of the decrease in metabolism, it is clear that if perimenopausal and postmenopausal women do not voluntarily decrease energy intake, the decline in energy expenditure is enough to result in significant weight gain over time. Furthermore, in addition to the changes in energy expenditure, Lovejoy et al also observed a decrease in 24-hour fat oxidation after menopause of nearly 30 g/d (~33%), which was not seen at follow-up in women who remained premenopausal (56). This suggests it may be particularly important for postmenopausal women to limit dietary fat intake to avoid excess fat storage.

Menopause and Body Fat Distribution

Although weight gain at menopause may have important health implications for older women, sex hormone changes at menopause appear to exert a stronger effect on body fat distribution, which also profoundly influences health risk. A number of studies using dual-energy X-ray absorptiometry (DEXA) or computed tomography (CT) scan to assess body fat distribution have reported an increased in abdominal fat accumulation in postmenopausal women relative to premenopausal women (5,54,58–60). It is well-known that abdominal fat distribution is associated with increased metabolic and cardiovascular risk and the shift in fat distribution at menopause may in part explain the increased health risks in older women. In fact, Zamboni et al (60) have demonstrated that, after statistically adjusting for the amount of visceral fat present, there were no difference in fasting or 2-hour glucose or triglyceride values between older and younger women.

Estrogen is known to influence adipose tissue lipoprotein lipase (LPL) activity and lipolysis. Therefore, changes in body fat distribution associated with declining estrogen are likely due to changes in adipose tissue metabolism. For example, higher adipose tissue LPL activity (promoting fat storage) has been observed in femoral adipocytes compared with abdominal adipocytes in premenopausal women but not in postmenopausal, estrogen-deficient women (61). Thus, unlike premenopausal women, postmenopausal women do not preferentially deposit fat in the periphery (ie, femoral adipose depot), but pre- and postmenopausal women are equally likely to deposit fat in adipose depots in the trunk. Furthermore, treatment with estrogen in postmenopausal women restores the lipoprotein lipase activity of the femoral adipocytes and attenuates lipolytic response in subcutaneous adipocytes but not in abdominal adipocytes (62,63).

Exogenous Estrogens and Obesity

As might be expected given the effects of estrogen on adipose tissue metabolism, several studies have confirmed that postmenopausal women taking estrogen replacement therapy (ERT) have a smaller increase over time in abdominal fat compared with those who are not taking estrogen (6,64,65). The effects of ERT on total body fat or body weight are less clear, but several large studies, including the Postmenopausal Estrogen/Progestin Intervention (PEPI) trial and SWAN study, have reported that ERT users gain less weight and have lower BMIs on average compared with postmenopausal women who do not use ERT (55,66). In contrast, the Rancho Bernardo population study found no significant different in BMI after 15 years of follow-up in ERT users vs non-users after the analysts adjusted data for confounding variables (67).

It is worth noting that, in contrast to the beneficial effects of estrogen on abdominal fat in women, androgens increase abdominal visceral fat in women. This raises a significant concern about testosterone-containing postmenopausal hormonal therapy in terms of its effect on fat distribution and visceral-fat-related health risks (4).

Consistent with the findings that suggest hormonally related declines in energy expenditure at menopause, several studies suggest that postmenopausal ERT use increases energy expenditure. Reimer et al compared resting energy expenditure (REE) in premenopausal women to postmenopausal ERT users and non-users (68). REE was significantly lower in postmenopausal women not taking ERT compared with premenopausal women, but there was no difference between ERT users and premenopausal women. Conversely, pharmacologic suppression of estradiol by GnRH antagonist administration in premenopausal women reduced REE by 5% (~70 kcal/d) (69). Together, these studies suggest that exogenous estrogen maintains higher energy expenditure whereas estrogen-deficiency reduces energy expenditure in healthy women.

In summary, menopause does seem to cause significant weight gain in some women, although the changes in weight may be minimal for others. Women who do not decrease their energy and/or fat intake to compensate for decreased energy expenditure and fat oxidation may be particularly at risk for excess weight gain. If energy balance is maintained, women should be able to maintain a healthy body weight throughout the menopausal transition. On the other hand, the estrogen-related shift in body fat distribution from lower-body/peripheral to upper-body/abdominal is less likely to be influenced by dietary habits and physical activity. Women who choose to take ERT for other reasons may experience a smaller gain in abdominal fat after menopause, however, for those who do not use ERT the emphasis should be on maintaining a healthy body weight overall and accepting that some redistribution of fat is likely to occur.

CONCLUSION

Sex-hormone influences on food intake, energy expenditure, and body composition likely play an important role in the current epidemic of obesity among women. Women must be aware of the potential impact of pregnancy and menopause on body weight so they can work with nutrition experts to plan specific strategies to avoid excess weight gain during these times. Of particular concern is the disproportionate burden of obesity and its health risks borne by minority women and poor women, particularly because the risk for pregnancy-associated weight retention appears higher in these populations. Aggressive strategies to limit excess pregnancy weight gain may be required. With regard to menopause, awareness of the hormonally induced shifts in body fat distribution may help women achieve greater acceptance of their bodies during the aging process, leading to greater psychological well-being.

An additional factor in regards to obesity and women's health is the effect of stress on body fat deposition and distribution. As postulated a number of years ago by Bjorntorp (70), increased stress causes neuroendocrine changes that promote the development of obesity and abdominal fat distribution. Again, it is essential that women and their health care teams understand how to proactively reduce the deleterious effects of environmental stressors in combination with hormonal changes. Through education and appropriate interventions, the burden of obesity on women's health can be diminished.

References

1. Ogden CL, Carroll MD, Curtin LR, McDowell MA, Tabak CJ, Flegal KM. Prevalence of overweight and obesity in the United States, 1999–2004. *JAMA*. 2006;295: 1549–1555.
2. Wang Y, Beydoun MA. The obesity epidemic in the United States—gender, age, socioeconomic, racial/ethnic, and geographic characteristics: a systematic review and meta-regression analysis. *Epidemiol Rev*. 2007;29:6–28.
3. National Institutes of Health. Clinical guidelines on the identification, evaluation, and treatment of overweight and obesity in adults—the evidence report. *Obes Res*. 1998;6(Suppl 2):51S–209S.
4. Lovejoy JC, Bray GA, Bourgeois MO, Machiavelli R, Rood JC, Greeson C, Partington C. Exogenous androgens influence body composition and regional body fat distribution in obese postmenopausal women. *J Clin Endocrinol Metab*. 1996;81: 2198–2203.
5. Svendsen OL, Hassager C, Christiansen C. Age- and menopause-associated variations in body composition and fat distribution in healthy women as measured by dual-energy X-ray absorptiometry. *Metabolism*. 1995;44:369–373.
6. Haarbo J, Marslew U, Gotfredsen A, Christiansen C. Postmenopausal hormone replacement therapy prevents central distribution of body fat after menopause. *Metabolism*. 1991;40:1323–1326.

7. Carmichael AR. Obesity as a risk factor for development and poor prognosis of breast cancer. *BJOG*. 2006;113:1160–1166.

8. Modesitt SC, van Nagell JR. The impact of obesity on the incidence and treatment of gynecologic cancers: a review. *Obstet Gynecol Surv*. 2005;60:683–692.

9. Gesink Law DC, Maclehose RF, Longnecker MP. Obesity and time to pregnancy. *Human Reprod*. 2007;22:414–420.

10. Sheldon JH. Maternal obesity. *Lancet*. 1949;2:869.

11. Williamson DF, Madans J, Pamuk S, Flegal KM, Kendrick JS, Serdula MK. A prospective study of childbearing and 10-year weight gain in US white women 25 to 45 years of age. *Int J Obes Relat Metab Disord*. 1994;18:561–569.

12. Lewis CE, Smoth DE, Caveny JL, Perkins LL, Burke GL, Bild DE. Associations of body mass and body fat distribution with parity among African-American and Caucasian women: the CARDIA study. *Obes Res*. 1994;2:517–525.

13. Ohlin A, Rössner S. Maternal body weight development after pregnancy. *Int J Obes*. 1990;14:159–173.

14. Walker LO. Managing excessive weight gain during pregnancy and the postpartum period. *J Obstet Gynecol Neonatal Nurs*. 2007;36:490–500.

15. Lederman SA. The effect of pregnancy weight gain on later obesity. *Obstet Gynecol*. 1993;82:148.

16. Olson CM, Strawderman MS, Hinton PS, Pearson TA. Gestational weight gain and postpartum behaviors associated with weight change from early pregnancy to 1 y postpartum. *Int J Obes Relat Metab Disord*. 2003;27:117–127.

17. Rossner S. Pregnancy, weight cycling and weight gain in obesity. *Int J Obes Relat Metab Disord*. 1992;16:145.

18. Rooney BL, Schauberger CW. Excess pregnancy weight gain and long-term obesity: one decade later. *Obstet Gynecol*. 2002;100:245–252.

19. Amorim AR, Rossner S, Neovius M, Lourenco PM, Linne Y. Does excess pregnancy weight gain constitute a major risk for increasing long-term BMI? *Obesity*. 2007;15:1278–1286.

20. Institute of Medicine. *Nutrition During Pregnancy, Part I: Weight Gain*. Washington, DC: National Academies Press; 1990.

21. Olafsdottir AS, Skuladottir GV, Thorsdottir I, Hauksson A, Steingrimsdottir L. Maternal diet in early and late pregnancy in relation to weight gain. *Int J Obes Relat Metab Disord*. 2006;30:492–499.

22. Gunderson EP, Abrams B, Selvin S. The relative importance of gestational gain and maternal characteristics associated with the risk of becoming overweight after pregnancy. *Int J Obes Relat Metab Disord*. 2000;24:1660–1668.

23. Keppel KG, Taffel SM. Pregnancy-related weight gain and retention: implications of the 1990 Institute of Medicine guidelines. *Am J Public Health*. 1993;83:1100–1103.

24. Lederman SA, Alfasi G, Deckelbaum RJ. Pregnancy-associated obesity in black women in New York City. *Matern Child Health*. 2002;6:37–42.

25. Siega-Riz AM, Adair LS, Hobel CJ. Institute of Medicine maternal weight gain recommendations and pregnancy outcome in a predominantly Hispanic population. *Obstet Gynecol*. 1994;84:565–573.

26. Goldberg GR, Prentice AM, Coward WA, Davies HL, Murgatroyd PR, Wensing C, Black AE, Harding M, Sawyer M. Longitudinal assessment of energy expenditure

in pregnancy by the doubly labeled water method. *Am J Clin Nutr.* 1993;57: 494–505.

27. Butte NF, Wong WW, Treuth MS, Ellis KJ, O'Brian Smith E. Energy requirements during pregnancy based on total energy expenditure and energy deposition. *Am J Clin Nutr.* 2004;79:1078–1087.

28. Muscati SK, Gray-Donald K, Koski KG. Timing of weight gain during pregnancy: promoting fetal growth and minimizing maternal weight retention. *Int J Obes Relat Metab Disord.* 1996;20:526–532.

29. Lovejoy JC. The influence of sex hormones on obesity across the female life span. *J Womens Health.* 1998;7:1247–1256.

30. Dewey KG. Impact of breastfeeding on maternal nutritional status. *Adv Exp Med Biol.* 2004;554:91–100.

31. Wosje KS, Kalkwarf HJ. Lactation, weaning and calcium supplementation: effects on body composition in postpartum women. *Am J Clin Nutr.* 2004;80:423–429.

32. Kac G, Benicio MHDA, Velasquez-Melendez G, Valnte JG, Struchiner CJ. Breastfeeding and postpartum weight retention in a cohort of Brazilian women. *Am J Clin Nutr.* 2004;79:487–493.

33. Dewey KG, Heinig MJ, Nommsen LA. Maternal weight loss patterns during prolonged lactation. *Am J Clin Nutr.* 1993;58:162–166.

34. Sarkar NR, Taylor R. Weight loss during prolonged lactation in rural Bangladeshi mothers. *J Health Popul Nutr.* 2005;23:177–183.

35. Linne Y, Dye L, Barkeling B, Rossner S. Weight development over time in parous women—the SPAWN study: 15 years follow-up. *Int J Obes Relat Metab Disord.* 2003;27:1516–1522.

36. Li R, Jewell S, Grummer-Strawn L. Maternal obesity and breastfeeding practices. *Am J Clin Nutr.* 2003;77:931–936.

37. Amir LH, Donath S. A systematic review of maternal obesity and breastfeeding intention, initiation and duration. *BMC Pregnancy Childbirth.* 2007;7:9.

38. Lovelady CA, Stephenson KG, Kuppler KM, Williams JP. The effects of dieting on food and nutrient intake of lactating women. *J Am Diet Assoc.* 2006;106: 908–912.

39. Driul L, Cacciaguerra G, Citossi A, Martina MD, Peressini L, Marchesoni D. Prepregnancy body mass index and adverse pregnancy outcomes. *Arch Gynecol Obstet.* 2008;278:23–26 (2007 Dec 11 [ePub]).

40. Metwally M, Ong KJ, Ledger WL, Li TC. Does a high body mass index increase the risk of miscarriage after spontaneous and assisted conception? A meta-analysis of the evidence. *Fertil Steril.* 2008;90:714–726 (2007 Dec 6 [ePub]).

41. Chu SY, Kim SY, Schmid CH, Dietz PM, Callaghan WM, Lau J, Curtis KM. Maternal obesity and risk of cesarean delivery: a meta-analysis. *Obes Rev.* 2007;8: 385–394.

42. Chu SY, Kim SY, Lau J, Schmid CH, Dietz PM, Callaghan WM, Curtis KM. Maternal obesity and risk of stillbirth: a meta-analysis. *Am J Obstet Gynecol.* 2007;197: 223–228.

43. Hedderson MM, Williams MA, Holt VL, Weiss NS, Ferrara A. Body mass index and weight gain prior to pregnancy and risk of gestational diabetes mellitus. *Am J Obstet Gynecol.* 2008;198:409.e1–e7 (2008 Feb 20 [ePub]).

44. Villamor E, Cnattingius S. Interpregnancy weight change and risk of adverse pregnancy outcomes: a population-based study. *Lancet*. 2006;368:1164–1170.

45. Shankar K, Harrell AM, Liu X, Gilchrist JM, Ronis MJ, Badger TM. Maternal obesity at conception programs obesity in the offspring. *Am J Physiol (Regul Integr Comp Physiol)*. 2008;294:R528–R538 (2007 Nov 21 [ePub]).

46. Taylor PD, Poston L. Developmental programming of obesity in mammals. *Exp Physiol*. 2007;92:287–298.

47. Rodriguez A, Miettunen J, Henriksen TB, Olsen J, Obel C, Taanila A, Ebeling H, Lennet KM, Moilanen I, Jarvelin MR. Maternal adiposity prior to pregnancy is associated with ADHD symptoms in offspring: evidence from three prospective pregnancy cohorts. *Int J Obes Relat Metab Disord*. 2008;32:550–557 (2007 Oct 16 [ePub]).

48. Polley BA, Wing RR, Sims CJ. Randomized controlled trial to prevent excessive weight gain in pregnant women. *Int J Obes Relat Metab Disord*. 2002;26: 1494–1502.

49. Claesson IM, Sydsjo G, Brynhildsen J, Cedergren M, Jeppsson A, Nystrom F, Sydsjo A, Josefsson A. Weight gain restriction for obese pregnant women: a case-controlled intervention study. *BJOG*. 2008;115:44–50.

50. Stotsenburg JM. The effect of spaying and semi-spaying young albino rats (*mus norvergicus albinus*) on the growth in body weight and body length. *Anat Rec*. 1913;7:183–194.

51. Asarian L, Geary N. Modulation of appetite by gonadal steroid hormones. *Philos Trans R Soc Lond B Biol Sci*. 2006;361:1251–1263.

52. Wing RR, Matthews KA, Kuller LH, Meilahn EN, Plantinga PL. Weight gain at the time of menopause. *Arch Intern Med*. 1991;151:97–102.

53. Pasquali R, Casimirri F, Labate AM, Tortelli O, Pascal G, Anconetani B, Gatto MR, Flamia R, Capelli M, Barbara L. Body weight, fat distribution and the menopausal status in women. The VMH Collaborative Group. *Int J Obes Relat Metab Disord*. 1994;18:614–621.

54. Toth MJ, Tchernof A, Sites CK, Poehlman ET. Effect of menopausal status on body composition and abdominal fat distribution. *Int J Obes Relat Metab Disord*. 2000;24:226–231.

55. Matthews KA, Abrams B, Crawford S, Miles T, Neer R, Powell LH, Wesley D. Body mass index in mid-life women: relative influence of menopause, hormone use, and ethnicity. *Int J Obes Relat Metab Disord*. 2001;25:863–873.

56. Lovejoy JC, Champagne CM, de Jonge-Levitan L, Xie H, Smith SR. Increased visceral fat and decreased energy expenditure during the menopausal transition. *Int J Obes Relat Metab Disord*. 2008;32:949–958.

57. Heymsfield SB, Gallagher D, Poehlman ET, Wolper C, Nonas K, Nelson D, Wang ZM. Menopausal changes in body composition and energy expenditure. *Exp Gerontol*. 1994;29:377–389.

58. Kotani K, Tokunaga K, Fujioka S, Kobatake T, Keno Y, Yoshida S, Shimomura I, Tarui S, Matsuzawa Y. Sexual dimorphism of age-related changes in whole-body fat distribution in the obese. *Int J Obes. Relat Metab Disord* 1994;18:207–212.

59. Hunter GR, Kekes-Szabo T, Trueth MJ, Williams MJ, Goran M, Pichon C. Intra-abdominal adipose tissue, physical activity, and cardiovascular risk in pre- and post-menopausal women. *Int J Obes Relat Metab Disord*. 1996;20:860–865.

60. Zamboni M, Armellini F, Harris T, Micciolo R, Bergamo-Andreis IA, Bosello O. Effects of age on body fat distribution and cardiovascular risk factors in women. *Am J Clin Nutr.* 1997;66:111–115.

61. Rebuffe-Scrive M, Eldh J, Hafstrom L-O, Bjorntorp P. Metabolism of mammary, abdominal, and femoral adipocytes in women before and after menopause. *Metabolism.* 1986:35:792–797.

62. Lindberg UB, Crona N, Silfverstople G, Bjorntorp P, Rebuffe-Scrive M. Regional adipose tissue metabolism in postmenopausal women after treatment with exogenous steroids. *Horm Metab Res.* 1990;22:345–351.

63. Pedersen SB, Kristensen K, Hermann PA, Katzenellenbogen JA, Richelsen B. Estrogen controls lipolysis by up-regulating α2A-adrenergic receptors directly in human adipose tissue through the estrogen receptor α. Implications for the female fat distribution. *J Clin Endocrinol Metab.* 2004;89:1869–1878.

64. Sites CK, Brochu M, Tchernof A, Poehlman ET. Relationship between hormone replacement therapy use with body fat distribution and insulin sensitivity in obese postmenopausal women. *Metabolism.* 2001;50:835–840.

65. Munoz J, Derstine A, Gower BA. Fat distribution and insulin sensitivity in postmenopausal women: influence of hormone replacement. *Obes Res.* 2002;10:424–431.

66. Espeland MA, Stefanick ML, Kritz-Silverstein D, Fineberg SW, Waclawiw MA, James MK, Greendale GA. Effect of postmenopausal hormone therapy on body weight and waist and hip girths. *J Clin Endocrinol Metab.* 1997;82:1549–1556.

67. Kritz-Silverstein D, Barrett-Connor E. Long-term postmenopausal hormone use, obesity, and fat distribution in older women. *JAMA.* 1996;275:46–49.

68. Reimer RA, Debert CT, House JL, Poulin MJ. Dietary and metabolic differences in pre- versus post-menopausal women taking or not taking hormone replacement therapy. *Physiol Behav.* 2005;84:303–312.

69. Day DS, Gozansky WS, van Pelt RE, Schwartz RS, Kohrt WM. Sex hormone suppression reduces resting energy expenditure and beta-adrenergic support of resting energy expenditure. *J Clin Endocrinol Metab.* 2005;90:3312–3317.

70. Bjorntorp P: Visceral obesity: a "civilization syndrome." *Obes Res.* 1993;1:206–222.

INDEX

Page number followed by *b* indicates box; *f,* figure; *t,* table.